Adaptation, Coping, and Resilience in Children and Youth

A Comprehensive Occupational Therapy Approach

Adaptation, Coping, and Resilience in Children and Youth

A Comprehensive Occupational Therapy Approach

Editors

Lenin C. Grajo, PhD, EdM, OTR/L

Washington University in St. Louis
School of Medicine
St. Louis, Missouri

Angela K. Boisselle, PhD, OTR

Cook Children's Health Plan
Fort Worth, Texas

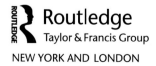

Routledge
Taylor & Francis Group

NEW YORK AND LONDON

First published in 2022 by SLACK Incorporated

Published in 2024 by Routledge
605 Third Avenue, New York, NY 10158

and by Routledge
4 Park Square, Milton Park, Abingdon, Oxon, OX14 4RN

Routledge is an imprint of the Taylor & Francis Group, an informa business

© 2022 Taylor & Francis Group

Cover Artist: Lori Shields

Library of Congress Control Number: 2022932492

ISBN: 9781630918545 (pbk)
ISBN: 9781003522515 (ebk)

DOI: 10.4324/9781003522515

DEDICATION

I can be changed by what happens to me, but I refuse to be reduced by it.

—Maya Angelou

This body of work is dedicated to
all the children and families we have worked with.
Your strength and resilience, and the many smiles along the way,
are the reasons we do what we do.

To Elnora and Essie, our mothers:
This body of work is in remembrance of both of you
and the profound love you have given us.

Contents

ACKNOWLEDGMENTS

We would like to thank our colleagues and friends at SLACK Incorporated: Brien Cummings, Kayla Whittle, Jennifer Cahill, and Allegra Tiver, and their teams. Thank you to Jamie Lief, Columbia University OT MS student, for her work as research assistant for the book, and to Aliya Boisselle for her assistance with the final chapter.

The majority of this text was written by outstanding educators, scholars, and clinicians during the peak of the 2020 global novel coronavirus pandemic. We are so grateful to these contributing authors for their own adaptation, coping, and resilience, and their generosity and patience in writing this important text amidst the chaos, professional and personal transitions, and life situations during these extremely challenging times.

Specific Words of Gratitude from Dr. Lenin C. Grajo

Every day I feel grateful for the many children and families I have worked with as a pediatric occupational therapist over the years. Their stories and experiences have made me the scholar and clinician I am today.

I am also grateful for the many colleagues and doctoral students I have worked and continue to work with. Their collaboration, support, and passion for the profession give me a sense of purpose. The research projects and innovations of my doctoral students inspire me every day. The change they hope to bring in the profession and practice of occupational therapy is truly remarkable. Thank you especially to my colleagues, peers, and students at Columbia University.

I dedicate this book to my sister Marijo, whose own struggles, experiences, narratives, and own adaptation, coping, and resilience continue to make me a better person. Lastly, I dedicate this work to my mother Elnora, who we lost in 2021. I am everything I am, because of the immeasurable love you have given me. I miss you every day.

Specific Words of Gratitude from Dr. Angela K. Boisselle

It has been an interesting time to write a book about adaptation, coping, and resilience: during a global pandemic and uncertain times for our country. One thing that struck me is the tenacity of the human spirit. I witnessed great strength and endurance of parents, children, health care workers, and service industry workers who kept on going even in the face of near-insurmountable odds. The connecting element that seemed fundamental throughout it all was the ability to adapt and carry on with occupations. Many discovered new occupations, while others rediscovered those long forgotten in order to simply pass the time in quarantine or, at the very least, maintain a semblance of normalcy. The lessons I learned throughout this time will not be lost. I dedicate this book to all of those affected over the recent years. I also attribute this work to the spirit of art, science, and human connection, for without those three things I would not have the blessed life that I lead.

Finally, I would like to thank my sisters and brother-in-law who are always in my corner and my friends who make me laugh until I cry. I would especially like to thank my amazing daughters, Marlee and Aliya. You are my everything. I love you.

ABOUT THE EDITORS

Lenin C. Grajo, PhD, EdM, OTR/L, is Associate Professor of Occupational Therapy and Psychiatry (PEFA), Director of the Division of Professional Education, and Associate Director of the Program in Occupational Therapy at Washington University in St. Louis School of Medicine. He has been a pediatric occupational therapist for 19 years and has practiced in the Philippines and the United States. He was previously on faculty in the Programs in Occupational Therapy at Columbia University in New York City. His research has focused on the application of Occupational Adaptation theory in instrument development and testing the effectiveness of interventions for children with specific learning disabilities, with particular focus on children with reading difficulties.

Dr. Grajo has published several peer-reviewed research articles, book chapters, and online continuing education programs related to interventions for children and youth and the Occupational Adaptation model. He is a certified therapist on the Cognitive Orientation to daily Occupational Performance (CO-OP) intervention approach. He has presented nationally and internationally on the role of occupational therapy in supporting children's literacy development.

Angela K. Boisselle, PhD, OTR, has more than 21 years experience as a pediatric occupational therapist and administrator. She currently works at Cook Children's Health Plan as a Utilization Management Therapy Manager. Her role involves operationalizing value-based payment models with therapy providers, establishing and overseeing medical necessity criteria for authorization of therapy services for pediatric Medicaid clients, and coordination of educational opportunities for therapy providers to promote quality therapy practices.

Dr. Boisselle's practice, service, and research background includes pediatric complex care, occupational adaptation, cerebral palsy, interprofessional collaboration, creativity, assistive technology and accessible design. She has served as research consultant, methodology committee member, peer reviewer, author, and editor. She is also a Clinical Instructor of Occupational Therapy in the Programs in Occupational Therapy at Columbia University Irving Medical Center.

CONTRIBUTING AUTHORS

Susan L. Bazyk, PhD, OTR/L, FAOTA (Foreword)
Professor Emerita
Occupational Therapy Program
Cleveland State University
Founding Director
Every Moment Counts, LLC
Cleveland, Ohio

Tammy Bruegger, OTD, MSE, OTR/L, ATP (Chapter 10)
Assistant Professor
Occupational Therapy Program
Rockhurst University
Assistive Technology Practitioner
The Children's Center for the Visually Impaired
Kansas City, Missouri

Susan M. Cahill, PhD, OTR/L, FAOTA (Chapter 7)
Director of Evidence-Based Practice
American Occupational Therapy Association
North Bethesda, Maryland

Catherine Candler, OTR, PhD, BCP (Chapter 5)
Professor
Abilene Christian University
Department of Occupational Therapy
Abilene, Texas

Anne Cronin, PhD, OTR, FAOTA, ATP (Chapter 4)
Professor
Department of Human Performance, Division of Occupational Therapy
West Virginia University
Morgantown, West Virginia

Rebecca Crossland, OTR, MOT (Chapter 5)
Occupational Therapist
Pediatric Occupational Therapy Department
West Texas Rehabilitation Center
San Angelo, Texas

Elaina DaLomba, PhD, OTR/L, MSW (Chapter 6)
Associate Professor
Occupational Therapy Department
Samuel Merritt University
Oakland, California

Lisa Griggs-Stapleton, PhD, OTR/L (Chapter 6)
Assistant Professor
Occupational Therapy Program
University of St. Augustine for Health Sciences
Dallas, Texas

Julia M. Guzmán, EdD, OTD, OTR/L (Chapter 3)
Assistant Professor
Department of Occupational Therapy
School of Health and Medical Sciences
Seton Hall University
Nutley, New Jersey

Douglene Jackson, PhD, OTR/L, LMT, ATP, BCTS (Chapter 15)
Chief Executive Officer, Consultant
GIFTS Institute, LLC
Pembroke Pines, Florida

Kathleen Kauper, MOT, OTR/L (Chapter 14)
Hawaii Hand Rehabilitation Services, LLC
Honolulu, Hawaii

Karrie L. Kingsley, OTD, OTR/L (Chapter 12)
Associate Professor/Director of Diversity, Access, and Equity
Chan Division of Occupational Science and Occupational Therapy
University of Southern California
Los Angeles, California

Lauren E. Milton, OTD, OTR/L (Chapter 13)
Assistant Professor
Program in Occupational Therapy
Washington University School of Medicine
St. Louis, Missouri

Kristie K. Patten, PhD, OT/L, FAOTA (Chapter 2)
Vice Dean of Academic Affairs
Steinhardt School of Culture Education and Human Development
New York University
New York, New York

Jennifer S. Pitonyak, PhD, OTR/L, SCFES (Chapter 13)
Associate Professor and Director
School of Occupational Therapy
Pacific University
Hillsboro, Oregon

Debra Rybski, MSHCA, PhD, OTR/L (Chapter 14)
Associate Professor
Department of Occupational Science and Occupational Therapy
Doisy College of Health Sciences
Saint Louis University
St. Louis, Missouri

Jessica Sparrow, OTD, OTR/L, BCP (Chapter 9)
Lead Occupational Therapist
Rehabilitation Services
St. Jude Children's Research Hospital
Memphis, Tennessee

Laura Stimler, OTD, OTR/L, BCP, C/NDT (Chapter 9)
Associate Professor
Auerbach School of Occupational Therapy
Spalding University
Louisville, Kentucky

Christine Urish, PhD, OTR/L, BCMH, FAOTA, CCAP (Chapter 11)
Professor and Doctoral Capstone Coordinator
Department of Occupational Therapy
Drake University
Des Moines, Iowa

FOREWORD

"Raising children . . . is vastly more than fixing what is wrong with them.
It is about identifying and nurturing their strongest qualities,
what they own and are best at, and helping them find niches
in which they can best live out these strengths."
—Seligman & Csikszentmihalyi, 2000, p. 6

Occupational therapy was founded on a commitment to mind-body unity, resulting in a rich history of promoting mental and physical health through the use of meaningful and enjoyable occupations (Meyer, 1922). Despite this long-standing perspective, services addressing "mental health" have often focused heavily on healing pathology (Barry & Jenkins, 2007; Keyes, 2007). Over the past two decades, a public health approach to children's mental health, emphasizing the promotion of mental health as well as the prevention of, and intervention for, mental disorders, has been advocated for both internationally (World Health Organization, 2001) and in the United States (Atkins & Frazier, 2011; Miles et al., 2010). This multi-tiered mental health promotion, prevention, and intervention framework has been applied to the occupational therapy process with children and youth (Bazyk, 2011a, 2011b, 2011c, 2019a, 2019b). Use of this framework supports a change in thinking from the traditional, individually focused, deficit-driven model of service provision to a whole-population, strength-based approach (Bazyk, 2011b). Occupational therapy services are provided at a universal level to promote positive mental health in all youth with and without disabilities and/or mental health challenges, at the targeted level with youth at risk of participation and mental health challenges, and at an individual level with youth identified with participation challenges and mental disorders (Bazyk, 2011a). As a part of *Every Moment Counts*, this framework is applied to promote mental health and participation throughout the day during classroom, lunch, recess, and after-school leisure activities (Bazyk et al., 2015; see also www.everymoment-counts.org).

Adaptation, Coping, and Resilience in Children and Youth: A Comprehensive Occupational Therapy Approach is a timely textbook for pediatric occupational therapy practice because it reinforces and expands on the importance of health promotion, prevention, and intervention with youth experiencing or at risk of mental and/or physical health challenges. The overarching aim of this textbook is the application of the adaptation, coping, and resilience framework (Grajo, 2019; Grajo & Boisselle, 2019) to the occupational therapy process with at-risk children and youth. Chapter 1 provides foundational information about the occupational adaptation, coping, and resilience framework, emphasizing strength-based approaches, ecological perspectives, and occupational participation. The application of evidence-based and occupation-focused strategies to the process of evaluation and intervention is reinforced throughout the textbook. Chapters 2 through 15 focus on the application of this framework with populations at risk of occupational participation and mental health challenges due to developmental or mental health conditions (e.g., autism, learning disabilities, intellectual disabilities, mental health disorders, ADHD), medical conditions and physical disabilities (e.g., chronic illness, cerebral palsy, cancer and terminal illness, visual impairments), and those affected by environmental stressors (e.g., adverse childhood experiences, bullying). This textbook is unique in its focus on populations that have received little or no attention in available occupational therapy textbooks, such as children and youth who identify as LGBTQ and gender expansive, children and youth of migrant farmworkers, and children and youth of color. These chapters, in particular, raise awareness of the mental, physical, and occupational challenges that youth representing these populations may face in everyday life.

Application of the adaptation, coping, and resilience framework throughout this textbook aligns with current research related to mental health promotion and prevention. For example, mental health promotion efforts emphasize teaching competencies associated with positive mental health (e.g., social and emotional abilities, coping strategies); creating supportive school, home, and community environments (e.g., reducing stigma, discrimination, and attitudinal barriers); and developing a knowledgeable interdisciplinary workforce (Barry & Jenkins, 2007; Bazyk, 2011b). Prevention efforts focus on reducing the incidence of mental health challenges by diminishing risk factors (e.g., poverty, bullying, stigma) and enhancing protective factors (e.g., supportive relationships and friendship, accommodations to reduce activity demands, sensory-friendly environments, etc.; Barry & Jenkins, 2007; Bazyk, 2011c). These promotion and prevention strategies are reflected in this textbook's application of the adaptation, coping, and resilience framework with and emphasis on occupation-based practice, strength-based approaches, and environment-focused services.

Adaptation, which occurs during participation in meaningful and healthy occupations, promotes the development of competencies leading to coping (Grajo, 2019; Grajo & Boisselle, 2019). Innovative approaches such as the use of occupation-based coaching are presented as effective strategies for enhancing participation when working with parents of children with intellectual disabilities (see Chapter 4). Additionally, strength-based approaches are applied to the occupational therapy process in each chapter. This is reflected by tuning in to the individual's unique character strengths and interests and helping youth participate in meaningful occupations that align with and enhance strengths. A mixed-method study by Carter et al. (2015) found that youth (autistic and those with developmental disabilities) who participated in a higher number of community-based, after-school activities reported a higher number of personal and interpersonal strengths, suggesting that occupation-based practice provides a relevant context for developing and deepening strengths over time.

Coping is considered a dynamic and purposeful process that occurs in response to challenges that exceed personal resources (Grajo & Boisselle, 2019). This textbook addresses a wide range of situational stressors that may occur as a result of internal factors (e.g., developmental, learning, or mental health disorders; acute or chronic illness; gender-expansive issues) or environmental factors (e.g., stigma, discrimination, bullying, unsafe living conditions, trauma). Coping is enhanced by helping youth develop internal resources and competencies (e.g., the use of deep breathing to reduce anxiety, using cognitive-behavioral strategies, engaging in healthy habits). For children of migrant farmers, adaptation and coping may be enhanced by exposing them to occupations relevant to the new culture and helping them to develop new health-promoting routines and rituals specific to their temporary community (see Chapter 14). Further, a need for targeted services focused on independent health management (i.e., activities related to managing health through routines; AOTA, 2020) is important for participation and transition to adulthood, especially in youth experiencing complex medical needs. In this population, children need to acquire the knowledge and skills necessary to manage their condition by self-monitoring symptoms, problem-solve during challenges, and utilize resources from the environment (Chapter 7). Specific to gender expansion, coping during gender transition reflects changing aspects of gender expression to align with gender identity (Chapter 12).

Coping is also enhanced by modifying the environment. This textbook's emphasis on contextual factors is supported in current research. With environment-focused interventions, the therapist, youth, provider, and family collaborate to remove environmental barriers (e.g., limited access to healthy leisure activities; discrimination), provide the necessary supports (e.g., physical, social, activity-based), and build on strengths to enhance successful participation (Anaby et al., 2016). Chapter authors also emphasized the importance of advocating for accessible and inclusive school and community programs for promoting coping. Specific to children and youth of color, coping can be negatively affected by environmental factors such as health and education disparities, racial injustice, systemic racism, and economic factors. Occupational therapy practitioners also make up part of the social environment and can either enhance or diminish adaptation and coping in children and youth of color, depending on our cultural humility and the delivery of culturally centered practice (Chapter 15). In this chapter, Jackson calls for practitioners' ongoing self-reflection in order to understand our personal beliefs and implicit biases, and to recognize systemic practices and policies that negatively affect marginalized populations.

Resilience, the desired outcome of adaptation and coping, is needed to participate successfully in order to experience health and quality of life. As a part of environment-focused intervention for adverse childhood experiences (ACES), the Empower Action Model is provided as an example of a resilience framework of protective factors, drawing from socio-ecological and life course perspectives, to provide a map for action at the individual, family, organization, community, and policy levels (Chapter 13). In addition to applying the adaptation, coping, and resilience framework in each chapter, information specific to collaborating with families, interprofessional collaboration, and global perspectives is also provided.

It is my hope that occupational therapy students and practitioners will read and apply content from this book in order to promote adaptation, coping, and resilience in diverse groups of children and youth. Knowledge gained can be instrumental in shifting from a traditional medical-model deficit approach to an authentic occupation-focused and strength-based perspective. In addition to helping children with diverse needs develop personal resources, this textbook also demonstrates the importance of environment-focused intervention as an essential ingredient for enhancing occupational participation, health, and quality of life in at-risk children and youth.

—*Susan L. Bazyk, PhD, OTR/L, FAOTA*

References

American Occupational Therapy Association. (2020). Occupational therapy practice framework: Domain and process (4th ed.). *American Journal of Occupational Therapy, 74*(Suppl. 2), 7412410010. https://doi.org/10.5014/ajot.2020.74S2001

Anaby, D. R., Law, M. C., Majnemer, A., & Feldman, D. (2016). Opening doors to participation of youth with physical disabilities: An intervention study. *Canadian Journal of Occupational Therapy, 83*(2), 83-90. https://doi.org/10.1177/0008417415608653

Atkins, M. S., & Frazier, S. L. (2011). Expanding the toolkit or changing the paradigm: Are we ready for a public health approach to mental health? *Perspectives on Psychological Science, 6*(5), 483-487. https://doi.org/10.1177/1745691611416996

Barry, M. M., & Jenkins, R. (2007). *Implementing mental health promotion.* Churchill, Livingstone, Elsevier.

Bazyk, S. (Ed.). (2011a). *Mental health promotion, prevention, and intervention with children and youth: A guiding framework for occupational therapy.* AOTA Press.

Bazyk, S. (2011b). The occupational therapy process: A public health approach to promoting mental health in children and youth. In S. Bazyk (Ed.), *Mental health promotion, prevention and intervention in children and youth: A guiding framework for occupational therapy* (pp. 45-69). AOTA Press.

Bazyk, S. (2011c). The promotion of positive mental health in children and youth: A guiding framework for occupational therapy. In S. Bazyk (Ed.), *Mental health promotion, prevention and intervention in children and youth: A guiding framework for occupational therapy* (pp. 21-43). AOTA Press.

Bazyk, S. (2019a). Best practices in school mental health: Promotion, prevention and intensive services. In G. Frolek, C. Rioux, & B. Chandler (Eds.), *Best practices for occupational therapy in schools* (2nd ed., pp. 153-160). AOTA Press.

Bazyk, S. (2019b). Occupational therapy's role in school mental health. In C. Brown, V. Stoffel, & J. Munoz (Eds.), *Occupational therapy in mental health: A vision for participation* (pp. 809-837). F. A. Davis.

Bazyk, S., Demirjian, L., LaGuardia, T., Thompson-Repas, K., Conway, C., & Michaud, P. (2015). Building capacity of occupational therapy practitioners to address the mental health needs of children and youth: Mixed methods study of knowledge translation. *American Journal of Occupational Therapy, 69*, 6906180060p1-6906180060p10.

Carter, E. W., Boehm, T. L., Biggs, E. E., Annandale, N. H., Taylor, C. E., Loock, A. K., & Liu, R. Y. (2015). Known for my strengths: Positive traits of transition-age youth with intellectual disability and/or autism. *Research and Practice for Persons with Severe Disabilities, 40*(2), 101-119. https://doi.org/10.1177/1540796915592158

Every Moment Counts. (n.d.). About. https://everymomentcounts.org/view.php?nav_id=21

Grajo, L. (2019). Theory of occupational adaptation. In B. E. B. Schell & G. Gillen (Eds.), *Willard and Spackman's occupational therapy* (13th ed.). Lippincott Williams & Wilkins.

Grajo, L., & Boisselle, A. (2019). Occupational adaptation in occupational therapy theories and models. In L. C. Grajo & A. Boisselle (Eds.), *Adaptation through occupation: Multidimensional perspectives.* SLACK, Incorporated.

Keyes, C. L. M. (2007). Promoting and protecting mental health as flourishing: A complementary strategy for improving national mental health. *American Psychologist, 62*, 95-108.

Meyer, A. (1922). The philosophy of occupational therapy. *Archives of Occupational Therapy, 1*, 1-10.

Miles, J., Espiritu, R. C., Horen, N., Sebian, J., & Waetzig, E. (2010). *A public health approach to children's mental health: A conceptual framework.* Georgetown University Center for Child and Human Development, National Technical Assistance Center for Children's Mental Health.

Seligman, M. E. P., & Csikszentmihalyi, M. (2000). Positive psychology: An introduction. *American Psychologist, 55*, 5-14.

World Health Organization. (2001). *The World Health report: Mental health: New understanding, new hope.* Author.

1

Adaptation, Coping, and Resilience in Children and Youth

Definitions, Models, and the Critical Role of Occupational Therapy

*Lenin C. Grajo, PhD, EdM, OTR/L and
Angela K. Boisselle, PhD, OTR*

CHAPTER OBJECTIVES By the end of this chapter, the reader will be able to:
- Describe various theoretical models for understanding adaptation, coping, and resilience in children.
- Articulate the critical role of occupational therapy in supporting adaptation, coping, and resilience in children and youth using occupation-based models.
- Apply adaptation, coping, and resilience principles within the occupational therapy process.

ADAPTATION, COPING, AND RESILIENCE IN CHILDREN AND YOUTH

There has been extensive research defining and describing the mechanisms of and the relationship between adaptation, coping, and resilience factors in children over the past 50 years. In this chapter, we attempt to synthesize various definitions and models

*Grajo L. C., & Boisselle, A. K. (Eds.). Adaptation, Coping,
and Resilience in Children and Youth: A Comprehensive
Occupational Therapy Approach (pp. 1-16).
© 2022 Taylor & Francis Group.*

and how the interrelated constructs of adaptation, coping, and resilience influence occupational participation. We then assert and articulate the role of occupational therapy in supporting adaptation, coping, and resilience in children and youth.

Defining Adaptation

Grajo and colleagues (2018) attempted to operationalize the global construct of occupational adaptation. From an analysis of 74 articles in occupational therapy and the academic discipline of occupational science, *occupational adaptation* may be defined as the internal human process that is: (1) a product of engagement, finding meaning, and satisfaction during occupational participation; (2) a process that emerges during transaction with the environment; (3) a manner of responding to change, altered situations, and life transitions; and (4) a formation of a desired sense of self, competency, and identity. This framing of adaptation is not unique to occupational therapy. In fact, developmental psychology has similar framing of the construct. Mahoney and Bergman (2002) used the term *positive adaptation* to define a similar construct with occupational adaptation. We present the juxtaposition and similarities of these definitions in Table 1-1.

In essence, both the occupational therapy and developmental psychology perspectives highlight the transactional and dynamic nature of adaptation. Adaptation, even in children and adolescents, can primarily be defined as the overarching process and manner of responding to daily life challenges. It is not a fixed state, but rather a process that can be observed as humans interact with their environment. During transitional moments of stress, this adaptive functioning may be observed as a mechanism of coping with various challenging situations. Children and youth, throughout their development, experience many transitional moments and ever-changing contexts for occupational participation. Early in child development, parents and caregivers at home serve as primary social occupational environments, with play and basic self-care as primary occupations. As children grow, their environments expand to include peers and teachers as they participate in more complex school-related and leisure occupations. The demands placed on them by increasing complexities of schoolwork, ever-expanding social relationships, and shift toward a sense of self and independence also increase and necessitate a more complex adaptation process. Their day-to-day activities and challenges become a means of discovering how children cope with various stressors.

Defining Coping

Seminally, Lazarus and Folkman (1984) defined the process of coping as the use of constantly changing cognitive and behavioral mechanisms to manage various demands in the environment. This process becomes more apparent when the challenge exceeds the available resources of the person. Compas (1987) expanded this definition to describe coping styles and coping efforts. *Coping styles* are methods of coping that characterize the individual's reactions to stress, either across different situations or over time within a given situation. *Coping efforts* or *strategies* are cognitive or behavioral actions taken

Table 1-1

Adaptation From a Developmental Psychology and Occupational Therapy Perspective	
Positive Adaptation (Mahoney & Bergman, 2002)	Occupational Adaptation (Grajo et al., 2018)
Positive adaptation involves the interplay between multiple, interdependent processes over time. These processes involve the person and the person's interaction with multiple levels of the environment (e.g., from family and peers to school, neighborhood, and societal conditions).	Occupational adaptation is identified as a mechanism to manage and respond to the occupational environment and as a manner of receiving validation from the environment.
The processes involved in positive adaptation are organized, in part, by the active role of the organism.	Occupational adaptation is a process of selecting and organizing activities, as part of a process of altering the meaning of engagement and changing the occupation itself and as a construct to define occupation as meaningful and requiring active participation from the person.
Positive adaptation can be understood only with reference to individual functioning as a whole and not on the basis of isolated behaviors. Positive adaptation can only be assessed with reference to individuals' pattern of functioning over time, and with reference to their personal resources and available opportunities in life.	Occupational adaptation is defined in the literature as an ongoing, nonlinear process to achieve a desired sense of self; a manner of developing a sense of competence, self-efficacy, and identity in occupational participation; and a manner of reframing identity, competence, the environment, and the fit among all three.
Positive adaptation is seen during "unusually favorable" developmental trajectories, in the context of a holistic-interactionistic developmental perspective.	Occupational adaptation is described as a manner of coping, being resilient, and as a use of appropriate strategies in response to altered or changing life situations.

in the course of a particular stressful episode. Compas (1987) also highlighted several themes to describe the interrelated nature of adaptation and coping particularly in the study of coping in children. These themes present the dynamic nature of personal factors (neurocognitive and behavioral factors) and environmental factors (particularly the role of parents and caregivers) in shaping the adaptation and coping capacities of the child. These themes are presented in Table 1-2. The child's early development and patterns of interactions with parents and primary caregivers define early mechanisms of coping and adaptation and how these factors influence their resilience.

The contexts in which children encounter daily occupations they need and want to participate in become central in identifying their unique stressors and coping mechanisms. Children who have changing "home" environments, such as those who live with grandparents or who change between separated or divorced parents throughout the week, may

Table 1-2

Seminal Understandings Based on Early Empirical Studies on Adaptation and Coping in Children and Youth

Themes in Understanding Coping in Children and Youth	Early Findings From the Literature
Attachment and separation	An infant's first experiences of distress is understood from the infant's reactions to separation and reattachment from and to the mother or caretaker.
Social support	There is a direct relation between social support and adjustment and the interaction of life events and social support in relation to the child's well-being.
Interpersonal cognitive problem solving	During interpersonal relationships, cognitive problem solving and coping are best evidenced by a dynamic orientation to problem solving and the child's ability to generate alternative solutions, consider consequences of social acts, develop means-ends thinking, develop social causal thinking, and be sensitive to problems.
Coping in achievement contexts	Coping strategies are viewed as individuals' efforts to minimize distress and maximize performance. Mastery-oriented children are examples of effective copers, in that they sustain high levels of motivation, persist in attempts at problem solving, increase their concentration, and display enhanced performance. Helpless children display ineffective coping, as reflected by their reduced levels of effort, high levels of discouragement, and deteriorated performance.
Type a behavior pattern	Type A individuals are characterized by competitive achievement striving, a sense of time urgency and impatience, and aggressiveness-hostility.
Repression-sensitization	Children described as repressers are those who neglect or avoid information in threatening situations; sensitizers focus their attention on cues that indicate danger in such situations. Parental inconsistency, restrictiveness, and use of punishment were all related to repression-sensitization behaviors in children.
Resilience or invulnerability to stress	This pattern of research has led to what is known as *protective factors*, seminally defined as attributes of persons, environments, situations, and events that appear to temper predictions of psychopathology based on an individual's at-risk status.

Adapted from Compas, B. E. (1987). Coping with stress during childhood and adolescence. *Psychological Bulletin, 101*(3), 393-403. https://doi-org.ezproxy.cul.columbia.edu/10.1037/0033-2909.101.3.393

present different levels of stress compared to those who have more stable home environments. For children who have very unstable home environments, such as those who live in housing programs or who are homeless, the school environment may be a more stable and secure environment. Children who have learning difficulties may find schoolwork more daunting and stressful than do their typically developing peers. Children with physical or social differences may have less access to leisure, recreational, and peer-related social activities. These various factors provide a situational perspective from which to describe the level of adversity children face and, therefore, define the child's level of resilience.

Defining Resilience

The National Scientific Council on the Developing Child (NSCDC) and the Harvard Center on the Developing Child are some of the leading institutions that have studied children's resilience over the past three decades. The NSCDC describes six key features in defining resilience (2015, p. 1):

- The capacity of a dynamic system to adapt successfully to disturbances that threaten its function, viability, or development.
- The ability to avoid deleterious behavioral and physiological changes in response to chronic stress.
- The capacity to resume positive functioning following adversity.
- A measure of the degree of vulnerability to shock or disturbance.
- A person's ability to adapt successfully to acute stress, trauma, or more chronic forms of adversity.
- The process of adapting well in the face of adversity, trauma, tragedy, threats, or significant stress.

The science of understanding resilience in children followed four waves of research over the past 60 years to become the concept as we know it today. O'Dougherty Wright and colleagues (2013) described these four waves, which clarify how we currently define and understand adaptation, coping, and resilience:

1. **First wave of research**: Identification of risk and protective factors that predispose or dampen the impact of adversity on a child's resilience;
2. **Second wave of research**: Understanding ecological perspectives and the impact of biological, social, and cultural processes on models and studies of resilience;
3. **Third wave of research**: Studies on effective interventions to promote resilience; and
4. **Fourth wave of research**: Understanding the genetic, neurobiological, and behavioral mechanisms of resilience.

These generations of studies have led to an understanding of the relationship among the constructs of adaptation, coping, and resilience. Compas et al. (2001) proposed this reframing (Figure 1-1):

> The primary distinction is that *coping* refers to processes of adaptation, *competence* refers to the characteristics and resources that are needed for successful adaptation, and *resilience* is reflected in outcomes for which competence and coping have been effectively put into action in response to stress and adversity (p. 89).

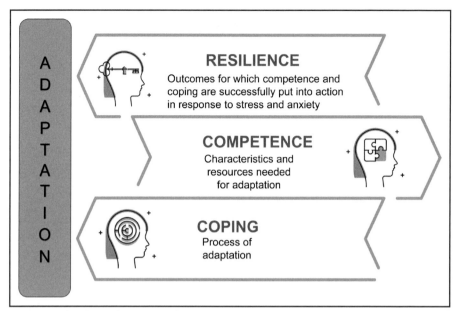

Figure 1-1. The relationship among adaptation, coping, and resilience. (Adapted from Compas, B. E., Connor-Smith, J. K., Saltzman, H., Thomsen, A. H., & Wadsworth, M. E. [2001]. Coping with stress during childhood and adolescence: Problems, progress, and potential in theory and research. *Psychological Bulletin, 127*[1], 87-127. https://doi-org.ezproxy.cul.columbia.edu/10.1037/0033-2909.127.1.87.)

Study for understanding adaptation, coping, and resilience in children and youth lends itself naturally to investigation of how occupational therapy as a profession can support and facilitate these three constructs. If adaptation, coping, and resilience are best understood within the transaction of the child and the environment during active doing and engagement in occupations (a very ecological perspective), why is it that there remains a lack of exploration of these constructs in the profession? In the next section, we assert that the constructs of adaptation, coping, and resilience are embedded in occupational therapy history and theories. A stronger reframing and articulation of how occupational therapy can support children's adaptation, coping, and resilience is warranted to facilitate the development of more research related to these constructs. We also present contemporary issues affecting children and youth that may influence current and emerging roles for occupational therapy.

THE ROLE OF OCCUPATIONAL THERAPY IN SUPPORTING ADAPTATION, COPING, AND RESILIENCE IN CHILDREN AND YOUTH

In her 1990 Eleanor Clarke Slagle Lecture, Sue Fine articulated various perspectives to describe the human experience of resilience. According to Fine, resilience becomes more apparent during traumatic and adverse experiences as the "hope and will to overcome"; resilience is more strongly sustained with "affiliation and recruitment of social support"; and is observed through various mechanisms, such as "finding meaning and purpose," having the "capacity to step back," "novel applications of problem-solving strategies," and "transforming dross into gold" (1991, pp. 497-499). More contemporary perspectives echo Fine's assertions that adaptation, coping, and resilience are embedded in what we do in occupational therapy.

Recent reconceptualizations of several occupational therapy conceptual models and theories have strongly described adaptation through the occupation process. The reconceptualization of these occupational therapy models now better reflects the nature of adaptation, coping, and resilience as best understood in the transaction with the occupational environment, manifested during life challenges and transitions and occupational participation, and requires the shifting of identity or understanding of the person as an occupational being (Grajo et al., 2018). Table 1-3 highlights some of these reconceptualized occupational therapy theories and how these can apply specifically to children and youth.

Evidence-based practice has shown the effectiveness of many activity- and participation-based and family- and child-centered interventions (e.g., Arbesman et al., 2013; Grajo et al., 2020; Kingsley et al., 2020) in improving life skills and participation of children and youth. We assert that it is the framing of the outcomes and process of occupational therapy that has to be shifted. Interventions must not only enhance client factors and performance skills, but also make sure that participation in occupations is facilitated in various meaningful contexts, and recognize that children and youth have the capacity to participate in occupations despite task-related, context-specific, and ability-dependent factors. This is the full manifestation of adaptation, and therefore contributes to effective and efficient coping and resilience. Thus, adaptation through occupation must be included as an outcome of occupational therapy interventions and must, therefore, be assessed and included in the process of occupational therapy.

Several occupational therapy documents now reflect the value and definition of adaptation through occupation. The revised Philosophical Base of Occupational Therapy (AOTA, 2018) defines *occupations* as "activities that bring meaning to the daily lives of individuals, families, communities, and populations and enable them to participate in society" and further adds that "participation in meaningful occupations is a determinant of health and *leads to adaptation*" (p. 1). The fourth edition of the Occupational Therapy Practice Framework used occupational adaptation in describing the outcomes of the occupational therapy process: "Occupational adaptation, or the client's effective and efficient response to occupational and contextual demands (Grajo, 2019a), is interwoven through all of these outcomes" (AOTA, 2020, p. 26). However, literature is scarce on the dynamic relationship of the facilitation of adaptation throughout the occupational therapy process to the impact on the child's or youth's capacity to cope and long-term resilience; this area requires further expansion and strengthening.

In this book, we aim to highlight how occupational therapists can continue using very similar assessment tools and intervention approaches, yet shift the perspective and broaden the process and outcomes of their therapy provision to include the facilitation of adaptation, coping, and resilience in children. We begin this text with the more common diagnoses of the children and youth whom occupational therapy services typically serve, which include various health-related, neurological, and developmental

Table 1-3

Adaptation as Explicitly Articulated in Some Occupational Therapy Models and Applications in Children and Youth

Occupational Therapy Model or Frame of Reference	Definition of Adaptation	Evaluation and Intervention Principles	Applications to Children and Youth
Occupational Adaptation (OA) Theory (Grajo, 2019b; Schkade & Schultz, 2003)	The internal normative process through which the person and occupational environment transact, during occupational participation; fully manifested when the person is faced with occupational challenges. A person manifests adaptation through the ability to plan, modify, and create new occupational responses to overcome daily-life challenges with a sense of mastery.	Adaptation is measured through the constructs of adaptive capacity and relative mastery. OA-guided intervention embraces the following principles: holistic assessment, focus and re-establishment of occupational roles; the client is the agent of change; facilitation of the occupational environment; occupations are central in eliciting adaptive responses; and focus on increasing adaptive capacity and relative mastery.	OA has been used as a guiding framework in school-based practice with children and youth with behavioral challenges, and, more recently, with children who have reading difficulties. The overall goal is to facilitate children's adaptive capacity and relative mastery so that they are able to participate and overcome challenges with school-related and daily occupations.
Model of Human Occupation (MOHO) (Bowyer, 2019)	A state of having a positive occupational identity and the corresponding occupational competence, constructed over time, through the dynamics of a constant interaction between personal factors and environmental impact.	Use of MOHO assessments to measure participation. Intervention with focus on Dimensions of Doing: support and building of occupational skills, occupational performance, and occupational participation.	The Short Child Occupational Profile (SCOPE; Bowyer et al., 2008) is a MOHO-based tool that can be used for children and adolescents to identify occupational strengths and challenges.

	Occupational adaptation occurs naturally as people pass through life phases. Adaptation can occur naturally, be the result of an unexpected occurrence, or be made consciously with an understanding of the possible implications of the decisions and choices made.	Outcomes of intervention are occupational identity, occupational competence, and occupational adaptation.	MOHO-based interventions aim at facilitating occupational competence of children and youth and, therefore, support development of their occupational identity and adaptation.
Ecology of Human Performance (EHP) (Dean, Wallisch, & Dunn, 2019)	Occupational adaptation is defined as a transactional process in which the person and the environment are both changed through participation in everyday life. Adaptation is a unique process understood from the range of everyday participation: a process facilitated or hindered by the transaction between the person, environment, and features of tasks.	Intervention uses a variety of approaches: Establish/restore, alter, adapt/modify, prevent, create	By analyzing factors within the person system, variables of the task, and factors in the environment, a child's performance range can be enhanced. Using a combination of the five EHP intervention approaches, a child's occupational performance can be enhanced.
Sensory Processing (Little & Dunn, 2019)	Adaptation is manifested as the neurobiological sensory processing abilities reflective of the transaction between individuals' biological traits and their contexts. Sensory processing abilities are linked to a person's activity participation and adaptive behavior.	Assessment and interventions are aimed at evaluating and promoting child development and use of strategies to allow individuals to meet and negotiate the demands of their contexts and environments to fully participate in occupations. Interventions to support participation include environment-focused approaches, collaborations with families, and understanding of sensory patterns.	Perhaps one of the most widely used frameworks in pediatric practice, sensory-based interventions are aimed at facilitating adaptive responses in children when navigating their occupational environments during participation in daily tasks.

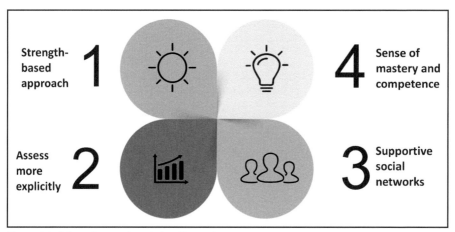

Figure 1-2. Adaptation, coping, and resilience themes.

conditions. We then expand the reach of occupational therapy by including contextual and personal factors that may present various risks for health disparities and developmental challenges. In particular, we include progressive perspectives and assert the role of occupational therapy in supporting children and youth who have undergone adverse childhood experiences, those who have experienced bullying, children and youth who identify as LGBTQ and gender expansive, children and youth of migrant farmworkers, and children and youth of color.

This chapter provides a broad overview of how we define adaptation, coping, and resilience in children and youth, and how these can be framed within the domain and process of occupational therapy. The specific chapters in this text apply these overarching definitions to various populations of children and youth and reframe how we can use an adaptation, coping, and resilience lens in how we deliver occupational therapy. The chapters in this text have common themes threaded among them, guided by best and evidence-based practice, on how to assert the role of occupational therapy to support adaptation, coping, and resilience in children and youth (Figure 1-2):

1. Shift the perspective from a deficit approach (biomedical model) to a strength-based approach.
2. Assess adaptation, coping, and resilience more explicitly.
3. Highlight an ecological perspective by building supportive social networks.
4. Build on adaptation by focusing on a sense of mastery and competence in occupational participation.

These four themes are threaded throughout the different chapters in this book. However, we present what this may look like in practice in this chapter using a case study.

Case Study 1-1

Max

Max is a second-grader in a private school in a suburban city. He was diagnosed with attention deficit disorders with an accompanying specific learning disability. His teachers have reported that he is often shy and withdrawn from peers during most of the morning academic activities, yet shows a more fun and engaging side during recess and other, more active class undertakings. He has recently been tested for reading difficulties and results reveal below-grade-level abilities. He has started working with an occupational therapist in the school setting.

Applying an Adaptation Coping, and Resilience Perspective With Max

Approach	How This May Look During Therapy Sessions
Shift from deficit-perspective to a strength-based approach	Max's occupational therapy comprehensive evaluation has identified sensory processing challenges, low average fine motor and coordination skills, and possible executive function challenges. Despite these challenges, his occupational profile has indicated that Max enjoys being in school, doing fun reading activities with his mom, baseball and other ball sports; likes everything related to Spider-Man and Marvel Universe characters; and is technologically savvy.
Assess adaptation, coping, and resilience explicitly	The occupational therapist included additional tools as part of the comprehensive evaluation: the Coping Inventory (Zeitlin, 1985) to identify coping and adaptive behaviors, the Short Child Occupational Profile (SCOPE; Bowyer et al., 2008) to identify strengths and barriers to occupational participation, and the Inventory of Reading Occupations-Pediatric version (Grajo, Candler, & Bowyer, 2019) to identify preferences and challenges related to daily reading activities.
Build supporting networks	As part of Max's intervention, the occupational therapist has asked his mom to log a reading journal. This log includes all peers, family members, and classmates with whom Max enjoys doing some reading activities. This has helped the occupational therapist identify fun reading activities and games that Max can do with family, friends, and classmates. Max's mom has started hosting Marvel Comic Book social activities with a few of Max's classmates. They borrow movies from the local library, which they get to watch after 1 hour of reading the comic books; Max has really enjoyed this activity. The occupational therapist has also communicated with Max's teacher to collaboratively problem-solve on strategies to encourage Max during more challenging reading tests and tasks in school.

(continued)

Case Study 1-1 (continued)

Approach	How This May Look During Therapy Sessions
Focus on sense of mastery and competence	Max's occupational therapist has focused on encouraging a feeling of mastery and increased self-esteem during therapy sessions (Figure 1-3). The occupational therapist used cognitive strategies to gradually increase the level of challenge and difficulty of reading tasks that Max is able to participate in. The goal for each goal-setting iteration is for Max to self-monitor the following: (1) number of sentences, paragraphs, or pages that Max is able to read; (2) set goals on how to identify strategies to mark errors during reading tasks and what strategies to use to avoid these mistakes; (3) make sure that there is fun and enjoyment in reading; and (4) identify self-reinforcing activities as a result of achieving the goal. This cognitive approach has empowered Max to realize that he can complete increasingly challenging reading tasks on his own; that he can develop and name his own strategies to use to overcome challenging reading tasks; and that he can have fun while completing difficult reading activities.

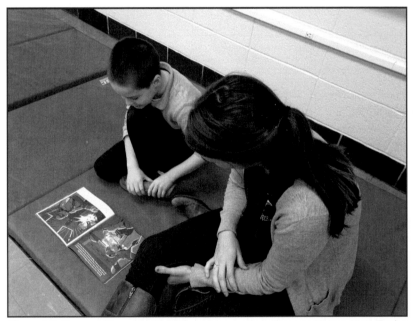

Figure 1-3. Max and his occupational therapist enjoying a Teenage Mutant Ninja Turtles story book.

CONTEMPORARY ISSUES AFFECTING CHILDREN'S ADAPTATION, COPING, AND RESILIENCE

Throughout this textbook, we present contemporary issues and contextual considerations with children and youth that are important for occupational therapists to address, as well as possible considerations for expanding the role of occupational therapy. These considerations and factors have impacts on children's adaptation, coping, and resilience. However, there are other factors that are of critical importance beyond what we can offer space for in this text. Here, we provide an overview of some of these pressing issues: immigration status, homelessness and poverty, the novel coronavirus (COVID-19) pandemic, increasing rates of domestic violence and other forms of violence and abuse, and racial injustice. Several of these issues are covered in some detail in some of the chapters (Chapter 11: children who have experienced bullying; Chapter 13: children who have encountered adverse childhood experiences; Chapter 15: children of color). Table 1-4 presents an overview of how these issues affect children's adaptation, coping, and resilience based on the literature.

Table 1-4

Contemporary Issues Affecting Adaptation, Coping, and Resilience of Children and Youth	
Contemporary Issues Affecting Children and Youth	Impacts on Adaptation, Coping, and Resilience
Immigration status of families	Literature supports that children of unauthorized immigrant parents face parental anxiety, fear of separation, and acculturative stress. Parent-child separations can be harmful to children's health, economic security, and long-term development. Early childhood exposure to stress and adversity can cause poor health and impaired development that may persist into adulthood. Anxiety and psychosocial stress are identified as risk factors for depression, substance abuse, cardiovascular diseases, and obesity (Hainmueller et al., 2017)
Homelessness and poverty	Children experiencing homelessness encounter high rates of psychosocial adversity and face risk for poor health and developmental problems. Many children in shelters have experienced stressful life events, including stressors directly related to residential instability (e.g., the loss of housing, community, and relationships), as well as other stressors such as witnessing domestic and community violence. These findings are more persistent for low-income and racial-minority groups (Cutuli et al., 2017).

(continued)

Table 1-4 (continued)

Contemporary Issues Affecting Adaptation, Coping, and Resilience of Children and Youth	
Contemporary Issues Affecting Children and Youth	**Impacts on Adaptation, Coping, and Resilience**
Global health pandemic	During the COVID-19 pandemic, parents' individual perception of the situation and challenges during quarantine is significantly associated with parents' stress and children's psychological problems. Interruption of academic and health care services may contribute to significant disruption of daily routines and occupations. The resulting increased level of stress may affect children's behavioral and emotional problems through the mediating role of parental stress. Additionally, confounding issues related to increased social isolation, increased caregiver burden, and potential familial financial challenges may place the child/youth at increased risk for abuse, neglect, and trauma (Spinelli et al., 2020; World Health Organization, 2020).
Exposure to violence and abuse	American estimates for exposure across the duration of childhood is 20% to 29% for bullying, 2% to 9% for dating violence, 5% to 19% for physical maltreatment, 7% to 33% for physical assault, 3% to 11% for sexual maltreatment/assault, and 13% to 27% for witnessing adults' domestic violence. Childhood violence and victimization are associated with risk for (a) many different kinds of psychiatric disorders, (b) comorbidity, (c) unfavorable course of illness, and (d) poor treatment response (Moffitt et al., 2013).
Racial injustice	Self-reported discrimination as well as expectations of discrimination by children and youth in minority groups are associated with depressive symptoms, low self-esteem/self-worth, and anxiety in adolescents and preadolescents. Perception of racism was shown to be associated with internalizing and externalizing behaviors, anger, conduct problems, and delinquent behaviors in adolescents and preadolescents (Pachter & Coll, 2009).
Social media use	One study in a systematic review found a positive correlation between depression and time spent on Facebook by adolescents. Major depression has been associated with adolescents who spent most of their time in online activities and performing image management on social networking sites (Karim et al., 2020).

SUMMARY

In this chapter, we recommend that occupational therapists evaluate and provide interventions to include a perspective on adaptation, coping, and resilience. This role and interventions are critically important to those working with children and youth and families. Beyond the typical medical and diagnostic groups that are often referred to receive occupational therapy services, we highlight progressive perspectives to include other at-risk groups of children who may typically not be referred for occupational therapy. By defining adaptation, coping, and resilience and the relationship of these constructs, we hope that this chapter introduces and sets the framework we propose and aids the reader to embrace the many assertions made by the different contributing authors throughout the textbook.

REFERENCES

American Occupational Therapy Association. (2018). Philosophy of occupational therapy education. *American Journal of Occupational Therapy, 72*(Suppl. 2), 7212410070. https://doi.org/10.5014/ajot.2018.72S201

American Occupational Therapy Association. (2020). Occupational therapy practice framework: Domain and process (4th ed.). *American Journal of Occupational Therapy, 74*(Suppl. 2), 7412410010. https://doi.org/10.5014/ajot.2020.74S2001

Arbesman, M., Bazyk, S., & Nochajski, S. M. (2013). Systematic review of occupational therapy and mental health promotion, prevention, and intervention for children and youth. *American Journal of Occupational Therapy, 67*, e120-e130. http://dx.doi.org/10.5014/ajot.2013.008359

Bowyer, P. (2019). Formation of identity and occupational competence: Occupational adaptation in the model of human occupation. In L. C. Grajo & A. Boisselle (Eds.), *Adaptation through occupation: Multidimensional perspectives.* SLACK Incorporated.

Bowyer, P. L., Kramer, J., Ploszaj, A., Ross, M., Schwartz, O., Kielhofner, G., & Kramer, K. (2008). *A user's manual for the Short Child Occupational Profile (SCOPE)* (v.2.2).Model of Human Occupational Clearinghouse. http://www.moho.uic.edu

Compas, B. E. (1987). Coping with stress during childhood and adolescence. *Psychological Bulletin, 101*(3), 393-403. https://doi-org.ezproxy.cul.columbia.edu/10.1037/0033-2909.101.3.393

Compas, B. E., Connor-Smith, J. K., Saltzman, H., Thomsen, A. H., & Wadsworth, M. E. (2001). Coping with stress during childhood and adolescence: Problems, progress, and potential in theory and research. *Psychological Bulletin, 127*(1), 87-127. https://doi-org.ezproxy.cul.columbia.edu/10.1037/0033-2909.127.1.87

Cutuli, J. J., Ahumada, S. M., Herbers, J. E., Lafavor, T. L., Masten, A. S., & Oberg, C. N. (2017). Adversity and children experiencing family homelessness: Implications for health. *Journal of Children & Poverty, 23*(1), 41-55. https://doi.org/10.1080/10796126.2016.1198753

Dean, E., Wallisch, A., & Dunn, W. (2019). Adaptation as a transaction with the environment: Perspectives from the ecology of human performance. In L. C. Grajo & A. Boisselle (Eds.), *Adaptation through occupation: Multidimensional perspectives.* SLACK Incorporated.

Fine, S. (1991). Resilience and human adaptability: Who rises above adversity?—1990 Eleanor Clarke Slagle Lecture. *American Journal of Occupational Therapy, 45*(6), 493-503. https://doi.org/10.5014/ajot.45.6.493

Grajo, L. (2019a). Theory of occupational adaptation. In B. E. B. Schell & G. Gillen (Eds.), *Willard and Spackman's occupational therapy* (13th ed.). Lippincott Williams & Wilkins.

Grajo, L. (2019b). Occupational adaptation as a normative and intervention process: Schkade and Schultz's legacy. In L. C. Grajo & A. Boisselle (Eds.), *Adaptation through occupation: Multidimensional perspectives.* SLACK Incorporated.

Grajo, L., & Boisselle, A. (2019). Occupational adaptation in occupational therapy theories and models. In L. C. Grajo & A. Boisselle (Eds.), *Adaptation through occupation: Multidimensional perspectives.* SLACK Incorporated.

Grajo, L., Boisselle, A., & DaLomba, E. (2018). Occupational adaptation as a construct: A scoping review of literature. *Open Journal of Occupational Therapy, 6*(1), Article 2. https://doi.org/10.15453/2168-6408.1400

Grajo, L., Candler, C., & Bowyer, P. (2019). The inventory of reading occupations—pediatric version. https://www.ps.columbia.edu/education/academic-programs/programs-occupational-therapy/faculty-innovations/ot-literacy

Grajo, L. C., Candler, C., & Sarafian, A. (2020). Interventions within the scope of occupational therapy to improve children's academic participation: A systematic review. *American Journal of Occupational Therapy, 74*, 7402180030. https://doi.org/10.5014/ajot.2020.039016

Hainmueller, J., Lawrence, D., Marten, L., Black, B., Figueroa, L., Hotard, M., Jimenez, T., Mendoza, F., Rodriguez, M., Swartz, J., & Laitin, D. (2017). Protecting unauthorized immigrant mothers improves their children's mental health. *Science, 357*, 1041-1044. https://doi.org/10.1126/science.aan5893

Karim, F., Oyewande, A. A., Abdalla, L. F., Chaudhry Ehsanullah, R., & Khan, S. (2020). Social media use and its connection to mental health: A systematic review. *Cureus, 12*(6), e8627. https://doi.org/10.7759/cureus.8627

Kingsley, K., Sagester, G., & Weaver, L. L. (2020). Interventions supporting mental health and positive behavior in children ages birth-5 yr: A systematic review (Table A.3). *American Journal of Occupational Therapy, 74*, 7402180050. https://doi.org/10.5014/ajot.2020.039768

Lazarus, R. S., & Folkman, S. (1984). *Stress, appraisal, and coping.* Springer.

Little, L., & Dunn, W. (2019). Adaptation from a sensory processing perspective. In L. C. Grajo & A. Boisselle (Eds.), *Adaptation through occupation: Multidimensional perspectives.* SLACK Incorporated.

Mahoney, J., & Bergman, L. (2002). Conceptual and methodological considerations in a developmental approach to the study of positive adaptation. *Applied Developmental Psychology, 23*, 195-217. https://doi.org/10.1016/S0193-3973(02)00104-1

Moffitt, T. E., & Klaus-Grawe 2012 Think Tank. (2013). Childhood exposure to violence and lifelong health: Clinical intervention science and stress-biology research join forces. *Development and Psychopathology, 25*(4, pt. 2), 1619-1634. https://doi.org/10.1017/S0954579413000801

National Scientific Council on the Developing Child. (2015). Supportive relationships and active skill-building strengthen the foundations of resilience (Working Paper 13). http://www.developingchild.harvard.edu

O'Dougherty Wright, M., Masten, A. S., & Narayan, A. J. (2013). Resilience processes in development: Four waves of research on positive adaptation in the context of adversity. In S. Goldstein & R. Brooks (Eds.), *Handbook of resilience in children* (2nd ed., pp. 15-55). Springer. https://doi.org/10.1007/978-1-4614-3661-4_2

Pachter, L. M., & Coll, C. G. (2009). Racism and child health: A review of the literature and future directions. *Journal of Developmental and Behavioral Pediatrics: JDBP, 30*(3), 255-263. https://doi.org/10.1097/DBP.0b013e3181a7ed5a

Schkade, J. K., & Schultz, S. (2003). Occupational adaptation. In P. Kramer, J. Hinojosa, & C. B. Royeen (Eds.), *Perspectives in human occupation: Participation in life* (pp. 181-221). Lippincott Williams & Wilkins.

Spinelli, M., Lionetti, F., Massimiliano, P., & Mirco, F. (2020). Parent's stress and children's psychological problems in families facing the COVID-19 outbreak in Italy. *Frontiers in Psychology, 11*, 1713. https://doi.org/10.3389/fpsyg.2020.01713

World Health Organization (2020). Disability considerations during the COVID-19 outbreak. https://www.who.int/publications/i/item/WHO-2019-nCoV-Disability-2020-1

Zeitlin, S. (1985). *Coping inventory manual observation form.* Scholastic Testing Service.

I

Developmental and Neurological Considerations

2

Autistic Children and Youth*
A Strength-Based Approach

Kristie K. Patten, PhD, OT/L, FAOTA

CHAPTER OBJECTIVES By the end of this chapter, the reader will be able to:

- Compare and contrast environments that are either supports or barriers to resilience, adaptation, and coping by autistic children and youth.
- Utilize evidence-based assessment and interventions that support inclusion and positive client-centered outcomes in work with autistic children and youth.
- Demonstrate how a strength-based practice can be part of an approach that fosters resilience, adaptation, and coping in autistic children and youth.

OVERVIEW OF THE POPULATION

Autism is a developmental condition characterized by social communication challenges and patterns of behavior, interests, or activities that may facilitate or hinder coping and adaptation. The most current prevalence rate of 1 in 54 in the United States

Grajo L. C., & Boisselle, A. K. (Eds.). Adaptation, Coping, and Resilience in Children and Youth: A Comprehensive Occupational Therapy Approach (pp. 19-44).
© 2022 Taylor & Francis Group.

(American Psychiatric Association, 2013; Maenner et al., 2020) is from data collected nationwide in 2016. Autism, diagnosed in early childhood up through adulthood, is over four times more prevalent among boys as compared to girls, with non-Hispanic white, non-Hispanic Black, and Asian/Pacific Islander children having approximately identical prevalence estimates; the prevalence is lower for Hispanic children (Maenner et al., 2020). Health disparities in early evaluation and diagnosis do exist, in that Black children are less likely to have an evaluation prior to age 36 months than are white children, and have a later median age of an autism diagnosis as compared to white children (48 months vs. 42 months; Maenner et al., 2020). The magnitude of these prevalence disparities has declined in recent years, and this is the first report by the Centers for Disease Control and Prevention (CDC) that has shown no overall difference in prevalence estimates. However, Black children with intellectual disabilities and autism receive a diagnosis at a later age, which may affect service provision and key outcomes (Maenner et al., 2020).

Occupational therapy practitioners work with autistic children and youth in early intervention, including home and community-based centers, schools, and private practices (Tomchek & Koenig, 2016). Children are referred for an occupational therapy evaluation and subsequent intervention in these settings and the occupational therapy evaluation process begins with the creation of an occupational profile (American Occupational Therapy Association [AOTA], 2020; Tomchek & Koenig, 2016) that documents the client's history; reason for referral; current occupations and difficulty with engagement in both individual and family occupations; daily routines; and social supports, as well as goals and priorities of the client and family. The occupational profile should identify the client's strengths, interests, and current coping strategies; it should also include environmental and contextual factors that either support or are a barrier to successful occupational engagement (Table 2-1; AOTA, 2020; Tomchek & Koenig, 2016).

The occupational profile essentially lays out the risk and protective factors as it identifies factors that enable or hinder occupational engagement. Resilience theory is the framework that proposes an interplay between risk and protective factors when faced with adversity (Bekhet & Matel-Anderson, 2017). *Risk factors* are factors that influence a person's ability to cope and predisposes them to stress. In the example in Table 2-1, an overwhelming chaotic environment would be identified as a risk factor, or as a barrier to occupational engagement when using occupational profile terminology. Protective factors, in contrast, can decrease the impact or effects of the risk factors, and lead to positive outcomes. The more protective factors an individual has, the higher the resiliency and the better the individual's ability to cope and adapt to environmental stress. In this example, sensory advocacy and awareness of potential sensory triggers could be viewed as a protective factor, as would understanding adults who have an awareness and would consider the sensory environment prior to exposure. The occupational therapist could work with the child to do a sensory scan and be aware of environments that are "sensory friendly" or, conversely, stress-producing. This is in line with Schkade and Schultz's (1992) and Grajo's (2019) view in the theory of occupational adaptation that the role of the occupational therapist is to "empower the person to develop their own sense of relative mastery in order to transact with the environment."

Table 2-1

Occupational Profile		
What aspects of the client's environments or context do they see as:		
	Supports to Occupational Engagement	Barriers to Occupational Engagement
Environment Physical	Sensory inclusive spaces, visual supports	Overwhelming sensory input, crowded physical spaces
Social	Opportunities to socialize around high-interest areas	Social demands and expectations that are set by non-autistic norms (e.g., heavy reliance on eye contact)
Context Cultural	Honesty and loyalty to groups, people, and causes	Denial of autistic culture and autistic-to-autistic communication
Personal	Self-advocacy skills that are explicitly taught	External demands to not engage in self-stimulatory or soothing actions (e.g., pacing, flapping)
Temporal	Strong desire for routine and a schedule	Unpredictable schedules or changes in plans
Virtual	Communicates more effectively via email or text	May not have access to technology for communication or proper training of support personnel, especially for non-speaking[1] individuals
Goals Targeted outcomes	• Increase self-regulation and self-advocacy skills • Increase functional communication skills • Increase participation in meaningful occupations • Identify and support sensory preferences	

[1] *Non-speaking* used in place of *nonverbal* as a more accurate description of communication challenges.

Adapted from American Occupational Therapy Association. (2014). Occupational therapy practice framework: Domain and process (3rd ed.). *American Journal of Occupational Therapy, 68*, S1-S48. https://doi.org/10.5014/ajot.2014.682006

Shifting to a Strength-Based Approach

It should be noted that empowering autistic clients to gain mastery is a crucial role for the occupational therapy practitioner to engage in, but that engagement should be done through a social model of disability vs. a medical model of disability (Shakespeare, 2013). This distinction must be made at the outset so that, as Grajo and colleagues outlined (2018), adaptation through occupation can result in a self-determined, desired sense of self. The medical model of disability would frame engagement in occupation, challenges to be overcome, and difficulties in life transitions differently than would a social model of disability. For example, the medical model highlights the challenges of autistic people and overlooks their potential strengths that may flourish in optimal contexts. These challenges then become the focus of intervention and the occupational therapist utilizes non-autistic norms as a desired outcome. When considering sensory processing, for example, occupational therapists quickly identify sensory processing issues through assessment and observation but often do not consider how auditory hypersensitivity or perceptual capacity may be a strength in meaningful occupations (e.g., listening to music, playing an instrument). By associating disability with deficits and weakness, the medical model promotes a negative portrayal of disability, which requires the individual to "overcome the disability" as a way to cope, adapt, and show resilience. This deficit-based model does not encourage autistic people, their families, and education and health professionals to identify clients' strengths and internal resources (Saleebey, 1996). With autism, the medical model may then run counter to building protective factors that promote adaptation, coping, and resilience.

Perhaps even more damaging, the medical model seeks to modify or normalize autistic traits and behaviors as a goal, which actually can be a risk factor and produce environmental stress (Hull et al., 2017). We do not ask our deaf clients to "hear more like me," or our wheelchair users to "walk more like me," but the medical model of autism asks the individual to "act and be more like me" every day, to align with non-autistic social norms, which can cause distress to autistic people. For example, atypical behaviors, such as lacking eye contact and engaging in repetitive behaviors, are considered undesirable in the medical model of autism. However, autistic self-advocates who are the experts of their own experience have been very clear when they describe eye contact (Higashida, 2013; Shore, 2003; Tammett, 2006). For autistic people, eye contact can lead to sensory overload and feelings of invasion; it is highly distracting and may negatively affect comprehension of auditory directions and provoke adverse emotional and physiological reactions, which further challenges their coping skills and adaptation. By avoiding eye contact, the individual may be actively coping with a stressful environment or social interaction and using an adaptive strategy to improve comprehension. This is why the way autism is framed—with the medical or social model of disability—will determine the roles and priorities the occupational therapists will adopt in relation to adaptation, coping, and resilience work. If autism is not framed as a deficit to be cured, then the occupational therapist can shift and begin to look at the stressors in the environment that are asking that child (and, by extension, the child's family) to "act more normal" (Kapp et al., 2019).

Research on family coping for parents of autistic children also supports this shift to a social model of disability (Hastings et al., 2005; Higgins et al., 2005). The stress that comes with parenting an autistic child is related to the everyday challenges, but it was when parents adopted escape or active avoidant strategies to cope with the stresses of raising a child with autism that more mental health issues and further stress resulted (Hastings & Johnson, 2001). When parents used positive reframing strategies and adopted a more strength-based view, rather than a deficit-based lens, family stress decreased. Interventions with parents might, on the basis of these findings, focus on "enhancing their positive perceptions of raising a child with autism" (Hastings et al., 2005). This reframing is in line with the social model of disability, which requires the occupational therapist to consider the environment, context, and attitudes that go beyond traditional interventions to facilitate adaptation, coping, and resilience (Patten Koenig, 2019). If adaptation is a transformative process that occurs while participating in, and as an outcome of participation in, occupation (Grajo et al., 2018), then how disability is interpreted is critical. The social model of disability demands the removal of contextual barriers in order to support participation (Bagatell, 2010; Imrie, 2009). A focus on strengths and interests is also central to support participation and transformation through meaningful occupation. McCrimmon et al. (2016) advocate for a resilience-oriented perspective as part of a strength-based model that would shift the focus away from deficiencies associated with a clinical disorder and toward individual experiences and achievements, as well as personal and environmental strengths that can support children who are under stress.

DEFINING ADAPTATION, COPING, AND RESILIENCE FOR AUTISTIC CHILDREN AND YOUTH

It is first important to understand the meaning of the construct of resilience in the context of autism. The term *resilience* usually refers to individuals who have a better than expected outcome in the face of some adversity (Masten, 2001). Individuals who have a "good" outcome in the face of such adversity are thought to be "resilient." Similar to the medical model of disability (which is individualistic), protective factors that account for resilience were originally considered traits of the autistic individual (such as high IQ or good social skills) that protected children from stress and adversity. Now, however, protective factors and resilience are thought to reflect not only individual but also relational, as well as contextual, variables in the environment, such as the availability of supportive adults and attitudes of non-autistic peers (Khanlou & Wray, 2014; Sasson et al., 2017; Ungar et al., 2013).

Coping in the autism literature is often based on the ability of the family to deal with a child diagnosed with autism (Bekhet & Matel-Anderson, 2017; Hastings et al., 2005; Higgins et al., 2005; Lee et al., 2019) and not on the adaptation, coping, and resilience skills of autistic children and youth themselves. This is in line with the medical model previously discussed, where the limitations lie within the child with a disability and the coping or adaptation is focused on how parents will cope and the stress they are under once they receive a diagnosis that their child is autistic. This is not to minimize the challenges: these are real for families and are discussed later in this chapter in relation to family collaboration. However, here the definitions of adaptation, coping, and resilience will be specifically applied to the autistic individual and what these constructs mean to their everyday lives.

As Compas et al. (2001) define it, *coping* is the process of adaptation that includes the behaviors and thoughts that are implemented by (in this case) autistic individuals when faced with stress. *Resilience* is the result of having the competence to mobilize coping responses that can be put into action effectively during times of stress and adversity. Lazarus and Folkman's (1984) classic definition of coping as "constantly changing cognitive and behavioral efforts to manage specific external and/or internal demands that

---

Case Study 2-1
Challenges in Adaptation and Coping: Thomas

Thomas is 9 years old and is in fourth grade in an inclusive classroom in the local public school. He is doing grade-level work in math and is hyperlexic in reading (reading at the eighth-grade level). He was diagnosed with autism at the age of 3 and has received early intervention services since then in an effort to address his atypical behavior, which includes flapping his hands, lack of eye contact, and restricted interest in bicycles (specifically, all kinds of wheels). He now receives occupational therapy as part of his Individualized Educational Plan (IEP). He struggles with handwriting, organizational skills, and self-regulation, and does not like transitions or unexpected changes in classroom plans. Thomas will often isolate himself during recess and lunch and will ask his teacher if he can have indoor recess on most days. He loves LEGO sets, especially wheeled vehicles, and spends much time putting them together in different types of trans-portation vehicles and drawing the vehicles he creates. He is in an inclusive classroom and often looks like he is not paying attention and is doodling, and mostly draws different sizes of wheels. He is referred for occupational therapy in order to improve his social skills and participation in group activities, as well as his self-regulation during transition times. His teachers have commented to Thomas that *"If you don't start participating, you will not have any access to your LEGO sets during recess, and they will have to be left at home."* Thomas is very stressed about this when he comes for the initial evaluation, repeatedly asking the occupational therapist if his LEGO sets are being taken away and getting increasingly more anxious as the evaluation proceeds.

---

are appraised as taxing or exceeding the resources of the person" (p. 141) is especially instructive for the autistic population, as much of the sensory and social environments in which autistic individuals find themselves are self-described as "taxing" or "overwhelming." Coping is the goal-oriented step to respond in order to reduce the stress. *Coping responses* are "intentional physical or mental actions in reaction to a stressor and directed toward the environment (problem-focused coping) or an internal state" (p. 88; emotion-focused coping; Compas et al., 2001). *Problem-focused coping* is defined as including responses such as seeking information, generating possible solutions to a problem, and taking actions to change the circumstances that are creating the stress. Emotion-focused coping involves such responses as expressing one's emotions, seeking solace and support from others, and trying to avoid the source of stress (Lazarus & Folkman, 1984). These coping mechanisms are part of the more global notion of *adaptive capacity* (Grajo, 2019), defined as the ability of the individual to identify, create, modify, and implement a variety of strategies to overcome daily-life challenges. The autistic individual must be able to utilize both their problem-solving skills as well as their emotional regulation to cope, and thus be more adaptive to environmental demands. These common environmental demands and challenges are presented in the mini-case study in Case Study 2-1.

The Role of Occupational Therapy: Best and Evidence-Based Practices for Assessment and Intervention

Conceptually, it is easy to understand why a strength-based approach to practice can foster adaptation, coping, and ultimately resilience. Putting it into daily practice may be much more difficult. A strength-based approach is grounded in the social model of disability and does not look at autism as something to be fixed. A discussion of autistic stakeholders, family members, and researchers on strength-based approaches to autism (Urbanowicz et al., 2019) yielded consensus that: a) strength-based language is used; b) strengths, interests, sensory preferences, and skills of the individual are recognized; and c) attributes that may be considered beneficial or detrimental are context dependent and largely socially constructed. However, we do not want to take everything that the autistic individual enjoys and turn it into a therapeutic approach; instead, we should consider a context-based approach that in combination with a strength-based approach addresses environmental barriers as well as builds on the person's strengths (den Houting, 2019; Urbanowicz et al., 2019). Both approaches will be considered in relation to the role of occupational therapy in assessment and intervention, but deficit-based approaches are not addressed here. A more comprehensive strength-based frame of reference for autistic children and youth can be found in Patten Koenig's (2019) chapter in Kramer, Hinojosa, and Howe's foundational text, *Frames of Reference for Pediatric Occupational Therapy*. Here, though, we highlight key assessment and intervention principles that the occupational therapist can directly apply to practice.

Assessments

If part of a resilience-oriented strength-based approach is truly understanding a client's strengths, then assessments must use that lens (Patten Koenig, 2019). Strength-based assessment (SBA) provides a method for identifying personal, familial, and broader contextual strengths (Cosden et al., 2006). SBA has been defined as the measurement of those "emotional and behavioral skills, competencies, and characteristics that create a sense of personal accomplishment; contribute to satisfying relationships with family members, peers, and adults; enhance one's ability to deal with adversity and stress; and promote one's personal, social, and academic development" (Epstein & Sharma, 1998, p. 3). Research outside the area of autism has found that SBA can be a useful addition to assessment protocols because it provides specific information on assets that can be incorporated into interventions. Further, SBA has the potential to affect the attitudes and beliefs of parents and educators involved in the assessment, creating greater hope about the child's ability to function well (Patten Koenig, 2019). From the beginning of the evaluation process, the practitioner transitions from problems to challenges, from pathology to strengths, and from a preoccupation with individual client factors to how the environment affects the person's ability to engage in meaningful occupation. This is a practice perspective radically different from the problem-focused approach.

There should be a deliberate use of standardized and nonstandardized assessments in occupational therapy practice with the goal of gaining an in-depth, as opposed to a superficial, understanding of an individual's strengths, talents, and interests in parallel with an assessment of the person's challenges. Table 2-2 highlights standardized assessments that can be used to explore strengths and protective factors for autistic children and youth. This list is small, but we may hope that it will grow as professionals from all fields realize the importance of SBA measures. The development of standardized SBA measures for children with autism and their families may be a critical link for enhancing the quality of life, self-determination, and autonomy of individuals with autism (Cosden et al., 2006).

In addition to assessments that look at the strengths, talents, and interests of the autistic individual, a key part of a resilience-oriented approach to assessment is the examination of the environment and context from a social model of disability to address factors that are hindering occupational engagement and adaptation. Even if the assessment has revealed strengths and abilities that have not previously been understood or considered, there also has to be an evaluation of how the environment supports or hinders these strengths. For example, if the practitioner views restricted interests as problematic, this attitudinal bias will determine if the strengths are even considered as such. Chen and Patten (2021) advocate for this expansion in role by suggesting that occupational therapy practitioners in school practice "shift attention from individual challenges to the external barriers and to create a supportive environment that promotes participation" (p. 2). This requires an expansion of occupational therapy practice from "student internal challenges to environmental barriers, including attitudes of peers, teachers, and school staff, teacher awareness of students' social needs and intervention strategies, and school practices and policies regarding inclusion" (Chen & Patten, 2021, p. 2).

Intervention

The focus of intervention then becomes threefold: first, building protective factors (sense of mastery, sense of relatedness); second, reducing risk factors (emotional reactivity); and third, the reduction and elimination of environmental and attitudinal barriers. A strength-based frame of reference with self-determination theory at its base can address building a sense of mastery and relatedness, and several interventions that occupational therapists already use can address challenges with emotional regulation. Environmental and attitudinal barriers that have an impact on the individual's ability to cope and adapt are much more entrenched and include negative associations that nonautistic individuals have toward autistic individuals (Sasson et al., 2017), neurotypical biases as to how interaction should occur and the stress those biases place on autistic individuals (Hull et al., 2017), and the failure to see that deficits in social communication are two-sided. Milton (2012) labeled this the "double empathy problem": a bidirectional phenomenon that highlights the difficulty that both autistic and non-autistic individuals have in understanding each other and having empathy for the other because of the different ways they experience the world. Unfortunately, as Milton (2012) points out, this misunderstanding stigmatizes autistic individuals because their perspectives are not

Table 2-2

Resilience and Coping: Strength-Based Assessments		
Assessment	Description	Strength-Based Information Provided
Resiliency Scales for Children and Adolescents (Prince-Embury, 2007)	Self-report for youth 9 to 19 years that assesses two domains of protective factors that support or enhance resilience and one risk factor that reduces resilience	• Sense of mastery (optimism, self-efficacy) • Sense of relatedness (trust, support, comfort) • Emotional reactivity
American Institutes for Research Self-Determination Scale (Wolman et al., 1994)	Parent, teacher, and student forms; each examines capacity and opportunity to apply knowledge, abilities, and perceptions toward becoming self-determined	• Identify and express own needs, interests, and abilities • Set goals • Make choices and plans for goal achievement
Child Occupational Self-Assessment (COSA; Kramer et al., 2014)	Self-assessment of occupational competence and value of everyday activities in children	• Identify interests • Self-report on competence • Identify goal areas
Canadian Occupational Performance Measure (COPM; Law et al., 2014)	Self-endorsed goals and satisfaction related to occupational performance in youth and adults	• Self-determined goals that indicate autonomy and individual goal priorities
Behavioral and Emotional Rating Scale: A Strength-Based Approach to Assessment Scale, Second Edition (BERS-2; Epstein, 2004)	Self-evaluation of strengths for children 11 to 18 years of age; parent evaluation of strengths for children 5 to 18 years of age; addresses relatedness and competence	• Interpersonal strengths • Family involvement • Intrapersonal strengths • School functioning • Affective strength • Career strength
The Survey of Favorite Interests and Activities (Smerbeck, 2017)	Identifies interests including potential benefits of interests in competence development and relationship building specific to autistic population	• Adaptive Coping subscale that looks at how interests foster happiness, emotional coping, and skill development
Vineland Adaptive Behavior Scales-II (VABS-II)—Adapting Subdomain (Sparrow et al., 2005)	Subdomain also referred to as the Coping subscale; examines how well individuals adapt to environmental demands	• Flexibility • Strengths such as adherence to rules

the dominant perspective within the environmental context of an educational system. The double-empathy problem then posits that the autistic individual must learn to cope and adapt to a world that does not understand their perspective and has pathologized it in most learning environments. If intervention is to be successful, then adaptation and coping skills must be developed in light of these differential perspectives: not all of the burden to cope must be placed on the autistic individual by having only that individual adapt to the non-autistic world. This is why it is critical to focus on the environmental pressures and demands that are often the biggest stressors.

Intervention Focus 1: Building Protective Factors

Interventions that build protective factors and foster resilience are interventions that foster self-determination (Patten Koenig & Shore, 2018). *Self-determination theory* (SDT; Deci & Ryan, 1985; Ryan & Deci, 2000, 2002, 2008) is a conceptual framework for understanding the psychosocial and contextual conditions that influence people's intrinsic and extrinsic motivation to learn. SDT proposes that goal achievement is directly related to a person's ability to satisfy three core psychological needs: autonomy, competence, and relatedness. These map directly onto the factors that have consistently been identified in the literature as building resilience.

- *Autonomy* is the feeling of control over one's own personal circumstances; agency, which is critical to build coping resources and is a necessary precursor to personal volition; or acting as the decision maker in one's own life (Deci & Ryan, 1985).
- *Competence* is the feeling associated with mastery and the experience that coincides with developing this mastery, which enhances self-esteem and resilience (Ryan & Deci, 2002). This mastery has direct ties to occupational adaptation or occupational dysadaptation, when the desire for mastery is lower, which is often the case with autistic students as their perceived capacities as persons are underestimated, and they are not perceived as competent (Grajo, 2019).
- *Relatedness* is the connection with others, having a sense of a reciprocal relationship and shared connection, experiences, and sense of purpose (Ryan & Deci, 2000). Gaining a sense of competence is facilitated by autonomy. Choice-making and agency must be a part of every session (Patten Koenig, 2019). A sense of connection, trust, and relatedness will result only if autistic ways of interacting and engaging with the world are viewed from a neutral or positive attribution standpoint (Patten Koenig, 2019).

Social and environmental contexts, including the therapeutic context, can either nurture or impede these three needs, which in turn can affect adaptation, coping, and resilience. See Table 2-3 on specific interventions to foster self-determination. Figures 2-1 to 2-3 illustrate some child-centered interventions to foster resilience.

Table 2-3

Interventions That Build Protective Factors and Reduce Risk Factors	
Building Protective Factors	**Interventions That Support Autonomy, Competence, and Relatedness**
	• Provide autonomy support and choice in goal setting and activity choice
	• Propose activity-based social groups for students with shared interests to participate in together
	• Follow the young child's interests and incorporate them into all aspects of intervention
	• Learn about autistic ways of knowing by reading self-advocates' writing or discussing directly with autistic individuals in order to better relate to how they experience the world
	• Foster self-advocacy skills
Reducing Risk Factors	**Interventions That Improve Emotional Regulation**
	• SCERTS Model[1], which works on two components of emotional regulation: self-regulation and mutual regulation (Prizant et al., 2006)
	• Zones of Regulation (Kuypers, 2011), designed to help autistic students recognize when they're in the different Zones (states of alertness/moods), and learn how to use strategies to regulate the Zone they are in
	• How Does Your Engine Run? (Willams & Shellenberger, 1996); can customize to use special interests (e.g., dinosaurs) to learn self-regulation strategies
	• Get Ready to Learn (2014), and other yoga-based programs that highlight self-regulation
	• Exercise and movement programs as stress-reduction programs
	• Augmentative and alternative communication (AAC) devices that offer functional ways to communicate
	• Visual supports and schedules to improve self-regulation and predictability

(continued)

Table 2-3 (continued)

Interventions That Build Protective Factors and Reduce Risk Factors	
Addressing Environmental and Attitudinal Barriers	**Interventions That Improve Context**
	• Ask for authentic autistic input for the design of the physical and sensory environment
	• Teach individual how to do a sensory scan of each environment, identify potential stressors, and then self-advocate or have a known alternative (e.g., bright lights: advocate to dim them or wear a baseball hat)
	• Suggest autistic affinity groups/support networks as children become adolescents
	• Propose class activities incorporating the client's interests to promote shared engagement
	• Address bullying or lack of reciprocal social interaction with peers
	• Provide peer awareness education for all students in collaboration with teachers and administrators (Chen & Patten, 2021)
	• Advocate for teacher education on strategies to support autistic students

[1] The acronym "SCERTS" refers to the model's focus on the following three domains: (1) social communication (SC), which refers to the development of spontaneous, initiated, functional communication, the development of secure and trusting relationships with children and adults, and an understanding of the conventions of different social situations; (2) emotional regulation (ER), which refers to the development of the ability to utilize specific strategies to cope with everyday stressors and to be most available for learning and interacting; and (3) transactional support (TS), which refers to the development and implementation of supports to help partners be highly responsive to an individual's needs and interests, modify and adapt the environment, and provide tools to enhance learning.

Intervention Focus 2: Reducing Risk Factors

Occupational therapy practitioners currently have available many therapeutic interventions that address reducing risk factors such as emotional reactivity, sensory processing issues, and self-regulation. These person factors and interventions are well documented in the occupational therapy literature. With autistic children and youth, emotional reactivity and subsequent difficulty with emotional regulation can be tied to overwhelming sensory input, or, conversely, a need for movement and sensory input, inability to communicate in reliable and consistent means, and unpredictability with task or environmental demands. Mirenda and Brown (2007) highlighted the need for intervention programs to focus on these stressors, by providing a more appropriate means of communication, using specific visual supports and schedules to reduce anxiety

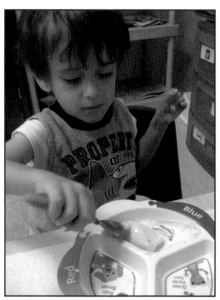

Figure 2-1. Child exploring different new foods.

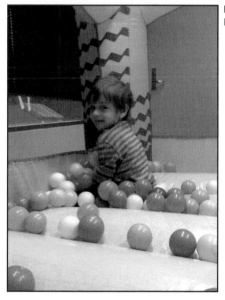

Figure 2-2. Child enjoying playing at the Bouncy House.

and develop adapting and coping strategies that help the autistic individual regulate their emotional responses. There are specific comprehensive programs, such as SCERTS (Prizant et al., 2006; Rubin et al., 2013), that emphasize both the development of emotional regulation and the development of communication to reduce problem behaviors; these reduce risk factors for autistic individuals. Table 2-3 presents specific interventions that reduce risk and foster emotional regulation in autistic children and youth.

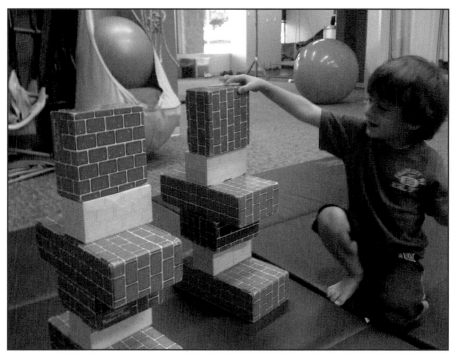

Figure 2-3. Child copying block patterns.

Intervention Focus 3: Reducing Environmental Barriers

Autistic ways of being and experiencing the world are often viewed through a negative lens. To begin to reduce barriers within the social and physical environment, the occupational therapist must first commit to viewing autistic ways of interacting and engaging with the world from a neutral or positive attribution (Patten Koenig, 2019). This involves presuming competence of the autistic individual, whether they have low- or high-support needs, or are able to speak or are non-speaking. This presumption of competence is in line with viewing autistic ways of interacting and experiencing the world as positive or neutral. The occupational therapist must then look at the environment as a place where the challenges, the deficits, and the weaknesses may not be as apparent as individual factors but may have the most significant impact. Examine strengths and weaknesses in the context of societal and environmental barriers so that they can be direct targets of intervention. Table 2-3 presents specific interventions that address environmental and attitudinal barriers.

COLLABORATIVE APPROACH
WITH FAMILIES

One of the most enduring evidence-based practices that support the development of resilience is access to social support (Masten, 2001; National Scientific Council on the Developing Child (NSCDC), 2015). Social support can come from a variety of sources, but it is most often associated with family support for autistic children and youth. How can the occupational therapist collaborate with families to build that social support system? Part of that collaboration can be imparting a strength-based lens on the first visit into the home as an early intervention provider. In a comparison study by Mossman Steiner (2010) of strength-based and deficit-based approaches, the words of the early interventionist mattered as clinicians either outlined areas of need or areas of strength, followed by the same suggestions for intervention and activity for the young autistic child. When the interventionist spoke from a deficit-based perspective (e.g. *"It seems like it is hard to get his attention," "He does not seem to focus on one thing for very long," "He moves from toy to toy," "One way to get his attention is . . ."*), all parents made numerous negative statements, and *never* made a positive statement about their child, displaying a more negative affect and decreased social interaction with their child (Mossman Steiner, 2010). By contrast, when the interventionist spoke from the strength-based approach (*"It seems like he has a lot of interests. That's a good sign," "Right now he seems interested in a couple of different toys. One way to get his attention is . . ."*), parents displayed more positive affect, had fewer negative statements, and engaged more playfully and more affectionately—and the children were more responsive to requests (Mossman Steiner, 2010). The therapists' perspective and approach contributed to increasing social support.

Working collaboratively with the family requires a recognition of the stress that they are experiencing. Using intervention models where family members are considered experts about their own child are critical (Prizant et al., 2006). Higgins et al.'s (2005) work on family coping found that caregivers of autistic children acknowledged high level of stress on families, with 41% reporting some form of physical, emotional, financial, or marital-relationship stress. Normal, spontaneous outings were difficult, not because of challenges arising from their child's behavior, but also, as one caregiver pointed out, from people's misinterpreting the child's behavior as "undisciplined"; this is due to lack of public awareness and indicates that the most challenging part of being a caregiver was dealing with others' perception of her child. Another participant indicated that "the real stress placed on me as a caregiver isn't so much from care for my child, but from the negative attitude and opinion of others who can't cope with an individual who is simply different than others" (Higgins et al., 2005, p. 135). This speaks to the social and environmental aspects being more disabling and less "protective."

Occupational therapists should collaborate with family members to provide interventions that help them articulate their ambitions for their children, and which tap into the children's strengths, competence, and mastery in order to build a meaningful life (Sirota, 2010). *No one builds their life on remediated weaknesses.* It is important to remember that simple statement from the minute the occupational therapist begins interacting and collaborating with a family to assist them in coping with the challenges they face as a family. Will everything be framed as a weakness to be remediated? Or will the occupational therapists embed strengths into their interactions and communications with family members? There is mounting evidence that the use of positive reframing of potentially traumatic and stressful events may be one of the only effective coping strategies where it is very difficult to act directly to reduce the impact of the stressor. Positive reframing, acceptance, and a strength-based approach to build upon skills can be powerful tools to building resilience as a family. This combination of supportive relationships, adaptive skill-building, and positive experiences is what constitutes the foundations of resilience.

Building Interprofessional Collaborations

The occupational therapy practitioner is usually a part of a multidisciplinary (may be intradisciplinary or transdisciplinary in early intervention) team, but primarily works with a speech and language pathologist, special educator and general educator (if the autistic student is in an inclusive classroom), paraprofessionals, behavioral specialists, and psychologists in the evaluation and intervention to which autistic children get referred. The occupational therapist can foster a collaborative approach by clearly explaining their role with autistic children and youth and advocating for a strength-based approach as a counter to traditional deficit-based approaches. One of the best collaborations that the occupational therapist can foster in order to accomplish this is to recruit and bring in autistic self-advocates who are young adults or older to discuss with families, staff, and/ or colleagues what is helpful in regard to coping and adaptation and what really hindered their ability to cope in school, at home, or in the community. This is a way to begin to gain a clearer understanding of an autistic way of being, and might be helpful to consider in your current interventions. For example, autistic adults may experience post-traumatic stress after many life events that may not be recognized as traumatic, and bullying and social isolation may have a more significant impact on their mental health (Rumball et al., 2020). Others have identified the harm that comes when they try to "mask" in order to act as non-autistic as they can during classes or in social situations to meet a non-autistic standard of behavior (Hull et al., 2017). This collaboration can engage the entire team in promoting a more resilience-based approach in their interventions.

A Global Perspective

Globally, the studies on coping and adaptation are in line with the research in the United States: they focus on parent and family coping and do not speak to building resilience from a strength-based perspective. Similarly, severity of autism as well as family resources are highlighted as predictors of stress and coping. In Jordan, a quantitative study conducted by Dardas and Ahmad (2014) examined the relationship between parents' characteristics and the coping strategies used in a sample of 184 Jordanian parents of autistic individuals. Parents with higher incomes used more diverse problem-solving coping strategies, and reported lower stress and higher quality of life. In Taiwan, Huang et al. (2014) found that parents of autistic children with milder support needs and behavior had lower stress than parents of children with more severe behaviors and higher support needs. In Iran, in what may be more indicative of gender roles, 58 mothers of autistic children had significantly higher stress scores than 45 fathers of children with ASD (Samadi et al., 2014).

Research teams in both the United Kingdom and Australia have demonstrated leadership with autistic-informed research that is focused primarily on autistic adults' mental health, coping, and stress, which is outside the scope of this chapter on autistic children and youth but notable among the international research community. These researchers, primarily using community participation or participatory action research methods, are guided by autistic individuals and seek to identify the stressors that autistic adults face, to reframe autistic behavior from first-person perspectives, and to highlight communication needs and mental health supports that would improve coping, adaptation, and quality of life (Crane et al., 2018; Cummins et al., 2020; Kapp et al., 2019). It is hoped that this research will provide guidance as to how communities can better support and accept autistic children and youth so that they can avoid the stressors that adults who did not have access to strength-based models endured. For example, occupational therapists often view "stimming" behavior (stereotyped or repetitive motor movements) as problematic and requiring intervention to reduce and normalize behavior, which often produces even more stress for the autistic child. Kapp and his colleagues (2019) interviewed 32 autistic adults and found that stimming is in fact a key self-regulatory mechanism, which helps the individual calm down during stressful times. According to the adults in the study, stimming was reported to be a very useful behavior that helped them contain, control, or express emotion, which is a critical coping strategy; however, the occupational therapist may previously have sought to extinguish such behavior based on a deficit-focused approach (Kapp et al., 2019). These adult studies can help inform practice with autistic children and youth.

ESSENTIAL CONSIDERATIONS FOR OCCUPATIONAL THERAPISTS TO BUILD ADAPTATION, COPING, AND RESILIENCE

Adopting a strength-based practice that builds adaptation, coping, and resilience is not rocket science, nor does it require advanced training. What it does require, which may be more difficult, is a fundamental shift in thinking. The "essential thinking" that must happen is outlined in Table 2-4. Once the occupational therapist makes this shift, their practice will become a more resilience-oriented practice that begins with a strength-based practice from initial evaluation and continues through discharge.

Table 2-4

Essential Considerations—Shifts in Thinking	
Traditional Thinking	Strength-Based Thinking
Assess for weaknesses in order to treat and build skills.	Assess for strengths in order to empower and build resilience.
Focus on developing typical social interaction.	Focus interactions on enrichment of and access to non-social interests as a goal.
Use social skill groups to increase competence in discrete social skills.	Use interest-based groups that autistic children and youth are autonomously motivated to participate in and develop natural connections and relationships that are meaningful.
Expand the repertoire of activities to avoid the restricted focus on interests at a higher level of intensity.	Incorporate strengths and interests into subject matter, routines, and social relationships. Intense interests may be related to information seeking and processing as well as foundations for relationships, and thus should be encouraged.
Work under the assumptions of neurotypical or non-autistic ways of knowing (e.g., eye contact indicates an attentive listener).	Work with autistic ways of learning, not against them. If eye contact is too distracting for the individual, acknowledge and understand that the individual's comprehension may not be affected by lack of eye contact.
Only use assessments that serve the purpose of evaluating weak areas that require remediation.	Purposefully use assessments that are designed to evaluate areas of strengths that require fostering in order to build resilience.
Interact with families as an expert occupational therapist in order to provide therapeutic intervention.	Because families and their autistic child are the experts, interact with them all to provide coaching and support to build on strengths, and use them to address challenges.

Case Study 2-2

In this case study, Annie is first presented from a typical deficit-based viewpoint. The assessment section will add specific testing but also reframe the deficit-based presentation from a strength-based approach to show the shift in thinking and how that then leads to different interventions that will affect adaptation, coping, and, ultimately, resilience.

Client Presentation

Annie is a 16-year-old female who attends a specialized school for autistic students; they are placed in small classrooms with a special education teacher and three paraprofessionals who are 1:1 aides for several students, including Annie. Annie is nonverbal and does not use gestures to communicate. She has

(continued)

Case Study 2-2 (continued)

a picture-exchange system, but it is not used consistently. Annie can respond, "yes," "no," and "I need help, please." She does demonstrate echolalia and will frequently say "Nashville" or "No Nashville" repeatedly. Annie perseverates on books on tape and country music, and she gets very agitated when staff try to remove her headphones. Annie engages in repetitive and stereotypical motor behavior, including hand flapping and rocking back and forth. When staff redirect her from her stimming, she tries to leave the room or asks to go to the bathroom. She will often walk back and forth in the back of the classroom. She demonstrates restricted interests, being especially attached to different pictures of Dolly Parton that she brings from home in a binder. This behavior interferes with her daily routines and she gets very agitated if she cannot flip through the book when she arrives in the morning.

Assessment

Initial Reframing of Deficit Presentation

Annie is able to understand directions, especially those related to her preferred activities. For communication, she uses a simple board with the responses "yes," "no," and "help," which she uses with 100% accuracy. She uses this board very quickly and often with a sense of humor, replying "yes" or "no" incorrectly as she smiles and laughs. Annie is sensitive to the visual world around her and enjoys listening to a variety of music. Annie knows how to set up her phone and play her music and operate her headphones and also has computer skills for internet searches and collecting information on her preferred interests. She is able to effectively use nonverbal cues to communicate with others and can easily pick up on the emotional state of another person. Annie can become totally absorbed in an activity and is able to pay close attention to details.

Testing and Observations

Traditionally, in this section of an assessment of Annie, we would see standardized testing, including IQ testing on which she would most likely score low given her inability to speak, followed by testing on additional assessments in order to produce a profile of deficits. The testing and observation section is a key place to shift to strength-based assessment. Recall that SBA has been defined as the measurement of those:

> *emotional and behavioral skills, competencies and characteristics that create a sense of personal accomplishment; contribute to satisfying relationships with family members, peers, and adults; enhance one's ability to deal with adversity and stress; and promote one's personal, social, and academic development* (Epstein & Sharma, 1998, p. 3).

So what are Annie's strengths? We begin to see the strengths that bear further exploration in the initial reframing. It will also be critical to see how the environment affects Annie's ability to engage in meaningful occupation. It is also critical to assess the amount of autonomy, competence, and relatedness Annie is feeling

(continued)

Case Study 2-2 (continued)

in her current environment, as these are powerful protective factors. Standard-ized testing is used only to elucidate Annie's strengths and interests, along with interviews of caregivers and teachers. Given that Annie is non-speaking, how do we bring her into an assessment process that doesn't just test and identify deficits? As Annie already uses a basic communication device with 100% accuracy and with a sense of humor, further investigation into her receptive ability with a device or cards or pictures that now also have answers related to her interest to country music (e.g., different singers, lyrics of Dolly Parton) should be done to expand reciprocal interaction with the presumption of competence. In addition to interviews with those who care about Annie, this is how the practitioner can begin to build a deeper understanding of meaningful occupation. Interviews with Annie's parents revealed her love of country music, a dedication to a tele-vision program regarding Nashville restaurants and homes that she does not re-quire any reminders to watch, and a vast collection of old country music album covers (without the records in them) in her room. Her parents have fostered this interest, and enjoy the reaction that Annie has when a new country song comes out; however, they are frequently told by school personnel at her IEP meetings, when they ask about it, that it is a perseverative interest that they should not foster, and it is not allowed in the classroom except for as a reward for good behavior. A sensory scan of the environment reveals a loud classroom with four adults in addition to the eight students. The adults in the classroom frequently talk to each other more than the students, many of whom are non-speaking. When related service providers enter the classroom for physical, occupational, or speech therapy sessions, the noise level increases. During these times, Annie can be observed to increase her pacing and rocking, which appear to be sooth-ing. The class is currently not engaging in any movement activities outside of the adaptive physical education once per week.

Going back to the concept of SBA, Annie's interest in country music and Nashville country-related items is the one thing that gives her a sense of personal accomplishment and contributes to a satisfying relationship with her parents. She is in a learning environment that does not value or recognize this as a strength. How, then, can she use her strengths and protective factors to cope during times of stress and adversity? The paradigm shift that has to happen can begin by using these interests to build resilience.

Interventions

Focus on Building Protective Factors

Autonomy and choice, as well as mastery and competence, are key to building protective factors. What choice does Annie currently have in her classroom set-ting? Her knowledge of country music is not recognized, but rather limited at the start of her day. Attitudinal barriers as to use of these interests will have to be addressed as an environmental barrier (see following discussion), but how would Annie's day look if her interests were followed and incorporated into all aspects of her day? More importantly, how would Annie's coping, resilience,

(continued)

Case Study 2-2 (continued)

Table 2-5

Minimize vs. Maximize Interests		
Interests	Minimize	Maximize
Audiobooks	Avoid letting Annie listen to audiobooks in the classroom	What is Annie listening to? What is the subject area? Build the content into other lessons. Build in reading time where she listens and uses pictures based on content to show what she learned or did during the reading time.
Country music	Let her listen to country music through her headphones only as a reward for good behavior	Build in country music throughout her day. Once she has identified times of stress with noise levels, give her access to headphones while working and not as a reward. Work with her interest, not against it.
Binder of Dolly Parton pictures	Take away the binder of pictures upon arrival and let Annie know she can get it back at the end of the day	Add to the binder of pictures and use it as an opportunity to work on computer skills as she builds an online collection and prints them out.
Nashville	Redirect her when she perseverates on the word "Nashville"	Use Nashville for geography, history, and functional skills. What would she have to search for online in order to plan a trip to Nashville? How much would it cost? Who would she invite?

and adaptation look throughout the day? Table 2-5 provides some initial ideas using the information given, but the ways to incorporate this meaningful occupation into Annie's day are only limited by the creative thought processes of those who interact with Annie in her school setting. Once Annie is secure in the knowledge that she has choice and autonomy in her interests, and that they are valued and seen as an integral part of who she is, she will be more readily able to adapt and cope in situations, knowing that she has access to activities that soothe as well as help grow her level of mastery—but only if they are reframed.

Focus on Reducing Risk Factors

Annie does display emotional reactivity to change, overwhelming sensory environments, and unpredictable requests. In addition, her inability to fully communicate in a reliable, universally understood manner is a source of frustration and stress. Building a predictable routine throughout the day, utilizing her interests, and addressing these risk factors will build self-regulation for Annie. Reduction of her stress level could be multi-pronged, including exercise and movement programs, visual supports and schedules, and expansion of her ability to communicate by providing a more expansive communication system. Specifically, Annie

(continued)

Case Study 2-2 (continued)

frequently paces in the back of the classroom. The occupational therapist could establish a walking routine with Annie and her 1:1 aide where regular walks with her music are integrated throughout the day. Visual support and schedules could be put in her Dolly Parton binder by using pictures of Dolly Parton that they find on the internet to indicate reading times, eating, exercise, computer use, etc. Because Annie wants to look at this binder every morning, including these items would give her the schedule and any changes in the schedule. The occupational and speech and language therapists could collaborate on utilizing Annie's interests as choices in an expanded AAC system that has word prediction or by typing out individual words. Annie could be asked to fill in song lyrics on the computer in order to assess her typing and different avenues for communication. All of these intervention suggestions will assist in reducing the risk factors as protective factors are built.

Focus on Environmental Barriers

The attitudinal barriers in the classroom will have to be addressed as the primary environmental barrier; it is one that is also easily ignored or felt to be an area that is not conducive to intervention. This has to change. The occupational therapist can be a change agent in articulating the concept of meaningful occupation and its relationship to interests. In-services and scheduled trainings can be used as an opportunity to explore this different paradigm, including bringing in self-advocates to discuss how interests can be used in meaningful ways in the classroom. An autistic adult telling educational professionals about the myriad of ways that their interests could have been utilized to foster relationships, build competence, and advance learning can be and has been a powerful transformational moment for many professionals.

Sensory issues are frequently seen as environmental barriers as well, and this case is no exception. The occupational therapist often takes the lead in providing a calming routine: sensory activities and movement programs that address the risk factors described previously. First, suggest working with Annie using picture cues and communication boards to identify times when the classroom is too noisy, and then collaborate with strategies to cope, where she is given a menu of choices and can choose her preferred method (e.g., headphone use, a computer search to look up five restaurants in Nashville and bring them back to the group). These can help Annie begin to self-advocate in what might be a very unpredictable environment.

As can be seen in this case study, by reframing, the occupational therapist can begin to generate a list of potential strengths that can provide a good starting point for intervention to build upon these strengths and utilize then to address challenging behaviors. Although it requires more observational skill and interpretation of these observations to reveal strengths and interests in a non-speaking individual, once found they are powerful ways to intervene and begin to develop a sense of autonomy, competence, and relatedness. By building these protective factors, reducing the risk factors associated with emotional reactivity and regulation, and addressing environmental barriers, the occupational therapist can truly increase the development of coping, adaptation, and resilience for the autistic individuals whom they serve.

REFERENCES

American Occupational Therapy Association. (2014). Occupational therapy practice framework: Domain and process (3rd ed.). *American Journal of Occupational Therapy, 68,* S1-S48. https://doi.org/10.5014/ajot.2014.682006

American Occupational Therapy Association. (2020). Occupational therapy practice framework: Domain and process (4th ed.). *American Journal of Occupational Therapy, 74*(Suppl. 2), 7412410010. https://doi.org/10.5014/ajot.2020.74S2001

American Psychiatric Association. (2013). *Diagnostic and statistical manual of mental disorders* (5th ed.). Author.

Bagatell, N. (2010). From cure to community: Transforming notions of autism. *Ethos, 38*(1), 33-55. https://doi.org/10.1111/j.1548-1352.2009.01080.x

Bekhet, A. K., & Matel-Anderson, D. (2017). Risk and protective factors in the lives of caregivers of persons with autism: Caregivers' perspectives. *Perspectives in Psychiatric Care, 53,* 199-207. https://doi.org/10.1111/ppc.12158

Chen, Y.-L., & Patten, K. (2021). The Issue Is—Shifting focus from impairments to inclusion: Expanding occupational therapy for neurodivergent students to address school environments. *American Journal of Occupational Therapy, 75,* 7503347010. https://doi.org/10.5014/ajot.2021.040618

Compas, B. E., Connor-Smith, J. K., Saltzman, H., Thomsen, A. H., & Wadsworth, M. E. (2001). Coping with stress during childhood and adolescence: Problems, progress, and potential in theory and research. *Psychological Bulletin, 127*(1), 87-127.

Cosden, M., Koegel, L. K., Koegel, R. L., Greenwell, A., & Klein, E. (2006). Strength-based assessment for children with autism spectrum disorders. *Research & Practice for Persons with Severe Disabilities, 31*(2), 134-143. https://doi.org/10.1177/154079690603100206

Crane, L. M., Adams, F., Harper, G., Welch, J., & Pellicano, E. (2018). 'Something needs to change': Mental health experiences of young autistic adults in England. *Autism, 23*(2), 477-493. https://doi.org/10.1177/1362361318757048

Cummins, C., Pellicano, E., & Crane, L. (2020). Autistic adults' views of their communication skills and needs. *International Journal of Language and Communication Disorders.* https://doi.org/10.1111/1460-6984.12552

Dardas, L. A., & Ahmad, M. M. (2014). Quality of life among parents of children with autistic disorder: A sample from the Arab world. *Research in Developmental Disabilities, 35*(2), 278-287. https://doi.org/10.1016/j.ridd.2013.10.029

Deci, E. & Ryan, R. (1985). *Intrinsic motivation and self-determination in human behavior.* Plenum. https://doi.org/10.1007/978-1-4899-2271-7

den Houting, J. (2019). Neurodiversity: An insider's perspective. *Autism, 23*(2), 271-273. https://doi.org/10.1177/1362361318820762

Epstein, M. H. (2004). *Behavioral and Emotional Rating Scale: A Strength-Based Approach to Assessment Scale* (2nd ed.). PRO-ED.

Epstein, M. H., & Sharma, J. (1998). *Behavioral and Emotional Rating Scale: A strength-based approach to assessment.* PRO-ED. https://doi.org/10.1177/073724770002500304

Gernsbacher, M. A. (2017). Editorial perspective: The use of person-first language in scholarly writing may accentuate stigma. *Journal of Child Psychology and Psychiatry, 58*(7), 859-861. https://doi.org/10.1111/jcpp.12706

Get Ready to Learn. (2014). Get Ready To Learn: Researched therapeutic yoga for home and school. http://home.getreadytolearn.net

Grajo, L. (2019). Occupational adaptation as a normative and intervention process: Schkade and Schultz's legacy. In L. C. Grajo & A. Boisselle (Eds.), *Adaptation through occupation: Multidimensional perspectives.* SLACK Incorporated.

Grajo, L., Boisselle, A., & DaLomba, E. (2018). Occupational adaptation as a construct: A scoping review of literature. *Open Journal of Occupational Therapy, 6*(1), Article 2. https://doi.org/10.15453/2168-6408.1400

Hastings, R. P., & Johnson, E. (2001). Stress in UK families conducting intensive home-based behavioral intervention for their young child with autism. *Journal of Autism and Developmental Disorder, 31,* 327-336. https://doi.org/10.1023/A:1010799320795

Hastings, R. P., Kovshof, H., Brown, T., Ward, N. J., Degli Espinosa, F., & Remington, B. (2005). Coping strategies in mothers and fathers of preschool and school-age children with autism. *Autism, 9*(4), 377-391. https://doi.org/10.1177/1362361305056078

Higashida, N. (2013). *The reason I jump: The inner voice of a 13 year old boy with autism.* Random House.

Higgins, D. J., Bailey, S. R., & Pearce, J. C. (2005). Factors associated with functioning style and coping strategies of families with a child with an autism spectrum disorder. *Autism, 9*(2), 125-137. https://doi.org/10.1177/1362361305051403

Huang, C., Yen, H., Tseng, M., Tung, L., Chen, Y., & Chen, K. (2014). Impacts of autistic behaviors, emotional and behavioral problems on parenting stress in caregivers of children with autism. *Journal of Autism and Developmental Disorders 44,* 1383-1390. https://doi.org/10.1007/s10803-013-2000-y

Hull, L., Petrides, K. V., Allison, C., Smith, P., Baron-Cohen, S., Lai, M. C., & Mandy, W. (2017). "Putting on my best normal": Social camouflaging in adults with autism spectrum conditions. *Journal of Autism and Developmental Disorders, 47*(8), 2519-2534. https://doi.org/10.1007/s10803-017-3166-5

Imrie, R. (2009). Rethinking the relationships between disability, rehabilitation, and society. *Disability and Rehabilitation, 19*(7), 263-271. https://doi.org/10.3109/09638289709166537

Kapp, S. K., Steward, R., Crane, L. M., Elliott, D., Elphick, C., Pellicano, E., & Russell, G. (2019). 'People should be allowed to do what they like': Autistic adults' views and experiences of stimming. *Autism, 23*(7), 1782-1792. https://doi.org/10.1177/1362361319829628

Kenny, L., Hattersley, C., Molins, B., Buckley, C., Povey, C., & Pellicano, E. (2016). Which terms should be used to describe autism? Perspectives from the UK autism community. *Autism, 20*(4), 442-462. https://doi.org/10.1177/1362361315588200

Khanlou, N., & Wray, R. (2014). A whole community approach toward child and youth resilience promotion: A review of resilience literature. *International Journal of Mental Health and Addiction, 12,* 64-79. https://doi.org/10.1007/s11469-013-9470-1

Kramer, J., ten Velden, M., Kafkes, A., Basu, S., Federico, J., & Kielhofner, G. (2014). *The Child Occupational Self-Assessment (COSA) Version 2.2.* Model of Human Occupation Clearinghouse, Department of Occupational Therapy, College of Applied Health Sciences, University of Illinois of Chicago.

Kuypers, L. M. (2011). *The zones of regulation: A curriculum designed to foster self-regulation and emotional control.* Think Social Publishing.

Law, M., Baptiste, S., Carswell, A., McColl, M. A., Polatajko, H., & Pollack, N. (2014). *Canadian Occupational Performance Measure* (5th ed.). Canadian Occupational Therapy Association.

Lazarus, R. S., & Folkman, S. (1984). *Stress, appraisal, and coping.* Springer.

Lee, G. K., Krizova, K., & Shivers, C. M. (2019). Needs, strain, coping, and mental health among caregivers of individuals with autism spectrum disorder: A moderated mediation analysis. *Autism, 23*(8), 1936-1947. https://doi.org/10.1177/1362361319833678

Maenner, M. J., Shaw, K. A., Baio, J., Washington, A., Patrick, M., DiRienzo, M., Christensen, D. L., Wiggins, L. D., Pettygrove, S., Andrews, J. G., Lopez, M., Hudson, A., Thaer Baroud, M., Schwenk, Y., White, T., Rosenberg, C. R., Lee, L.-C., Harrington, R. A., Huston, M., Hewitt, A., . . . Dietz, P. M. (2020). Prevalence of autism spectrum disorder among children aged 8 years—Autism and Developmental Disabilities Monitoring Network, 11 sites, United States, 2016. *MMMR Surveillance Summaries, 69*(SS-4), 1-12. http://dx.doi.org/10.15585/mmwr.ss6904a1

Masten, A. S. (2001). Ordinary magic: Resilience processes in development. *American Psychologist, 56,* 227-238. https://doi.org/10.1037//0003-066X.56.3.227

McCrimmon, A. W., Matchullis, R. L., & Altomare, A. A. (2016). Resilience and emotional intelligence in children with high-functioning autism spectrum disorder. *Developmental Neurorehabilitation, 19*(3), 154-161.

Milton, D. E. M. (2012). On the ontological status of autism: The 'double empathy problem', *Disability & Society, 27*(6), 883-887. https://doi.org/10.1080/09687599.2012.710008

Mirenda, P., & Brown, K. (2007). Supporting individuals with autism and problem behavior using AAC. *Perspective on Augmentative and Alternative Communication. 16*(2), 26-31. https://doi.org/10.1044/aac16.2.26

Mossman Steiner, A. (2010). A strengths-based approach to parent education for children with autism. *Journal of Positive Behavior Interventions, 13*(3). https://doi.org/10.1177/1098300710384134

National Scientific Council on the Developing Child. (2015). Supportive relationships and active skill-building strengthen the foundations of resilience: Working Paper 13. https://developingchild.harvard.edu/resources/supportive-relationships-and-active-skill-building-strengthen-the-foundations-of-resilience

Patten Koenig, K. (2019). A strength based frame of reference for autistic individuals. In P. Kramer, J. Hinojosa, & T. Howe (Eds.), *Frames of reference for pediatric occupational therapy* (4th ed.). Wolters Kluwer.

Patten Koenig, K., & Shore, S. (2018). Self-determination and a shift to a strengths based model. In R. Watling & S. Spitzer (Eds.), *Autism: A Comprehensive Occupational Therapy Approach* (4th ed.). AOTA Press.

Prince-Embury, S. (2007). *Resiliency scales for children and adolescents: A profile of personal strengths.* Pearson.

Prizant, B. M., Wetherby, A. M., Rubin, E., Laurent, A. C., & Rydell, P. J. (2006). *The SCERTS Model: Volume I Assessment; Volume II Program planning and intervention.* Brookes.

Rubin, E., Prizant, B. M., Laurent, A. C., & Wetherby, A. M. (2013). Social communication, emotion regulation, and transactional support (SCERTS). In S. Goldstein & J. Naglieri (Eds.), *Interventions for autism spectrum disorders*, 107-127. Springer.

Rumball, F., Happé, F., & Grey, N. (2020). Experience of trauma and PTSD symptoms in autistic adults: Risk of PTSD development following DSM-5 and non-DSM-5 traumatic life events. *Autism Research, 00*, 1-11. https://doi.org/10.1002/aur.2306

Ryan, R. M., & Deci, E. L. (2000). Self-determination theory and the facilitation of intrinsic motivation, social development and well-being. *American Psychologist, 55*, 68-78. https://doi.org/10.1037/0003-066x.55.1.68

Ryan, R. M., & Deci, E. L. (2002). Overview of self-determination theory: An organismic dialectical perspective. In E. L. Deci & R. M. Ryan (Eds.), *Handbook of self-determination research* (pp. 3-33). University of Rochester Press.

Ryan, R. M., & Deci, E. L. (2008). Self-determination theory and the role of basic psychological needs in personality and the organization of behavior. In O. P. John, R. W. Robbins, & L. A. Pervin (Eds.), *Handbook of personality: Theory and research* (pp. 654-678). Guilford Press.

Saleebey, D. (1996). The strengths perspective in social work practice: Extensions and cautions. *Social Work, 41*(3), 296-305.

Samadi, S. A., McConkey, R., & Bunting, B. (2014). Parental well-being of Iranian families who have children with developmental disabilities. *Research in Developmental Disabilities, 35*(7), 1639-1647. https://doi.org/10.1016/j.ridd.2014.04.001

Sasson, N. J., Faso, D. J., Nugent, J., Lovell, S., Kennedy, D. P., & Grossman, R. B. (2017). Neurotypical peers are less willing to interact with those with autism based on thin slice judgments. *Scientific Reports, 7*, 40700. https://doi.org/10.1038/srep40700

Schkade, J. K., & Schultz, S. (1992). Occupational adaptation: Toward a holistic approach for contemporary practice, part 1. *American Journal of Occupational Therapy, 46*(9), 829-837. https://doi.org/10.5014/ajot.46.9.829

Shakespeare, T. (2013). The social model of disability. In L. J. Davis (Ed.), *The disability studies reader* (4th ed., pp. 214-221). Routledge.

Shore, S. M. (2003). *Beyond the wall: Personal experiences with autism and Asperger Syndrome* (2nd ed.). Autism Asperger Publishing.

Sirota, K. G. (2010). Narratives of transformation: Family discourse, autism and trajectories of hope. *Discourse and Society, 21*(5), 544-564. https://doi.org/10.1177/0957926510373992

Smerbeck, A. (2017). The survey of favorite interests and activities: Assessing and understanding restricted interests in children with autism spectrum disorder. *Autism*, 1-13. https://doi.org/10.1177/1362361317742140

Sparrow, S. S., Cicchetti, D., & Balla, D. A. (2005). *Vineland Adaptive Behavior Scales, Second Edition (Vineland-II).* Pearson. https://doi.org/10.1037/t15164-000

Tammett, D. (2006). *Born on a blue day: Inside the extraordinary mind of an autistic savant.* Free Press.

Tomchek, S. D., & Koenig, K. (2016). Occupational therapy practice guidelines for individuals with autism spectrum disorder. AOTA Press.

Ungar, M., Ghazinour, M., & Richter, J. (2013). Annual research review: What is resilience within the social ecology of human development? *Journal of Child Psychology and Psychiatry, 54*, 348-66. https://doi.org/10.1111/jcpp.12025

Urbanowicz, A., Nicolaidis, C., den Houting, J., Shore, S. M., Gaudion, K., Girdler, S., & Savarese, R. J. (2019). An expert discussion on strength-based approaches in autism. *Autism in Adulthood, 1*(2), 82-89. https://doi.org/10.1089/aut.2019.29002.aju

Williams, M. S., & Shellenberger, S. (1996). *How does your engine run?* Therapyworks.

Wolman, J., Campeau, P., DuBois, P., Mithaug, D., & Stolarski, V. (1994). *AIR Self-Determination Scale and User Guide.* American Institute of Research.

3

Children and Youth With Specific Learning Disabilities*

Lenin C. Grajo, PhD, EdM, OTR/L and
Julia M. Guzmán, EdD, OTD, OTR/L

CHAPTER OBJECTIVES By the end of this chapter, the reader will be able to:

- Describe the strengths and challenges of children with learning disabilities in terms of their adaptation, coping, and resilience.
- Apply an occupational adaptation and empowering lens in developing an occupational profile for children with learning disabilities.
- Identify best and evidence-based practices in supporting the adaptation, coping, and resilience of children with learning disabilities using an empowering framework.
- Describe how collaboration with families and an interprofessional team can strengthen interventions geared toward supporting adaptation, coping, and resilience in children with learning disabilities.

---

*Authors' Note

In this chapter we interchangeably use the terms *children with specific learning disabilities (SLD)* and *children with learning disabilities or learning disorders (LD)* to reflect both the contemporary use of the term (SLD as indicated in the *Diagnostic and Statistical Manual of Mental Disorders, Fifth Edition* [*DSM-5*]) and terms used in seminal and more global literature (LD). We use these terms without major distinction throughout.

Grajo L. C., & Boisselle, A. K. (Eds.). *Adaptation, Coping, and Resilience in Children and Youth: A Comprehensive Occupational Therapy Approach* (pp. 45-72).
© 2022 Taylor & Francis Group.

OVERVIEW OF THE POPULATION

Specific learning disability (SLD) is a neurodevelopmental disorder that is diagnosed by low educational competence in the early primary school years (American Psychiatric Association [APA], 2013). Children who encounter difficulties in the major childhood occupation of academic learning are often identified as having LD (Burtner et al., 2002). An SLD, according to the Individuals with Disabilities Education Act (IDEA, 2004) is a developmental disorder that can result in the inability to listen, think, speak, write, spell, or perform mathematical calculations. Although children with SLD face different challenges in everyday occupations, such as activities of daily living, social participation, play, leisure, and academic achievement, only academic concerns have received notice (Rosenblum & Weintraub, 2007).

Diagnosis

Learning disorders can only be diagnosed after formal education starts. A diagnosis is made through a combination of observation, interviews, family history, and school reports. Neuropsychological testing may be used to assist in finding the best way to help the individual with a specific learning disorder (Hale et al., 2010). To be diagnosed with a specific learning disorder, a person must meet four criteria (APA, 2013):

a. Have difficulties in at least one of the following areas for at least 6 months despite targeted help:
    - Difficulty reading (e.g., inaccurate, slow, and only with much effort)
    - Difficulty understanding the meaning of what is read
    - Difficulty with spelling
    - Difficulty with written expression (e.g., problems with grammar, punctuation, or organization)
    - Difficulty understanding number concepts, number facts, or calculation
    - Difficulty with mathematical reasoning (e.g., applying math concepts or solving math problems)
b. Have academic skills that are substantially below what is expected for the child's age and cause problems in school, work, or everyday activities.
c. The difficulties start at school age even if some people do not experience significant problems until adulthood (when academic, work, and day-to-day demands are greater).
d. Learning difficulties are not due to other conditions, such as intellectual disability, vision or hearing problems, a neurological condition (e.g., pediatric stroke), adverse conditions such as economic or environmental disadvantage, lack of instruction, or difficulties speaking/understanding the language.

For a more detailed discussion on the different subtypes of SLD and their clinical presentation, readers are encouraged to review Grajo, Guzman, Szklut, and Philibert (2020). Under federal law—the Individuals with Disabilities Education Act (IDEA, 2004)—students with LD are eligible for special education services. The law requires that if a child is suspected of having an LD, the school must provide an evaluation, and those found to have LD are eligible for special education services. A team, including school personnel and parents, will develop an Individualized Education Plan (IEP) for the student. Parents should specifically ask for an evaluation if they are concerned. The federal law also requires that free appropriate public education (FAPE) be offered to all students, including those requiring special education (Hale et al., 2010). The Every Student Succeeds Act (ESSA) is a U.S. law passed in December 2015 that governs the United States' K-12 public education policy and emphasizes "personalized learning." Personalized learning models can give each student differentiated learning experiences based on their needs, interests, and strengths; this includes students with disabilities, which benefits students with SLD (ESSA, 2015).

Special education services can help children with LD improve in reading, writing, and math. Effective interventions involve systematic, intensive, individualized instruction that may improve the learning difficulties and/or help the individual use strategies to compensate for the disorder. Education for a person with LD often involves multimodal teaching involving multiple senses (Hale et al., 2010). Students with LD also benefit from accommodations, such as additional time on tests and written assignments, using computers for typing rather than writing by hand, and smaller class size. Successful interventions, strategies, and accommodations for a child may change over time as the child develops and academic expectations change (Rosenblum, 2016). Children with a diagnosis of an LD who have mild or moderate deficits in the areas of visual motor, graphomotor, and/or fine motor skills that affect their performance with handwriting skills may be referred by either caregivers and/or teachers for assessment. Occupational therapists have typically defined their roles in evaluating children with LD using assessments for underlying mechanisms that support academics, such as fine motor and visual perceptual skills (Tseng & Chow, 2000).

There remains a gap in research on how occupational therapists support the adaptation, coping, and resilience of children with LD. This chapter aims to highlight literature from various disciplines and use this to synthesize best practices and propose a framework for a distinct role of occupational therapy. This framework is presented in later sections and highlighted to draft essential considerations for practice.

Defining Adaptation, Coping, and Resilience in Children and Youth With Specific Learning Disabilities

The psychosocial adaptation, coping, and resilience of children and youth with SLD have been thoroughly researched and discussed in the special education literature, including studies with longitudinal and phenomenological designs. Because of learning challenges, children with SLD are more vulnerable to stress, have feelings of lesser competence and success than peers in various contexts of daily life, and experience many challenges that may significantly affect their feelings of confidence, self-worth, and accomplishment (Mather & Ofiesh, 2013). In a seminal exhaustive review of earlier studies, Morrison and Cosden (1997) found five factors related to coping and resilience in children and youth with LD. The researchers found that children and youth with LD: (1) tend to have comorbid emotional problems; (2) have family environments that can be both protective or risk factors for child development; (3) have higher rates of school dropout; (4) are more likely to experience juvenile delinquency; and (5) are more likely to be exposed to substance use. Table 3-1 summarizes how each of these factors can both be protective or risk factors for the resilience and adaptation of children and youth with SLD.

Morrison and Cosden's study (1997) on factors affecting adaptation and resilience in children with SLD is supported by more contemporary studies. The National Center for Learning Disability's "State of Learning Disabilities" report yields very similar findings (Horowitz et al., 2017):

- Nearly one in five students (19%) with IEPs misses three or more weeks of school each year, compared to about one in eight students (13%) without IEPs. School aversion and chronic absenteeism can be a sign of unidentified or inadequately addressed learning and attention issues.
- Students with disabilities are more than twice as likely to be suspended as students without disabilities, and the loss of instructional time increases the risk of repeating a grade and dropping out. In 2013-2014, 65% of all special education disciplinary removals involved students with SLD and other health impairments.
- In 2013–2014, 18.1% of students with SLD dropped out, nearly three times the rate of all students (6.5%).
- Failure to address learning and attention issues too often leads to students being incarcerated, which further disrupts their education and contributes to high dropout and recidivism rates. Some studies indicate that a third or more of incarcerated youth have LD, and an even greater proportion may show signs of ADHD.

Another seminal review of the literature supports the substantial research on the cognitive and neuropsychological processing difficulties that underlie LD in children that can be associated with their adaptation, coping, and resilience. Greenham (1997) found that children with LD are more likely to be rejected by their peers, have been reported to engage in fewer social interactions, to initiate these interactions less, and to be less tactful and cooperative than their typically achieving peers; also, individuals with LD misinterpret verbal and, in particular, nonverbal cues more often than do their non-LD peers. Greenham (1997) also found evidence that children with LD possess the same amount of social knowledge as do children without LD, but fail to use this knowledge spontaneously. These psychosocial factors can then put children and youth with SLDs at greater risk for nonresilience, anxiety, and depression. In a study from Canada, Panicker and Chelliah (2016) found that children and youth with SLDs have lower resilience scores on standardized tests and, more often, have higher levels of stress and anxiety. The researchers also found that children with reading disorders were more likely to be depressed than those without reading disorders, and are more likely to be emotionally affected by their academic difficulties.

Table 3-1

Factors Influencing Adaptation, Coping, and Resilience in Children With Learning Disabilities		
Factors Related to Adaptation, Coping, and Resilience in Children With Learning Disabilities	Protective Factors	Risk Factors
Emotional adjustment Children with SLD tend to have comorbid emotional problems and LD.	Self-esteem and self-awareness may function as protective factors in the sense that they may facilitate lower levels of anxiety.	Depression and anxiety are the result of high levels of frustration and perceived lack of control and predictability. Lower levels of autonomy and higher levels of anxiety are perceived in students with LD than in those without disabilities.
Family adaptation The family environment has been identified as a key factor that can provide both risks (e.g., discord, inconsistent discipline) and protection (e.g., a supportive adult relationship, cohesive family functioning) for the developing child.	Families that effectively respond to the needs of children with LD are those that are cohesive and flexible, and utilize coping skills at home and during interactions in schools.	Hyperactivity is a noted risk for family functioning. The presence of behavior problems, particularly in boys with LD, also appears to contribute to the experience of parental stress. Parental expectations and disappointments and patterns of enmeshment, overprotection, and rigidity result in higher dysfunction.
School dropout Dropout rates in children with LD are higher compared to those without disabilities.	Successful dropout prevention programs, such as small class size with low student-teacher ratios, responsive educational programming, individualized attention, basic skill instruction, and parent involvement	Risk factors include prior school attendance, discipline problems, reading ability, socioeconomic status, and family intactness; school transfers, suspensions, and expulsions. School practices that lead to student alienation, disengagement, and loss of commitment also contribute to the dropout problem.

(continued)

Table 3-1 (continued)

Factors Influencing Adaptation, Coping, and Resilience in Children With Learning Disabilities		
Factors Related to Adaptation, Coping, and Resilience in Children With Learning Disabilities	Protective Factors	Risk Factors
Juvenile delinquency Youth with LD are more likely to be adjudicated delinquent than those without disabilities; delinquents with LD had a greater likelihood of recidivism and parole failure.	Positive attachment to teachers and peers, positive engagement with and experiences in school tasks Increased academic skill levels and reduction of psychological distress	Students with LD are more likely than typically achieving peers to fail in school and to develop negative self-image (which is correlated with school dropout and delinquent activity). Children with LD may possess personality characteristics (e.g., impulse control challenges, problem-solving difficulties, social perception problems, lower self-esteem, suggestibility) that may make them more susceptible to delinquent activity. The association between juvenile delinquency and LD is strongest with hyperactivity and conduct disorders.
Substance abuse Youth with LD are more likely to have substance dependence than those without.	Not described	Low self-esteem Hyperactivity Environmental risks including early and persistent behavior problems, low commitment to school, peer rejection in elementary school, experience of school failure
Synthesized from Morrison, G., & Cosden, M. (1997). Risk, resilience, and adjustment of individuals with learning disabilities. *Learning Disability Quarterly, 20*(1), 43-50. https://doi.org/10.2307/1511092		

Despite the numerous challenges in psychosocial adaptation faced by children and youth with SLDs, contemporary perspectives advocate using a more empowering or strength-based approach in framing the adaptation, coping, and resilience of this population. A summary of this empowering perspective is listed in Table 3-2. The empowering paradigm supports seminal findings on the protective factors that are listed in Table 3-1. Case Study 3-1 provides a case illustration to help understand the challenges and strengths of a student with SLD.

Table 3-2

An Empowering Perspective on Adaptation, Coping, and Resilience of Children and Youth With Specific Learning Disabilities

Adaptation, Coping, and Resilience Factors	Empowering Perspective
Role of reciprocal and supportive relationships	Reciprocity in interpersonal relations was consistently found to be an important component of the social support construct with mediating impact. Reciprocity in peer relations is of unique importance, including a positive (special friends) as well as a negative impact (identified enemies).
	Special friendships marked the experiences of those who were resilient. They appeared to be able to identify individuals who would be compatible friends. They made use of these friendships to boost themselves when they were depressed or frustrated.
	Resilient students identified particular teachers or school personnel who either found ways to teach these students despite their LD or gave them extra attention.
	Supportive adults or mentors are able to foster trust and bolster the self-esteem of children with LD. Teachers in the school environment can serve as protective factors for children.
	Successful individuals with LD have at least one person in their lives who accepts them unconditionally and serves as a mentor.
Ability to identify particular areas of strength	Resilient students enthusiastically identified single areas of particular strength that they have and took pride in participating in these activities.
Self-determination	A distinctive element that has been described in previous research is a definite reach toward self-determination.
	The capacity to accomplish goals is influenced by the accuracy of one's self-knowledge and self-perceptions, and thus acts as an internal locus of control.
Using distinctive turning points	Often resilient individuals were able to identify and describe very specific times or events in life that they then or subsequently saw as turning points.
Embracing the disability	Students who demonstrated resilience found it useful to specifically acknowledge that they had LD and confront the way that those disabilities affected their achievements.

(continued)

Table 3-2 (continued)

An Empowering Perspective on Adaptation, Coping, and Resilience of Children and Youth With Specific Learning Disabilities	
Adaptation, Coping, and Resilience Factors	Empowering Perspective
Identifying success experiences	One of the most noticeable differences between the resilient and non-resilient students was the resilient students' ability to identify successful experiences and describe these experiences as deliberate steps in their success. Thus, they were able to both identify activities in which they might find success and use those activities to attain even more success.
Celebrating accomplishments in academic and non-academic domains	Students who received support in positive development in other areas of performance besides traditional school subjects were found to have more positive results in terms of coping and resilience.
	Another important consideration is to identify specific academic areas in which students with LD can be educated along with peers, using the same materials and procedures, to facilitate their sense of competence.

Adapted from Margalit, M. (2003). Resilience model among individuals with learning disabilities: Proximal and distal influences. *Learning Disabilities Research & Practice, 18*(2), 82-86; Mather, N., & Ofiesh, N. (2013). Resilience and the child with learning disabilities. In S. Goldstein & R. Brooks (Eds.), *Handbook of resilience in children* (2nd ed., pp. 239-255). Springer; and Miller, M. (2002). Resilience elements in students with learning disabilities. *Journal of Clinical Psychology, 58*(3), 291-298. https://doi.org/10.1002/jclp.10018.

THE ROLE OF OCCUPATIONAL THERAPY IN ASSESSMENT AND INTERVENTION WITH FOCUS ON ADAPTATION, COPING, AND RESILIENCE

In this section, we highlight and propose a framework, based on evidence and best practices, that uses an empowering approach to facilitate the adaptation, coping, and resilience of children and youth with SLD through an occupational therapy intervention process. This proposed framework, illustrated in Figure 3-1, emphasizes four critical perspectives based on synthesis of the literature to support children and youth: (1) emphasize strengths and protective factors rather than focusing on deficits and challenges; (2) use cognitive strategies to overcome daily challenges; (3) apply sociocultural and self-determination frameworks; and (4) focus on the development of mastery, self-confidence, and self-esteem. We will discuss these four perspectives within the evaluation and intervention processes of occupational therapy.

Case Study 3-1

Logan

Logan is a 13-year-old student in the eighth grade diagnosed with specific developmental reading disorder, low muscle tone, mixed receptive/expressive language disorder, fine motor impairment, lack of coordination, and other disorders of social-emotional development. Educational records indicate that Logan's academic skills are in the low range in all areas. He attends an inclusive classroom of 25 students and is reported to have improved his academic performance with the support of regular and special education teachers. Logan has a history of behavior difficulties. Logan reported that his favorite subject is math, and he enjoys karate and video games. He complains that reading assignments, especially those that require long readings, are very difficult for him.

Logan participates well in his classroom setting, according to his teacher. During the observation, Logan was engaged in completing previously assigned coursework. He interacted with a peer sitting next to him and frequently was inattentive to the work to be completed. During an interview, Logan shared that he "always gets tired and frustrated" when doing assignments that require written expression based on reading assignments. Essays, journaling, and book summary assignments are extremely hard for him. These assignments often cause a lot of tension between him and his mom, as he often avoids doing these assignments until the night before the deadline and then is uncooperative when his mom helps him complete these tasks. He is exploring the use of organizational assistive technologies to help him complete such assignments more efficiently. He does better when using text-to-speech technologies and having the assignment read to him by the software. However, he enjoys reading superhero comics and can write stories with graphic illustrations and complex plot lines.

Principle 1: Create an Occupational Profile That Focuses on Strengths and Protective Factors—Considerations for Occupational Therapy Evaluation

Margalit (2003), a proponent of using a resilience model for children with LD, has been one of the strongest advocates of shifting from a deficit to an empowering approach in the way interventionists address the needs of this population. Margalit has emphasized that most research concerning children with LD has been performed within a deficiency model that examined in depth the children's difficulties, causes, and outcomes in terms of maladjustment and intervention planning. We propose a shift in the way occupational therapy evaluations are conducted and analyzed. It is essential to use performance and skill-level assessments to gain a better understanding of client factors and performance skills that are challenging for the child with LD. However, participation-level and contextual assessments are also necessary to get an understanding of areas of strengths, preferences in terms of childhood occupations, and contextual factors that may serve as protective factors for daily life challenges that may facilitate adaptation,

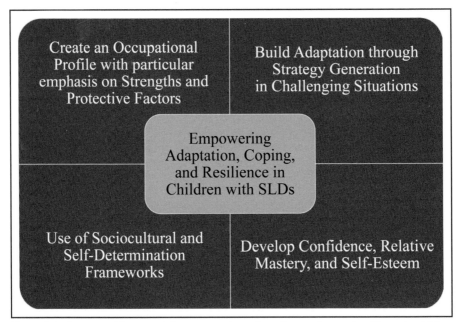

Figure 3-1. A proposed framework for empowering adaptation, coping, and resilience in children with LD.

coping, and resilience. Table 3-3 provides an overview of some measures that can be used to assess factors related to adaptation, coping, resilience, and occupational participation of children and youth with SLD.

Principle 2: Apply Sociocultural and Self-Determination Frameworks

There is a multitude of literature supporting the need to use sociocultural and self-determination frameworks to foster adaptation, coping, and resilience in children with LD. Schkade and Schultz (2003), as expanded by Grajo (2019), have asserted the role of eliciting the occupational environment and empowering the person as the primary agent of change to facilitate the internal, normative occupational adaptation process. When facilitating the occupational environment, using a framework that encourages a collaborative approach among the child, the child's family, teachers and mentors, and peers can help support adaptation, coping, and resilience. Mather and Ofiesh (2013) have documented evidence showing that supportive adults or mentors are able to foster trust and bolster the self-esteem of children with LD and that collaboration and nurturing relationships with teachers in the school environment can serve as protective factors for children. Mather and Ofiesh further elaborated that successful individuals with LD are those who have people in their lives who accept them unconditionally and serve as mentors. Tonkin and colleagues (2014) also documented that family values, preferences,

Table 3-3

Measures That Can Be Used to Assess Adaptation, Coping, Resilience, and Participation in Children and Youth With Learning Disabilities	
Measure	**Description**
Adolescent/Adult Sensory Profile (Brown & Dunn, 2002)	This self-questionnaire, for individuals 11 years of age or older, measures possible contributions of sensory processing to the person's daily performance patterns. The classification system is based on normative information (https://www.pearsonassessments.com/store/usassessments/en/Store/Professional-Assessments/Motor-Sensory/Adolescent-Adult-Sensory-Profile/p/100000434.html).
Canadian Occupational Performance Measure, Fourth Edition (Law et al., 2005)	This interview tool helps identify the family's priorities for their child with special needs and assists in developing therapy goals with the child's primary caregivers. Distributed by the Canadian Association of Occupational Therapy (http://www.caot.ca).
Child Occupational Self-Assessment (COSA; Keller et al., 2005)	A self-report that asks children to rate their performance competency and the importance of that activity. Available through the Model of Human Occupational Clearinghouse (http://www.moho.uic.edu).
Children's Assessment of Participation and Enjoyment (CAPE; King et al., 2004)	The CAPE is designed to explore an individual's day-to-day participation to allow planning of intervention or measure outcomes. The CAPE may be used independently or with the Preferences for Activities for Children (PAC; http://www.psychcorp.com).
Early Coping Inventory (Zeitlin et al., 1988)	This observation instrument is used to assess coping-related behavior, including sensorimotor organization, reactive behaviors, and self-initiated behaviors, in children functioning at the 4-month to 36-month developmental level (http://www.ststesting.com/early.html#EAR).
Home Observation for Measurement of the Environment (HOME; Caldwell & Bradley, 1984)	The initial version of this inventory, the Infant/Toddler HOME, was designed to measure the support available to a child from birth to 3 years of age in the home environment. The Early Childhood HOME (ages 3 to 6 years), the Middle Childhood HOME (ages 6 to 10 years), and the Early Adolescent HOME (ages 10 to 15 years) are also available (https://uwm.edu/mcwp/wp-content/uploads/sites/337/2015/12/HOME12-1-14.pdf).
Occupational Therapy Psychosocial Assessment of Learning (OT PAL; Townsend et al., 2001)	The OT PAL measures psychosocial factors that influence a child's learning. The tool uses observation and interview to assess volition, habituation, and environmental fit within the classroom of children aged 6 to 12 years.

(continued)

Table 3-3 (continued)

Measure That Can Be Used to Assess Adaptation, Coping, Resilience, and Participation in Children and Youth With Learning Disabilities	
Measure	**Description**
Pediatric Volitional Questionnaire (PVQ) 2.1 (Basu et al., 2008)	This observational assessment is designed to evaluate a young child's volition, including motivation, values, and interests, and the impact of environment. For children aged 2 to 7 years. Available through the Model of Human Occupational Clearinghouse (http://www.moho.uic.edu).
Preferences for Activities of Children (PAC; King et al., 2004)	The PAC is used to assess an individual's preference for activities. The PAC may be used independently or together with the CAPE (https://www.pearsonassessments.com/store/usassessments/en/Store/Professional-Assessments/Behavior/Adaptive/Children%27s-Assessment-of-Participation-and-Enjoyment-and-Preferences-for-Activities-of-Children/p/100000481.html).
School Function Assessment (SFA; Coster et al., 1998)	The SFA is a judgment-based questionnaire designed to measure a student's performance of functional tasks that support their participation in the academic and social aspects of an elementary school program (grades K–6). The SFA was designed to facilitate collaborative program planning for students with a variety of disabling conditions (https://www.pearsonassessments.com/store/usassessments/en/Store/Professional-Assessments/Behavior/Adaptive/School-Function-Assessment/p/100000547.html).
Sensory Processing Measure (SPM; Parham et al., 2007 [Home Form]; Miller-Kuhaneck et al., 2007 [School Form])	The SPM was developed to allow assessment of sensory processing, praxis, and social participation in the home, classroom, and other school environments, and to compare an individual child's performance with normative samples of other school-aged children.
The Short Child Occupational Profile (SCOPE) 2.2 (Bowyer et al., 2008)	This measure determines how volition, habituation, skills, and the environment facilitate or restrict a child's participation. Available through the Model of Human Occupational Clearinghouse (http://www.moho.uic.edu).
Test of Environmental Supportiveness (TOES; Bundy, 1999)	Assesses the extent to which the environment supports a child's play. This measure investigates the caregiver's actions, rules, and boundaries during the child's play; identifies peer, younger, and older playmates' use of cues and domination of interaction; describes natural and fabricated objects used during play; and describes the amount and configuration of space, the sensory environment, and the safety and accessibility of space. Available from Colorado State University, Department of Occupational Therapy.

(continued)

Table 3-3 (continued)

Measures That Can Be Used to Assess Adaptation, Coping, Resilience, and Participation in Children and Youth With Learning Disabilities

Measure	Description
The Inventory of Reading Occupations—Pediatric Version (IRO-Pedi; Grajo et al., 2019)	The IRO-Pedi is a two-part self-report and/or interview tool that can be used to develop a reading participation profile for a child/student in grades 1 to 3. The IRO-Pedi aims to identify what kinds of materials the child or student reads based on a list of 17 reading categories. The identification of reading materials can lead to the development of five reading participation goals for occupation-based literacy intervention. Public domain (https://www.ps.columbia.edu/education/academic-programs/programs-occupational-therapy/faculty-innovations/ot-literacy).

cohesiveness, and resources play a vital role in determining children's participation in meaningful activities. The researchers added that participation is best supported when a child lives in a region with accessible and supportive community-based programs, where the family has specific participation preferences and can provide social support. Margalit (2004) has also found that supportive peers play critical roles in enhancing participation. This research found that children with LD in inclusive placements reported more positive social and emotional functioning than their peers in self-contained classes. Children receiving in-class support were more popular, had higher self-perceptions of academic competence, and demonstrated fewer problem behaviors than children receiving resource-room support. Children in inclusive classes had more satisfying relationships with their best school friends, were less lonely, and had fewer problem behaviors than children in self-contained special education classes (Margalit, 2004). Though the findings were not exclusive to children with LD, a systematic review by Grajo, Candler, et al. (2020) found moderately strong evidence on the use of peer instruction and support from similarly aged peers to enhance literacy participation in school-aged children.

There is also strong supportive evidence on the value of using a self-determination framework in facilitating adaptation, coping, and resilience in children with SLDs. *Self-determination* is defined as a combination of attitudes, knowledge, and skills that enable individuals to engage in goal-directed, self-regulated, autonomous behavior (Luckner et al., 2020) and the capacity to accomplish goals as influenced by the accuracy of one's self-knowledge and self-perceptions (Mather & Ofiesh, 2013). Several meta-analyses and systematic reviews document the effectiveness of academic intervention using a self-determination framework in children with SLDs and developmental disabilities. Konrad et al. (2007) found, in 34 self-determination studies with 312 participants ages 9 to 13, that self-management interventions showed stronger positive effects when academic interventions combined self-management and goal-setting to increase productivity. Burke et al. (2020), in a meta-analysis of 34 studies that included 1200 children with LD,

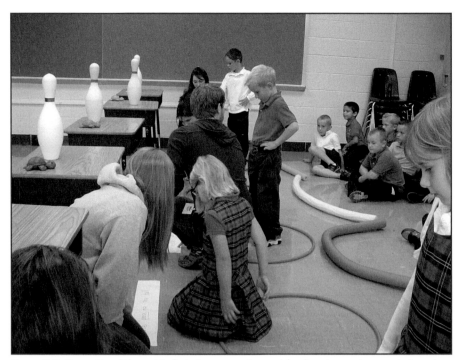

Figure 3-2. Occupational therapists fostering supportive and fun learning environments in a classroom to support literacy development.

found positive outcomes of intervention for overall self-determination or one or more skills associated with self-determined action. An exemplification of a self-determination approach embedded within an occupational adaptation framework is a level III study for children with reading disabilities by Grajo and Candler (2016a; Figure 3-2). This study found that integrating self-initiated choices in creative participation in reading activities during occupational therapy sessions in an 8-week program led to significant increases in perceived reading performance and satisfaction. As part of the intervention, participants were allowed to identify their occupation-based reading goals and to structure the format of the sessions.

Principle 3: Build Adaptation Through Strategy Generation

Strategy instruction has been documented as an evidence-based and best-practice tool for use in occupational therapy to support children with SLDs (Handley-More, 2019). In particular, the use of cognitive strategies may help children with LD to develop plans and action steps to overcome daily occupational challenges. The purpose of cognitive strategy use is to support learning or performance, so it can help a person deal with challenges to occupational performance (Toglia et al., 2012).

One evidence-based cognitive strategy protocol in occupational therapy is the Cognitive Orientation to daily Occupational Performance (CO-OP) approach (Polatajko & Mandich, 2004). Two specific pilot studies on the use of CO-OP for children with SLDs have documented its effectiveness. Karunakaran et al. (2018) found that in an intervention program for children with SLDs aged 10 to 14, CO-OP not only improved instrumental activities of daily living skills (specifically grocery shopping), but also made the children independent and confident in their task performance. Similarly, Grajo and Candler (2016a) used the CO-OP approach and occupational adaptation model in an intervention approach called the Occupation and Participation Approach to Reading Intervention (OPARI), and found increased reading participation, performance, mastery, and satisfaction in a group of school-aged children with reading disabilities. In the OPARI, the skillful use of facilitative techniques rather than direct instruction is emphasized to enable children to identify, test, refine, and use strategies that they have created and named on their own.

Client-centered goal setting is a critical principle of the CO-OP approach. Similar to principles of self-determination, goal-directed behavior in the CO-OP approach involves a dynamic decision-making process (Hunt & Reed, 2017). Clients are empowered to set meaningful occupational goals and skills they want to master. Generalization and transfer of learned skills in many different occupations are learned through a process of self-generation of strategies, which often includes the use of a global-strategy approach called Goal-Plan-Do-Check and domain-specific strategies (McEwen & Houldin, 2017; see Figures 3-2 to 3-5). Goal-Plan-Do-Check is an iterative process of facilitating the client to identify meaningful goals and skills to achieve (Goal), create a set of strategies and steps to perform the task or activity (Plan), perform the activity and use appropriate problem-solving strategies (Do), and assess the effectiveness of these strategies and whether the goal has been achieved (Check).

Principle 4: Develop Positive Behaviors, Confidence, Relative Mastery, Sense of Competence, and Self-Esteem

Self-esteem and confidence are crucial ingredients in giving people with LD a sense of well-being and of being valued members of a community (Goleniowska, 2014). In Table 3-4, we highlight some examples, as supported by the literature, of how occupational therapists can facilitate confidence, relative mastery, competence, and self-esteem to enhance participation and adaptation, coping, and resilience in children with SLDs.

Using this empowering framework, we propose that occupational therapists shift the paradigm in terms of assessment and intervention from just building and remediating deficient skills needed for academic and daily life participation. By using strengths and protective factors, occupational therapists may be able to address and facilitate better adaptation, coping, and resilience in children with SLDs, and thereby create more opportunities to participate in occupations and develop client factors and skills.

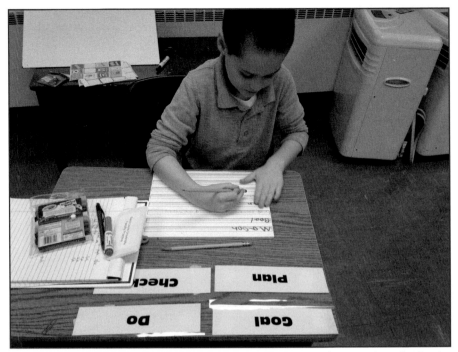

Figure 3-3. A child uses the Goal-Plan-Do-Check global strategy approach to complete schoolwork.

COLLABORATIVE APPROACH WITH FAMILIES

Child-centered care means working with the family to enhance the family members' abilities to care for and protect their child. The therapist focuses on the child's needs within the context of the child's family to build on the family's strengths and goals to achieve the best outcome. The collaborative approach includes empowering the family so they can better care for their child, including them in the interventions, focusing the interventions on family needs and goals, and building upon the family's capacities and strengths (O'Brien & Kuhaneck, 2020).

Occupational therapists can provide child-centered intervention through the purposeful consideration of how individual and family occupations interact with client factors and performance skills and patterns, considering the context and the environment (AOTA, 2020). Occupational therapists support a collaborative approach because they recognize the interrelationship of the client's skills, performance patterns, and environment, including the family and home environment (Kuhaneck et al., 2015). This collaborative approach is also emphasized in our proposed empowering framework.

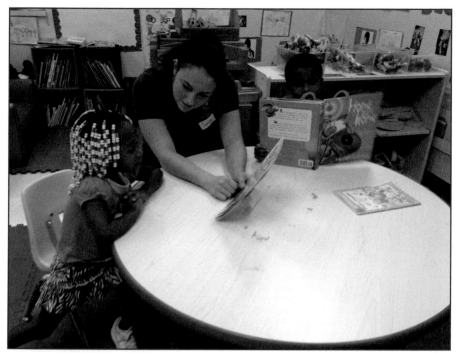

Figure 3-4. An occupational therapist facilitates self-monitoring strategies to empower students to complete reading tasks.

INTERPROFESSIONAL COLLABORATIONS

Occupational therapists work with a variety of professionals to support the needs of children and youth with SLDs. Grajo, Guzman, Szklut, and Philibert (2020) listed a team of specialists (Figure 3-6) that the occupational therapist may work with in school practice, outpatient and private practices, and home and community-based practice. While working collaboratively, it is essential that the occupational therapist advocate for the distinct value and role of our profession, not only in addressing the building and remediation of skills needed for daily living and education-related participation, but also in facilitating the child's adaptation, coping, and resilience through occupation-focused interventions.

GLOBAL PERSPECTIVES

There is great variation in how different countries define, develop laws and policies, and provide supports for children and youth with LD. Globally, inclusive education is embraced as practice; however, the availability of protections and guarantees for special education services vary greatly. Agrawal and colleagues (2019) conducted a systematic review analyzing how LD are defined and how services based on legislation are provided for children with SLDs in 10 different countries. We synthesize highlights of these findings in Table 3-5.

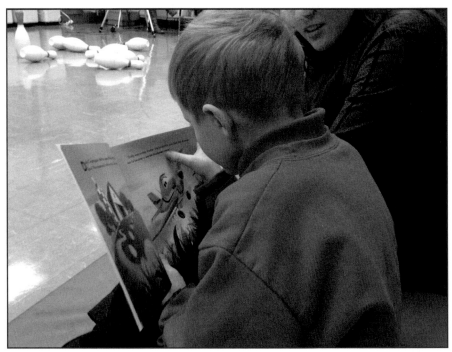

Figure 3-5. An occupational therapist uses facilitative prompting to enable a child identify strategies that will help overcome challenges in reading.

Table 3-4

Examples of Evidence-Supported Strategies to Support Positive Behaviors and Build Self-Esteem, Confidence, and Mastery in Children With SLDs	
Approach	**Use in Therapy**
Use facilitative techniques through guided questioning and strategies (Grajo & Candler, 2016b)	Provide opportunities for students to explore and identify strategies that may help overcome problems with school-related activities. During therapy, ask a series of questions to allow the student to identify effective and ineffective ways to complete structured school tasks.
Encourage self-monitoring (Handley-More, 2019)	Self-monitoring is an effective mechanism for students with SLD to address academic behaviors and measure productivity, accuracy, and successful strategy use. This may include helping students identify target behaviors, gather data to determine when self-monitoring can best be used, collaborating with the student to encourage self-monitoring, and training the student to identify target behaviors for academic success.

(continued)

Table 3-4 (continued)

Examples of Evidence-Supported Strategies to Support Positive Behaviors and Build Self-Esteem, Confidence, and Mastery in Children With SLDs

Approach	Use in Therapy
Social-skills training (Arbesman et al., 2013)	Social-skills training for disliked or rejected children and adolescents improves social interaction, peer acceptance, and social standing. Programming for at-risk, aggressive, or antisocial children and adolescents improves attention, peer interaction, and prosocial behaviors and reduces aggressive, delinquent, and antisocial behaviors. There is strong evidence that social-skills programming for children and adolescents with LD and ADHD improves communication and social and functional skills and reduces problem behaviors.
Strengthen parent-child interactions (Kingsley et al., 2020)	The use of a manualized parent-child interaction therapy provides specific training to parents in how to interact with their child to support positive behaviors. Interventions that develop child- and parent-directed interactions showed significant effect with large effect sizes on child behavior, including reducing externalized and challenging behaviors.

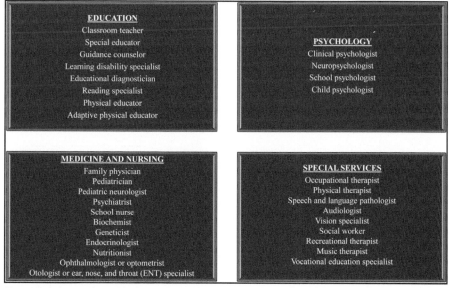

Figure 3-6. Team of specialists that may be involved in the care of children with SLDs. (Adapted from Grajo, L., Guzman, J., Szklut, S., & Philibert, D. [2020]. Learning disabilities and developmental coordination disorder. In R. Lazaro, S. Reina-Guerra, & M. Quiben [Eds.], *Umphred's neurological rehabilitation* [7th ed.]. Elsevier.)

Table 3-5

Global Perspectives on Specific Learning Disabilities		
Country	State of Learning Disabilities	Special Education Laws
Canada	LD is recognized but special education services are decentralized and up to local agencies.	Canadian Charter of Rights and Freedoms, an antidiscrimination bill, ensures that the civil rights of individuals with disabilities are protected.
China	LD not prominently recognized until the 2000s.	Following Compulsory Education Law in 1986, the Learning in Regular Classrooms initiative was launched to educate students with disabilities in regular schools.
Denmark	Until recently, no common practice for the identification of individuals with dyslexia or LD in reading existed in Denmark.	The Folkeskole Act (a general education law) was amended in 2012 to provide more realistic and concrete guidelines for inclusive education.
Germany	In addition to providing special-needs education for students with specific disabilities, students experiencing temporary learning difficulties (including reading and writing difficulties) are eligible for special-needs education.	Specific policies protecting students with disabilities are contained in the 1994 Recommendation on Special Education in the Schools of the Federal Republic of Germany.
Japan	The onus for identification of LD has been on teachers, who have limited understanding of characteristics and identification of students with LD and dyslexia.	A 2009 amendment of the School Education Act charged schools with providing students who have visual and hearing impairments, behavioral disorders, intellectual disabilities, physical limitations, and/or health-related impairments with the appropriate skills and knowledge to improve daily living and promote independence.
Mexico	LD is not recognized as a distinct disability category in Mexico; however, a provision stating that LD is a temporary disability that requires services in public schools exists.	Special education policy under the General Education Law discourages the use of a parallel curriculum model (i.e., separate but equal) and favors inclusive or "integrated" practices within the general education classroom.

(continued)

Table 3-5 (continued)

Global Perspectives on Specific Learning Disabilities		
Country	State of Learning Disabilities	Special Education Laws
Netherlands	Laws have existing definitions primarily for dyslexia.	Inclusive Education Act of 2014 requires each local school board to provide adequate education for every student regardless of educational needs and support required.
Singapore	The Ministry of Education defines LD as difficulties in reading, writing, spelling, remembering, and organizing information.	Education for children with mild disabilities has been recognized and services for these students were established in the 1970s.
Taiwan	The definition and criteria are very similar to those used in the United States.	Special Education Act revised in 2014 defines 13 categories of disability and 6 categories of giftedness and talents.
United Kingdom	The term *learning disability* is used in a way that the term *intellectual disability* is used in the United States; *learning difficulty* is the term used to define what is an LD in the United States.	Several laws and provisions (prior to Brexit) linked the UK with the European Union on the provision of special education.
Synthesized from Agrawal, J., Barrio, B., Kressler, B., Hsiao, Y., & Shankland, R. (2019). International policies, identification, and services for students with learning disabilities: An exploration across 10 countries. *Learning Disabilities: A Contemporary Journal, 17*(1), 95-114. https://files .eric.ed.gov/fulltext/EJ1218057.pdf		

ESSENTIAL CONSIDERATIONS

In Table 3-6, we highlight key discussions and essential considerations for occupational therapists based on our proposed empowering framework to support adaptation, coping, and resilience in children with SLDs.

Table 3-6

Essential Considerations for Occupational Therapists Using an Empowering Framework	
Perspectives Based on Proposed Empowering Framework to Support Adaptation, Coping, and Resilience in Children With SLDs	Essential Consideration for Occupational Therapists
Use of a strength-based and empowering approach	When developing an occupational profile during assessment, highlight more than the skill- and participation-related deficits of the child. Choose participation-related assessments that will also illuminate the child's preferences and strengths and use those as mechanisms for motivation and engagement during intervention.
Strategy use	Facilitate the use and naming of cognitive strategies that can be transferred and generalized across different contexts of occupational participation. When a child names and develops their own strategies, these will facilitate strategy use during challenging situations and occupations. This may empower adaptation, coping, and resilience.
Use of sociocultural and self-determination frameworks	Collaborate and identify family members, friends, peers, and teachers who may become supportive networks for the child with SLD. Allow the child to set their own goals, determine valuable occupations, and provide opportunity to gain control in the therapeutic relationship.
Emphasis on building mastery, self-esteem, and confidence	Elicit adaptive responses by modifying and enabling the activities and occupational environment so the child feels a sense of mastery and self-esteem when completing challenging daily occupations.

Case Study 3-2

Using an Empowering Framework With Eric

In this case study, we apply the empowering framework to understand and provide intervention in the case of Eric. We also apply terminologies and constructs from the *Occupational Therapy Practice Framework, Fourth Edition* (OTPF-4; AOTA, 2020).

Eric is an 8-year-old student who was re-evaluated at the request of his parents due to concerns with his emotional regulation, self-care, and academic skills. Eric is in the third grade and is currently eligible for special education and related services under the classification of SLD with concomitant diagnoses of

(continued)

Case Study 3-2 (continued)

attention deficit hyperactivity disorder and specific anxiety disorders, including obsessive compulsive spectrum disorder. Initially, Eric had support from a shared aide; however, because of scheduling and Eric's academic needs, the shared support was increased to 1:1 support. Eric participates in a self-contained program for language arts and math, and the general education class with in-class resource support for science and social studies. Related services include group/individual counseling, occupational therapy, and group speech therapy.

Occupations in Which Eric Is Successful

Eric's social-emotional and behavioral functioning and acquisition of adaptive skills indicate the following: his communication skills are a relative strength; his daily living/self-care skills are emerging well; his socialization, including conversational skills and interpersonal relating, is a relative weakness. Eric is independent with all dressing skills, and he is able to use most classroom tools and materials. His reading and writing skills show challenges, but he is able to follow multistep directions.

Personal Interests and Values

Eric enjoys watching sports, especially baseball, and participates in karate, yoga, and dance. Eric enjoys attending school and, by his own admission, would attend school year-round if he could.

Aspects of the Client's Environments That Are Seen as Either Supports or Barriers to Occupational Engagement

Eric has a younger brother. Parental and sibling relationships are described as positive. The household is described as extremely structured with a consistent routine. His mother describes Eric as a "good-natured, sweet, nonjudgmental, motivated, [and] friendly" child who wants to do well in school. He has presented with behavioral issues, addressed via a behavior plan and counseling in and out of school, which continue to be of concern: occasional high levels of agitation/anger in reaction to change; unsafe behavior, including threatening and perseveration on emergency equipment/processes; and socially inappropriate/provocative gestures and commentary. He continues to grow in differentiating how he should relate to adults vs. peers; he understands that some commentary is "too personal" and can make others "feel uncomfortable." He knows that he needs academic support and relies heavily on his 1:1 paraprofessional. While he continues to have a negative view of the self-contained settings in which he was placed in the past, he acknowledged that the small group setting is quieter and allows him to focus better; he does not have to rush because his pace is slow, and he really appreciates that the teacher has more time to work with him.

Client's Priorities and Desired Targeted Outcomes

Eric described himself as "smart, intelligent, kind, [and] sweet." He reported a good relationship with his parents and with his younger brother. His mother is most concerned about Eric's "lack of typical peer relationships, academic challenges, [and] future independence." Eric shares the same goals as his parents:

(continued)

Case Study 3-2 (continued)

to continue to promote his social-emotional development (including relating with peers and adults), to refine his adaptive skills, and to address his sometimes-problematic behavior and foster his self-awareness and self-regulation in all settings of the school environment. Eric will continue to receive occupational therapy services to address self-care, self-regulation, and fine motor skills for improved participation in the school setting.

Assessment

Specific and Global Mental Functions. *Mental functions* are specific affective, perceptual, and cognitive functions required to be able to effectively focus and attend to meaningful tasks and occupations. The Coping Inventory was used to assess Eric's self-coping skills. That tool assesses his abilities to cope with his self and with the environment in three dimensions (Zeitlin, 1985):

1. **Productive/Non-Productive**: Productive coping behaviors are socially responsible, enhance self-esteem, and produce desirable results. To be effective, the person must respond to the social demands to which they are exposed. This involves an ability to influence what happens and to have some control of personal needs and environmental demands.
2. **Flexible/Rigid**: Flexibility is the capacity to respond differentially to various situations and demands. Flexible copers demonstrate the ability to shift plans appropriately or reformulate ideas already held.
3. **Active/Passive**: Active copers initiate and sustain action, whether mental or physical. They have more opportunities to develop relationships or interests, more choices, and more possibilities of finding a substitute to handle their frustration.

Eric's Adaptive Behavior Index score is 2.5, meaning that his coping mechanisms are minimally effective in most situations. He is categorized in the assessment as having a Non-Productive, Passive, and Somewhat Rigid adaptive behavior index.

Eric's **most adaptive behaviors** include:	Eric's **least adaptive behaviors** include:
• Ability to balance independence with sufficient dependence. • Plays with other children and appears curious. • Demonstrates capacity for fun, zest, delight, and pleasure.	• Gets frustrated easily. • Cannot handle anxiety. • Cannot cope with high-stress situations. • Easily gets discouraged. • Unable to find a way of handling difficult or challenging situations.

Level of Participation Using the School Function Assessment

SFA Part I: Participation. This section best describes the student's current level of participation in school settings. Continued areas of need for Eric in this section include frequent redirection during structured game playing, following rules, and playing cooperatively with peers. He also requires frequent supervision in the areas of transportation, transitions from one area or activity to the

(continued)

Case Study 3-2 (continued)

next, and tasks associated with mealtime (which includes organizational skills and management).

SFA Part II: Tasks Supports. This section best describes the student's needs for additional help or for modifications to perform school-related functional tasks. Continued areas of need for assistance or adaptation include maintaining a seated position during the length of an activity or event.

SFA Part III: Occupation-Based Performance (Functional Assessment).

Written Work: When engaged in copying five-word sentences or three sentence paragraphs from a near point source, Eric demonstrates inconsistent letter sizing, line regard, and spacing throughout his work. Eric's classroom teacher utilizes a behavior modification program to which Eric responds, but sometimes inconsistently. Eric is observed to respond to immediate gratification, and his occupational therapist is working toward delaying gratification in order to increase participation and work production.

Tasks Behavior/Completion: Eric required constant verbal cues for redirection in order to redirect focus during the assessment. Eric was easily distracted by his peers and environment. He continuously greeted every student/adult who passed the testing area and asked, "How are you doing?" or was observed to stare at what they were doing. Eric constantly demonstrated behaviors to avoid performing tasks at hand, such as tapping his pencil, singing, making noises, or attempting to talk to the therapist about various other topics. Throughout reassessment, Eric required constant verbal cues to initiate, carry out, and complete tasks.

Applying an Empowering Framework on Intervention

The occupational therapist working with Eric in an outpatient setting embraced a strength-based empowering approach. Despite Eric's behavioral and task-related challenges, the therapist viewed Eric as extremely motivated to succeed and willing to foster deep friendship with peers. The therapist's first recommendation is the use of a Learning Pod. In collaboration with Eric's mom, they were able to identify two classmates who are very friendly with Eric, and with enthusiasm from the parents of those students, they created a pod that meets every day to do homework together for 2 hours after school. The Learning Pod takes turns hosting the group of three students, serving tasty snacks, and following the rules for the Learning Pod that were collaboratively identified by the occupational therapist, Eric, and his mom: (1) independent reading and focused time for homework for 45 minutes; (2) group collaboration and problem-solving for 45 minutes; (3) fun and games for the last 30 minutes if they complete all work on time. The parents of each child hosting the Learning Pod take responsibility for maintaining the pod rules. Initially, Eric had challenges focusing during the independent reading time, but with encouragement and modeling from supportive peers, Eric is learning to structure his time well and is mostly successful in completing many homework tasks during pod time. His mom has to supplement structured time during occasions when Eric needs more help to complete assignments.

The occupational therapist started using the framework of Goal-Plan-Do-Check when working with Eric on highly structured school tasks. They use a

(continued)

Case Study 3-2 (continued)

whiteboard to set timed goals to complete assignments and developed a variety of strategies to help Eric during written composition activities and reading tasks that can be challenging for him. The therapist also trained Eric's mom to use the general approach of Goal-Plan-Do-Check for doing work at home. Instead of a whiteboard, Eric chose to create a Strategy Notebook where he can write his strategies for writing and reading assignments.

The occupational therapist also started corresponding with Eric's school teacher to identify topics that Eric is interested in for independent book reading and written expression assignments. Instead of teacher-assigned books, the teacher has allowed Eric to send a list of 20 books and stories that he is interested in and excited about. The teacher reviews Eric's list and draws from this list to align educational goals for reading and writing and assign him homework and projects.

Eric continues to make slow but steady progress in terms of improving task-related behaviors. His small Learning Pod now includes five classmates and Eric is showing progress on being able to establish friendships with his pod-mates, and also in learning to be independent and productive with homework. He feels supported by his parents and friends and his teacher and has shared joy in the progress that he is making.

REFERENCES

Agrawal, J., Barrio, B., Kressler, B., Hsiao, Y., & Shankland, R. (2019). International policies, identification, and services for students with learning disabilities: An exploration across 10 countries. *Learning Disabilities: A Contemporary Journal, 17*(1), 95-114. https://files.eric.ed.gov/fulltext/EJ1218057.pdf

American Occupational Therapy Association. (2020). Occupational therapy practice framework: Domain and process (4th ed.). *American Journal of Occupational Therapy, 74*(Suppl. 2), 7412410010. https://doi.org/10.5014/ajot.2020.74S2001

American Psychiatric Association. (2013). *Diagnostic and statistical manual of mental disorders* (5th ed.). Author. https://doi.org/10.1176/appi.books.9780890425596

Arbesman, M., Bazyk, S., & Nochajski, S. M. (2013). Systematic review of occupational therapy and mental health promotion, prevention, and intervention for children and youth. *American Journal of Occupational Therapy, 67*(6), e120-e130. http://dx.doi.org/10.5014/ajot.2013.008359

Basu, S., Kafkes, A., Schatz, R., Kiraly, A., & Kielhofner, G. (2008). *A user's manual for the Pediatric Volitional Questionnaire* (2.1 ed.). Model of Human Occupational Clearinghouse. http://www.moho.uic.edu

Bowyer, P. L., Kramer, J., Ploszaj, A., Ross, M., Schwartz, O., Kielhofner, G., & Kramer, K. (2008). *A user's manual for the Short Child Occupational Profile (SCOPE)* (v.2.2). Model of Human Occupational Clearinghouse. http://www.moho.uic.edu

Brown, C., & Dunn, W. (2002). *Adolescent/Adult Sensory Profile: User's manual*. Psychological Corporation.

Bundy, A. C. (1999). Test of Environmental Supportiveness (TOES). Colorado State University.

Burke, M., Raley, S., Shogren, K., Hagiwara, M., Mumbardo-Adam, C., Uyanik, H., & Behrens, S. (2020). A meta-analysis of interventions to promote self-determination for students with disabilities. *Remedial and Special Education, 41*(3), 176-188. https://doi.org/10.25384/sage.c.4256012.v1

Burtner, P. A., Ortega, S. G., Morris, C. G., Scott, K., & Quails, C. (2002). Discriminative validity of the Motor-Free Visual Perceptual Test Revised in children with and without learning disabilities. *Occupational Therapy Journal of Research, 22*(4), 161-163. https://doi.org/10.1177/153944920202200405

Caldwell, B. M., & Bradley, R. H. (1984). *Home observation for measurement of the environment*. University of Arkansas.

Coster, W. J., Deeney, T., Haltiwanger, J., & Haley, S. (1998). *School Function Assessment (user's manual).* The Psychological Corporation, Therapy Skills Builders.

Every Student Succeeds Act, 20 U.S.C. § 6301 (2015). https://www.congress.gov/bill/114th-congress/senate-bill/1177

Goleniowska, H. (2014). The importance of developing confidence and self-esteem in children with a learning disability. *Advances in Mental Health and Intellectual Disabilities, 8*(3), 188-191. https://doi.org/10.1108/AMHID-09-2013-0059

Grajo, L. (2019). Occupational adaptation as a normative and intervention process: Schkade and Schultz's legacy. In L. C. Grajo & A. Boisselle (Eds.), *Adaptation through occupation: Multidimensional perspectives.* SLACK, Incorporated.

Grajo, L., & Candler, C. (2016a). An Occupation and Participation Approach to Reading Intervention (OPARI) part I: Defining reading as an occupation. *Journal of Occupational Therapy, Schools and Early Intervention, 9*(1), 74-85. http://dx.doi.org/10.1080/19411243.2016.1141082

Grajo, L., & Candler, C. (2016b). An Occupation and Participation Approach to Reading Intervention (OPARI) part II: Pilot clinical application. *Journal of Occupational Therapy, Schools and Early Intervention, 9*(1), 86-98. http://dx.doi.org/10.1080/19411243.2016.1141083

Grajo, L., Candler, C., & Bowyer, P. (2019). The Inventory of Reading Occupations—Pediatric version (IRO-Pedi). https://www.ps.columbia.edu/education/academic-programs/programs-occupational-therapy/faculty-innovations/ot-literacy

Grajo, L., Candler, C., & Sarafian, A. (2020). Interventions within the scope of occupational therapy to improve children's academic participation: A systematic review. *American Journal of Occupational Therapy, 74*(2), 7402180030p1-7402180030p32. https://doi.org/10.5014/ajot.2020.039016

Grajo, L., Guzman, J., Szklut, S., & Philibert, D. (2020). Learning disabilities and developmental coordination disorder. In R. Lazaro, S. Reina-Guerra, & M. Quiben (Eds.), *Umphred's neurological rehabilitation* (7th ed.). Elsevier.

Greenham, S. (1997). Learning disabilities and psychosocial adjustment: A critical review of literature. *Child Neuropsychology, 5*(3), 171-196. https://doi.org/10.1076/chin.5.3.171.7335

Hale, J., Alfonso, V., Berninger, V., Bracken, B., Christo, C., Clark, E., Davis, A., Decker, S., Denckla, M., Dumont, R., Elliott, C., Feifer, S., Fiorello, C., Flanagan, D., Fletcher-Janzen, E., Geary, D., Gerber, M., Gerner, M., Goldstein, S., . . . Yalof, J. (2010). Critical issues in response-to-intervention, comprehensive evaluation, and specific learning disabilities identification and intervention: An expert white paper consensus. *Learning Disability Quarterly, 33*(3), 223-236. https://doi.org/10.1177/073194871003300310

Handley-More, D. (2019). Best practices in supporting students with specific learning disabilities. In G. Frolek Clark, J. Rioux, & B. Chandler (Eds.), *Best practices for occupational therapy in schools* (2nd ed., pp. 305-312). AOTA Press.

Horowitz, S. H., Rawe, J., & Whittaker, M. C. (2017). *The state of learning disabilities: Understanding the 1 in 5.* National Center for Learning Disabilities.

Hunt, A., & Reed, N. (2017). Goal setting in the CO-OP approach. In D. Dawson, S. McEwen, & H. Polatajko (Eds.), *Cognitive orientation to daily occupational performance in occupational therapy: Using the CO-OP approach to enable participation across the lifespan.* AOTA Press.

Individuals with Disabilities Education Act, 20 U.S.C. § 1400. (2004). https://sites.ed.gov/idea

Karunakaran, M., Sugi, S., & Rajendran, K. (2018). Effectiveness of cognitive orientation to daily occupational performance to improve shopping skills in children with learning disability. *Indian Journal of Occupational Therapy, 50*, 92-97. https://doi.org/10.4103/0445-7706.244551

Keller, J., Kafkas, A., Basu, S., Federico, J., & Kielhofner, G. (2005). *Child Occupational Self-Assessment (COSA).* Model of Human Occupational Clearinghouse. http://www.moho.uic.edu

King, G. A., King, S., Rosenbaum, P., Kertoy, M., Law, M., & Hurley, P. (2004). Children's Assessment of Participation and Enjoyment (CAPE) and Preferences for Activities of Children (PAC). Harcourt Assessment.

Kingsley, K., Sagester, G., & Weaver, L. L. (2020). Interventions supporting mental health and positive behavior in children ages birth-5 yr: A systematic review (Table A.3). *American Journal of Occupational Therapy, 74*(2), 7402180050. https://doi.org/10.5014/ajot.2020.039768

Konrad, M., Fowler, C., Walker, A., Test, D., & Wood, W. (2007). Effects of self-determination interventions on the academic skills of students with learning disabilities. *Learning Disability Quarterly, 30*(2), 89-113. https://doi.org/10.2307/30035545

Kuhaneck, H. M., Madonna, S., Novak, A., & Pearson, E. (2015). Effectiveness of interventions for children with autism spectrum disorder and their parents: A systematic review of family outcomes. *The American Journal of Occupational Therapy, 69*(5), 1-12A. https://doi.org/10.5014/ajot.2015.017855

Law, M., Baptiste, S., Carswell, A., McColl, M. A., Polatajko, H. J., & Pollock, N. (2005). *Canadian Occupational Performance Measure* (4th ed.). CAOT.

Luckner, J., Banerjee, R., Movahedazarhouligh, S., & Millen, K. (2020). A systematic review of replicative self-determination intervention studies. *The Journal of Special Education, 54*(1), 29-39. https://doi.org/10.1177/0022466919850188

Margalit, M. (2003). Resilience model among individuals with learning disabilities: Proximal and distal influences. *Learning Disabilities Research & Practice, 18*(2), 82-86.

Margalit, M. (2004). Second-generation research on resilience: social-emotional aspects of children with learning disabilities. *Learning Disabilities Research & Practice, 19*(1), 45-48. https://doi.org/10.1111/j.1540-5826.2004.00088.x

Mather, N., & Ofiesh, N. (2013). Resilience and the child with learning disabilities. In S. Goldstein & R. Brooks (Eds.), *Handbook of resilience in children* (2nd ed., pp. 239-255). Springer.

McEwen, S., & Houldin, A. (2017). Generalization and transfer in the CO-OP approach. In D. Dawson, S. McEwen, & H. Polatajko (Eds.), *Cognitive orientation to daily occupational performance in occupational therapy: Using the CO-OP approach to enable participation across the lifespan.* AOTA Press.

Miller, M. (2002). Resilience elements in students with learning disabilities. *Journal of Clinical Psychology, 58*(3), 291-298. https://doi.org/10.1002/jclp.10018

Morrison, G., & Cosden, M. (1997). Risk, resilience, and adjustment of individuals with learning disabilities. *Learning Disability Quarterly, 20*(1), 43-50. https://doi.org/10.2307/1511092

O'Brien, J. C., & Kuhaneck, H. (2020). *Case-Smith's occupational therapy for children and adolescents* (8th ed.). Mosby/Elsevier.

Panicker, A. S., & Chelliah, A. (2016). Resilience and stress in children and adolescents with learning disability. *Journal of the Canadian Academy of Child and Adolescent Psychiatry, 25*(1), 17-23.

Parham, L. D., Ecker, C., Miller-Kuhaneck, H., Henry, D. A., & Glennon, T. J. (2007). *Sensory Processing Measure (SPM): Manual.* Western Psychological Services.

Polatajko, H. J., & Mandich, A. (2004). Enabling occupation in children: The Cognitive Orientation to daily Occupational Performance (CO-OP) approach. CAOT Publications ACE.

Rosenblum, S. (2016). Handwriting features and executive control among children with developmental dysgraphia. *American Journal of Occupational Therapy, 70*(4, Suppl. 1), 7011500040. https://doi.org/10.5014/ajot.2016.70S1-PO4054

Rosenblum, S., & Weintraub, N. (2007). Learning disabilities and occupational therapy: Review of research and practice as reflected in the IJOT. *Israel Journal of Occupational Therapy*, (16), H137-H158.

Schkade, J. K., & Schultz, S. (2003). Occupational adaptation. In P. Kramer, J. Hinojosa, & C. B. Royeen (Eds.), *Perspectives in human occupation: Participation in life* (pp. 181-221). Lippincott Williams & Wilkins.

Toglia, J. P., Rodger, S. A., & Polatajko, H. J. (2012). Anatomy of cognitive strategies: A therapist's primer for enabling occupational performance. *Canadian Journal of Occupational Therapy, 79*(4), 225-236. https://doi.org/10.2182/cjot.2012.79.4.4

Tonkin, B., Ogilbie, B., Greenwood, S., Law, M., & Anaby, D. (2014). The participation of children and youth with disabilities in activities outside of school: A scoping review. *Canadian Journal of Occupational Therapy, 8*(14), 226-236. https://doi.org/10.1177/0008417414550998

Townsend, S. C., Carey, P. D., Hollins, N. L., Helfrich, C., Blondis, M., Hoffman, A., Collins, L., Knudson, J., & Blackwell, A. (2001). Occupational Therapy Psychosocial Assessment of Learning (OT PAL). Model of Human Occupational Clearinghouse. http://www.moho.uic.edu

Tseng, M. H., & Chow, S. M. K. (2000). Perceptual-motor function of school-age children with slow handwriting speed. *American Journal of Occupational Therapy, 54*(1), 83-88. https://doi.org/10.5014/ajot.54.1.83

Zeitlin, S. (1985). *Coping inventory manual observation form.* Scholastic Testing Service.

Zeitlin, S., Williamson, G. G., & Szczepanski, M. (1988). *Early Coping Inventory: A measure of adaptive behavior.* Scholastic Testing Service.

4

Children and Youth With Intellectual and Developmental Disabilities*

Anne Cronin, PhD, OTR, FAOTA, ATP

Chapter Objectives By the end of this chapter, the reader will be able to:

- Describe common patterns in adaptive behavior and occupational engagement in children and youth with intellectual and developmental disability of different levels of severity.
- Summarize how both a growth mindset and a strength-based perspective can support the role of occupational therapy in addressing the adaptation, coping, and resilience of persons with intellectual and developmental disabilities.
- Using current evidence and theory, defend and emphasize the need for environmental modification and accommodations in occupational therapy interventions for children and youth with intellectual and developmental disabilities.

***Author's Note**

This chapter is dedicated to Victoria, who made a huge difference in the lives of many.

Overview of the Population

Intellectual disability is the diagnostic term replacing "mental retardation" in the *Diagnostic and Statistical Manual of Mental Disorders, Fifth Edition* (*DSM-5*; American Psychological Association [APA], 2013). In this conception, an intellectual disability is

Grajo L. C., & Boisselle, A. K. (Eds.). *Adaptation, Coping, and Resilience in Children and Youth: A Comprehensive Occupational Therapy Approach* (pp. 73-101).

a subtype of the broader category of developmental disorders. One challenge associated with describing this clinical population is the variability in the use of diagnostic labels for the same condition, both over time and across geographic regions. The most used diagnostic label for this population in the United States is intellectual and developmental disability (IDD). The labels "learning disability" and "mental retardation" are widely used in other areas of the world. In most cases, IDD is identified in individuals before the age of 10. Children with more severe IDD are usually identified in the first two years of life (Boat & Wu, 2015). Standardized tests of intelligence are one tool commonly used for assessment and in assignment of the diagnostic label of IDD. Another aspect of the diagnosis of IDD is *adaptive behavior*. Adaptive behaviors include all activities of daily living (ADLs), such as eating, getting dressed, and managing toileting, as well as some components of instrumental activities of daily living (IADLs), such as safety awareness, following school rules, and cleaning up a workspace. Adaptive behavior also includes the ability to engage at an age-appropriate level in the occupations of education, work, and social participation.

Focusing on the strengths of the person rather than the impairment is central to the occupational therapy process. Occupational therapists rely on the assessment of daily function and the performance of adaptive behaviors as the most appropriate evaluation of intellectual ability. A child with an IDD will be unlikely to keep up with similarly aged peers in terms of either adaptive behavior or academic performance skills. Although the intellectual deficits present in this population are considered permanent, and the deficits often prevent the child from reaching developmental milestones at a typical rate, occupational therapists must take a strength-based approach.

Occupational engagement is the mental process that motivates the person both to attempt tasks and to persist in performing them. The *Occupational Therapy Practice Framework: Domain and Process, Fourth Edition (OTPF-4)* defines *occupational engagement* as "the performance of occupations as the result of choice, motivation, and meaning within a supportive context (including environmental and personal factors). Engagement includes objective and subjective aspects of clients' experiences and involves the transactional interaction of the mind, body, and spirit" (American Occupational Therapy Association [AOTA], 2020, pp. 5-6). Although skill acquisition may not occur at the same pace as with their typical peers, the person with IDD can learn complex tasks. In the case of Victoria, presented in Table 4-1, she has successfully embraced all of the age-typical roles of a high school senior, with an individualized educational path to accommodate her moderate IDD. The definitions and implications of the different levels of severity of IDD are presented in the next section.

PREVALENCE OF INTELLECTUAL AND DEVELOPMENTAL DISABILITIES

Because data often include individuals with other types of developmental disabilities, statistics on the prevalence of IDD are unclear. The National Health Interview Survey 2014–2016 included four possible diagnostic choices—autism spectrum disorder, intellectual disability, developmental disability, and other developmental delays—and reported that the prevalence of intellectual disability is about 1.34% of the United

Table 4-1

Occupational Profile of Victoria

Reason the Client Is Seeking Service and Concerns Related to Engagement in Occupations

Now in her senior year of high school, Victoria has continued to attend school while undergoing cyberknife procedures and chemotherapy for metastatic osteosarcoma. Victoria and her family are committed to keeping her engaged in all of the activities she loves, such as swimming, running, and cooking, while working around the impact of cancer treatments.

Occupations in Which the Client Is Successful

Victoria is a good athlete, participating on the high school swim team. She is independent in ADLs and requires only standby support in many IADLs. Victoria has good interpersonal skills and has been successful in community activities with her age peers.

Personal Interests and Values

Victoria's favorite class right now is her culinary class. She participates in a weekly yoga class and swims on the high school swim team, practicing nightly with them (from 8:30 p.m. to 9:45 p.m.). Victoria wants the senior year that her sisters had, including her senior celebration from varsity sports participation and attending the prom. Victoria loves listening to music and she loves Disney movies.

Occupational History (i.e., life experiences)

Victoria, the youngest of three sisters, was born with Down syndrome. Her parents report that they feel blessed they had both the education and social support to advocate for Victoria, and eventually, to build supports for all children with special needs in her home state. Until she was 13 years old, when she was diagnosed with osteosarcoma, Victoria lived a charmed life full of friends, family, and many extracurricular activities. Since her cancer diagnosis, she has undergone extensive, often painful, treatment. She received her "fancy foot," a below-knee prosthetic foot, 1 year after her cancer diagnosis.

When Victoria started high school, she became a manager of the volleyball team, co-treasurer of Family, Career and Community Leaders of America (FCCLA), a Best Buddies member, and a varsity member of the swim team. She volunteers in her community and is active in her church.

Performance Patterns (i.e., routines, roles, habits, and rituals)

Victoria manages her morning and evening ADL routines independently. In her new cancer treatment regimen, she has to take at least 12 pills per day, and her parents provide oversight of her medication management. Because of her chemotherapy, Victoria needs to stay very hydrated, and needs prompting from her family in managing this.

She attends high school and swim practice every weekday. She has weekly appointments at the infusion center for her chemotherapy and attends church with her parents on Sundays.

(continued)

Table 4-1 (continued)

Occupational Profile of Victoria

Aspects of the Client's Environments That Are Seen as Either Supports or Barriers to Occupational Engagement

Victoria is a very social and active young woman who, because of her cancer treatment, is immune-suppressed and restricted from participation in many loved activities. For example, she was unable to volunteer at the summer camp where she helped in the crafts tent. She has a supportive family and social community that includes school staff and students, her faith community, and the staff at the hospital where she receives her treatments.

Client's Priorities and Desired Targeted Outcomes

Victoria wants to engage in all of the celebrations that mark the graduation from high school. She wants to continue to gain skills as a cook. Victoria, with the help of her sisters, has a social media presence to raise funds for cancer research. Victoria is very proud of her role in this and wants to continue with it (Figures 4-1 to 4-6).

Figure 4-1. Victoria.

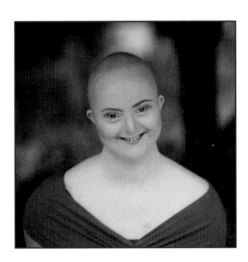

States population (Zablotsky et al., 2017). The worldwide prevalence of IDD is slightly higher, at 2% to 3% of the population (Percy et al., 2017). Genetic syndromes account for 30% to 50% of IDD (Zablotsky et al., 2017). The three most common of these genetic syndromes worldwide are Down syndrome, 22q11.2 deletion syndrome, and fragile X syndrome. Down syndrome is by far the most common of these, occurring four to five times as often as the next most common. Fragile X and 22q11.2 deletion syndromes have a similar incidence in girls, but fragile X is the more common of these two in boys. As the technology for identifying genetic disorders improves and becomes more widely used, it is likely that more of the persons with IDD of unknown etiology will be identified as having a disorder with a genetic basis. IDD often co-occurs with other developmental conditions such as attention deficit/hyperactivity disorder (ADHD), cerebral palsy,

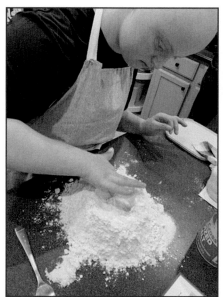

Figure 4-2. Victoria making homemade pasta in culinary class.

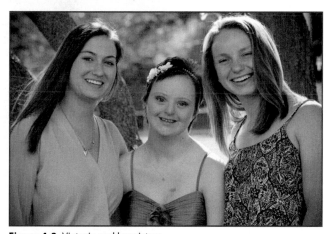

Figure 4-3. Victoria and her sisters.

autism spectrum disorder, and genetic conditions that include other physical and physiological impairments. For example, impairments in hearing (rates of loss are 40 times higher) and vision (8.5 times higher) are common in people with IDD (Percy et al., 2017). The American Association on Intellectual Developmental Disabilities (AAIDD, 2010) identifies four categories of factors that cause or contribute to IDD: biomedical, social, behavioral, and educational. Social factors may provide an underlying cause or serve to broaden the impact of existing individual impairments (Percy et al., 2017). Educational factors and social factors often interact and contribute to rather than cause IDD (AAIDD, 2010).

Figure 4-4. Victoria at the prom.

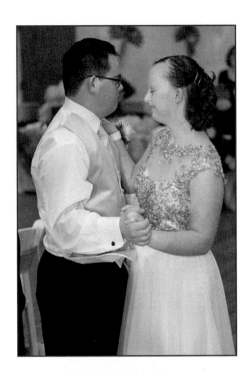

Figure 4-5. Victoria with the university dance group.

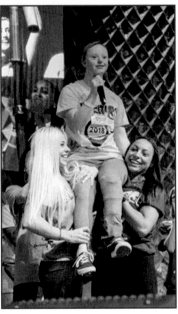

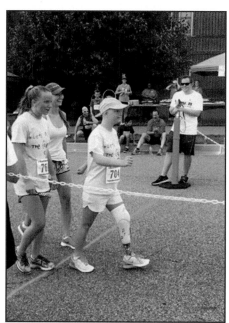

Figure 4-6. Victoria in a cancer 5K marathon.

CLASSIFICATIONS OF SEVERITY

Classifications of severity in IDD reflect the degree of impairment in both intellectual functioning and adaptive behavior. These classifications are important to understand because they offer the occupational therapist much more insight into the individual than the larger diagnostic label of IDD. Related to the construct of adaptive behavior, *functional cognition* is the ability to use and dynamically integrate intellectual function to support the performance of desired skills. Distinct from traditional views of intelligence, functional cognition includes contextually relevant skill performance that can be scaffolded so that the person can accomplish complex everyday activities and occupations (Giles et al., 2020). Together, functional cognition, occupational engagement, and adaptive behaviors form the basis for the person's ability to recognize the need to try alternate strategies to achieve a goal: the person's *adaptive capacity*. See Table 4-2 for an overview of classifications of intellectual disability severity based on the *DSM-5*.

ENGAGEMENT IN OCCUPATIONAL BEHAVIORS FOR CHILDREN AND YOUTH WITH IDD

Limits in adaptive capacity, paired with low social expectations and previous experiences with performance failures, often result in low motivation for task performance and limited occupational engagement. The construct of *occupational engagement* is operationalized as inclusive of behavioral, cognitive, and social-emotional facets. Observable

Table 4-2

DSM-5 Classifications of Intellectual Disability Severity		
Severity Category	Approximate Distribution	Severity Classified on the Basis of Occupational Engagement
Mild	85%	Mild IDD may not be identified until the person starts school (Sulkes, 2018). Learning occurs at a slower rate than that of their age peers, yet persons with mild IDD are able to learn basic academic foundations often up to a grade 6 academic level (Mancini & Greco, 2012). As adults, persons with IDD can engage in typical adult occupations with minimal levels of support.
Moderate	10%	Early identification of IDD is common among children with moderate IDD because their impairments are more extensive, and this markedly slows learning. These persons will require extensive support to benefit from the school environment. They often have limited speech and need support in the use of alternative communication strategies to make their needs and wants known. Some can learn up to grade 2 reading, writing, and counting skills, but have poor comprehension of the concepts and difficulty applying the skills in novel situations (Mancini & Greco, 2012).
		People in this category can learn self-care skills with some supervision but often demonstrate impaired social functioning, distractibility, and difficulty working independently.
		With accommodations, most adults with moderate IDD can take basic care of themselves, build friendships, travel to familiar places in their community, engage productively in a structured work setting, and learn necessary skills related to safety and health.
Severe/ profound	5%	These two categories are presented together because they are usually comorbid with other impairments or conditions, and from a functional perspective can be challenging to isolate from one another. Movement impairments are common in persons with severe and profound IDD, and these impairments negatively affect the development of both functional cognition and adaptive skills in early childhood. On the higher performance end of this range, individuals may have the ability to understand speech but have limited expressive communication skills (Sattler, 2002).
		With supervision, many adults with severe IDD can function in structured, supportive employment settings. A person with profound IDD typically needs total support in self-care and has very restricted participation in occupations (Mahoney, 2020).

behavioral aspects of engagement are orientation to a task, task persistence, and application of physical effort (Eklund & Bejerholm, 2017). Functional cognition incorporates metacognition, executive function, performance skills, and performance patterns (Giles et al., 2020).

In some instances, persons with IDD have functional limitations that are far greater than would be predicted based on their intelligence testing. Impairments in adaptive capacity, lack of opportunity for engagement at an optimal challenge level, past experiences of failure, and low expectations can reduce engagement in occupation for children and youth with IDD. Failure to engage in occupations limits opportunities for learning and magnifies the level of disability that manifests in the person with IDD. Important to note is that there are also instances of persons with IDD, such as the case of Victoria (presented in Table 4-1), who function far above predicted levels, because they have had opportunity for engagement.

WHAT ARE TYPICAL ROLES AND EVIDENCE FOR THE ROLE OF OCCUPATIONAL THERAPY FOR CHILDREN AND YOUTH WITH IDD?

Historically, many of the occupational therapy services provided to children and youth with IDD have focused on changing any underlying impairment or skill deficits. Interventions targeting changes in body structures and functions are not effective to increase participation in this population (Adair et al., 2015). Although the intellectual impairment is chronic and not altered significantly by interventions targeting intellectual deficits, focusing on the person's strength and supports for functional performance of adaptive behaviors can lead to improved occupational performance and appropriate role acquisition.

Mastery motivation is the intrinsic press to become competent in the world and is expressed through persistent striving on a preferred task where accomplishment involves a performance challenge (Gilmore & Cuskelly, 2017). In typically developing children, mastery motivation emerges in early childhood and is a precursor to self-determination and independent function. *Self-determination* is a mindset that each person has the right to direct their own life choices (Bremer et al., 2003). The combination of mastery motivation and learning provides the fundamental underpinning for self-determination. For a person with IDD, self-determination is the ability to make choices, learn to solve problems effectively, and cope with the consequences of personal decision making.

Based on a longitudinal study of persons with Down syndrome, Gilmore and Cuskelly (2017) found that mastery motivation made a unique and positive contribution to functional outcomes that was distinct from the effects of cognitive ability. Environmental modification and accommodations help support a mastery mindset for children and youth with IDD by increasing their opportunities for occupational engagement and their experience of successful performance. The severity of each child's intellectual disability is a "client factor" in the language of the *OTPF-4* (AOTA, 2020).

Individuals who are more severely impaired may benefit from the interventions described to support the performance patterns of early childhood, even when they have chronologically aged beyond this developmental period.

Evidence for the Role of Occupational Therapy in the Performance Patterns of Early Childhood

Significant delays in the attainment of sensorimotor skills, including difficulties in initiating and executing goal-directed movements, are often the first indicators of IDD (Shaw & Jankowska, 2018). Motor abilities are learned in tandem with cognitive abilities in early childhood. Although a focus on interventions targeting skills deficits does not increase participation (Adair et al., 2015), sensorimotor skill delays can limit opportunities for learning and further contribute to intellectual impairment due to this relationship (Houwen et al., 2016). Kim and colleagues (2016) reported that improvement in fine motor skills significantly and positively predicted improvements in cognitive skills for children with IDD. Improvements in gross motor skills did not significantly contribute to improvements in either cognitive skills or social skills in this study. Because the child's primary deficits are in intellectual abilities, aggressive support of strategies to optimize this early childhood period of nervous system plasticity in support of cognitive development is an essential focus of occupational therapy intervention.

Children with IDD, especially those with significant and multiple disabilities, demand intense family accommodations from birth onward (Wilder & Granlund, 2015). Interventions chosen for each child in the early childhood period are designed to support the child's eventual transition to a classroom environment. Occupational therapy guidance in the construction of an environmental context that is modified to accommodate the child's strengths and is grounded in family routines will be supportive of both the family system and occupational engagement.

Morgan and colleagues (2015) described an early intervention program based on motor learning concepts. This type of coordinated approach, which actively includes parents during interventions and in-home program development, shows the most promise for young children with IDD. Determining when a motor impairment is due to a difficulty in learning, rather than motor function, guides clinical reasoning and intervention strategies (i.e., focusing on motor learning and parent coaching), and intervention will thus be more effective in improving motor skills.

Socioemotional learning (SEL) is the process of acquiring critical skills in "the recognition and management of emotions, the establishment and achievement of positive goals, the appreciation of the other's perspective, the establishment and maintenance of positive relationships, responsible decision making, and constructive control of interpersonal situations" (Faria et al., 2019, p. 457). SEL is gained through the metacognitive organization of emotional knowledge and requires perception and judgment. Children with IDD are likely to have difficulty acquiring emotional knowledge. Strategies widely recommended to support SEL are the teaching of specific fostering socioemotional competencies through explicit instruction (Faria et al., 2019). Case-Smith (2013) reported that different interventions were effective for children at different developmental levels. For example, effective interventions for infants primarily involved coaching parents and included touch-based interventions such as massage and parent training in strategies to increase joint attention. Effective interventions for preschool-age clients continue to include parent coaching, and add direct instruction that uses the behavioral techniques of modeling, rehearsal, and practice, prompting, and positive reinforcement embedded in play activities in natural environments. Indirect occupational therapy intervention in support of teachers and students in inclusive education settings is likely to increase the success of the child's participation in the classroom.

Social participation requires specific performance skills that include the use of both verbal and nonverbal skills to communicate. Communication interventions are clearly within the scope of speech-language pathology, but occupational therapists need to understand communication development to support the motor skills needed for gesturing or device use, the behavioral self-regulation necessary for turn-taking and peer interaction, the body awareness required for rules of proximity, and other rules of pragmatic communication and social interaction. Occupational therapists also need to recognize and reinforce unconventional communication strategies to help motivate the child to be a communicator.

Evidence for the Role of Occupational Therapy in Performance Patterns in Primary Education

Environmental modification and accommodation are an essential role of occupational therapy in facilitating mastery, self-determination, and occupational performance patterns in a classroom learning environment. Selanikyo et al. (2017) report that students with IDD do not participate fully in school activities and depend significantly on others to maximize participation. The goal of occupational therapy in the school setting is to allow the student with IDD to participate as fully—and as developmentally appropriately—as possible.

Finally, all occupational therapy interventions should be designed to teach and support self-determination. Mumbardó-Adam and colleagues (2017) report that students with lower levels of intellectual function often also have lower levels of self-determination. Despite this link between intellectual function and self-determination, these authors report that there is also evidence that environmental opportunities to make meaningful decisions are more important than IQ in predicting self-determination.

Basic to the development of self-determination is the development of *behavioral self-regulation:* the learned ability to use executive functions in daily problem solving, emerging linguistic capabilities, and social-emotional learning (Erdmann & Hertel, 2019). Common behavioral targets for intervention in school settings are increasing on-task behaviors in both daily living skills and classroom activities, improving the ability to attend to classroom instruction selectively, increasing the ability to follow directions, improving the ability to work productively with peers, and increasing the use of context-appropriate functional communication. These behavioral targets will maximize a student's ability to learn and benefit from the educational setting. As the student transitions from primary to secondary education, the ability for behavioral self-regulation, social interaction, and a sense of self-determination are increasingly essential.

Evidence for the Role of Occupational Therapy in Performance Patterns in Secondary Education

Secondary education for youth with IDD involves a change in emphasis for many students. Those students with IDD who have the capacity to participate in postsecondary education will continue with an academic focus to their educational goals. Still, for many students with IDD, the focus shifts to work readiness. Functional communication skills become even more important as an intervention focus in support of work, education, and leisure occupations (Eismann et al., 2017).

The occupation of work is "labor or exertion related to the development, production, delivery, or management of objects or services" (AOTA, 2020, p. 33). Work includes a broad array of supporting readiness skills, including both advocating for oneself and identifying and selecting work opportunities consistent with personal interests, abilities, and goals. Connecting occupational therapy interventions to postsecondary education and employment goals is recommended to support the process of transition out of secondary education (Eismann et al., 2017).

Increasingly, occupational therapists include technology-based approaches to teach secondary students with IDD functional skills (Waldman-Levi et al., 2019). Smart devices and wearable technology are widely accepted by persons in this age group and can offer powerful supports to independent function. Interventions embedded in natural environments and using collaboration in environmental analysis can give students the knowledge, skills, and attitudes needed to request accommodations for themselves.

EVIDENCE-DRIVEN OCCUPATIONAL THERAPY STRATEGIES FOR CLIENTS WITH IDD

Children are seldom referred to occupational therapy simply because they are diagnosed with an IDD; instead, referrals to occupational therapy result from a child's inability to effectively participate in expected or desired occupations, rather than because of a diagnosis. General, evidence-driven occupational therapy strategies for children and youth with IDD include the use of a strength-based perspective, engagement in occupation, family-centered practices, team collaboration, and the use of natural environments. These strategies are described in Table 4-3.

Table 4-3

General Evidence-Driven Occupational Therapy Strategies
Use a Strength-Based Rather Than a Deficit-Based Perspective
Strength-based perspectives focus on the person-environment fit rather than on patterns of impairment. Each person has a unique profile of strengths and limitations that influences their functioning across different environments (Shogren et al., 2017). Assessment in a strength-based approach examines not only the individual but also the individual's environment to identify any constraints that limit learning. A strength-based perspective encourages practitioners to consider the potential and dreams of an individual and the dreams and goals of that individual's family support network.
Achievement of Health, Well-Being, and Participation in Life Through Engagement in Occupation
Persons with IDD often have unique and distinctive patterns of interests and limited capacity to engage in occupations without accommodation. Health and quality of life are supported when individuals with IDD can engage in home, school, workplace, and community life to the highest degree desired. Occupational engagement is a positive outcome of the occupational therapy process for persons with IDD (AOTA, 2020).
Family-Centered and Culturally Appropriate Practices
Family-centered practices are effective with individuals with IDD because of their ongoing need for support, and because the complexity of their health and educational issues requires collaboration to achieve positive outcomes. The family forms the learning context in which most children learn ADL and IADL skills. Family education in environmental modification and accommodations supports this skill development (Shaw & Jankowska, 2018).
Team Collaboration
Occupational therapists work in teams with the individual, parents, other caregivers, teachers, and other professionals to coordinate services and to plan and implement strategies that capitalize on the strengths, interests, and goals of both the individual with IDD and the family/social support system of the individual with IDD (Rosner et al., 2020). Including the person with IDD in the team collaboration to the greatest extent possible supports self-determination and increases the likelihood that the goals will address the needs and concerns of the individual (Shaw & Jankowska, 2018).
Use Natural Environments
Natural environments provide the best context for interventions for individuals with IDD. Skill acquisition by individuals with IDD often fails to generalize across environments because the behavior of the learners comes under the control of irrelevant features of the environment, such as a particular room layout or a particular piece of furniture. The generalization of learned skills to multiple environments is the ideal, but not always within the capability of the individual with IDD. The use of natural environments limits the impediment caused by the poor generalization of learned skills.

Table 4-4

Performance Patterns and Performance Skills			
Performance Patterns		**Performance Skills**	
Characteristics of Children With IDD		*Characteristics of Children With IDD*	
Habits	Often require explicit teaching and use of schedules as prompts.	Motor skills	Delays are present in psychomotor skills, including reaction time, skilled hand use, and motor planning.
Routines	Limited in complexity and often require explicit teaching. They have limited temporal processing. Routines may be co-occupations rather than individual performances.	Process skills	Impairments are present in the ability to organize objects, time, and space. They have limited adaptive capacity for applying knowledge and adapting performance.
Roles	Limited in complexity and often require explicit teaching. They are restricted in variety.	Social-interaction skills	Impairments are present in both verbal and nonverbal communication skills. There is impairment in understanding of communication pragmatics.
Rituals	They are usually addressed as co-occupations.		Because rituals have a strong affective component, children with IDD may feel extra pressure or distress in these situations. This extra affective pressure may serve to either support or hinder occupational performance.

The behavioral science frames of reference, which include interventions for social learning and cognitive-behavioral intervention approaches as well as applied behavioral analysis (Cronin & Graebe, 2018), offer evidence-based strategies to support learning. "Acquisitional learning theories" reflect an integration of social learning theory and a developmental perspective and are particularly relevant for guiding the occupational therapy process for this population (Howe et al., 2020). Focused activity analysis and the use of behavioral strategies to increase motivation are interventions that can support the learning of these target performance patterns and skills in context (Waldman-Levi & Erez, 2015). Performance patterns and performance skills typically observed in children with IDD are listed in Table 4-4.

Defining Adaptation, Coping, and Resilience in Children and Youth With IDD

Adaptation and Occupational Engagement

Adaptation is a process of change through which a person becomes better able to participate in desired occupations in a manner that is both successful and rewarding (Grajo, 2019). An intrinsic desire for mastery of the environment through participation in occupations is one of the overarching principles of occupational adaptation. As noted earlier in this chapter, mastery motivation results from successes in occupational engagement that results in the completion of desired tasks or challenges. For example, if a parent intercedes during dressing because the child is slow and has limited problem-solving capabilities, the child may become disinterested, making completion of the activity challenging for both the child and the family. Parental intercession could support dependent behavior, interfere with the development of adaptive behaviors, and limit self-determination. Rather than interceding, using task analysis to build a scaffold of sub-tasks supports mastery motivation without lowering the standards for task performance set by the family. In motivating task engagement and persistence, mastery motivation also supports the process of adaptation.

A strength of many children with IDD is that the skills they have learned can become very strong. This strength can also present some challenges. Children with IDD learn social rules regarding greetings, personal space, and physical contact in early childhood. It is typical for young children to enthusiastically practice greetings in public settings through greeting strangers, and to hug or be more physical in their greeting than the average adult. Over years of development, the typically developing child refines and narrows this behavior so that greetings are customized to social context. Persons with IDD may continue to use the "early childhood" form of the social behavior into adulthood. The adult who enthusiastically greets and hugs strangers in public places is intrusive and inappropriate at best. At worst, such persons can become a target for social and even sexual exploitation. Persons with IDD often find it challenging to adaptively alter previously learned behaviors in response to a new social context (Barrett et al., 2012). A supportive environment and context for occupational performance that include customized strategies to repair problems in activity sequence or social interactions can provide opportunities for situated learning that can make a challenging task achievable. Interventions and coaching in age-appropriate contexts will support social-emotional learning related to the current activity demands of the individual. For example, the ability to access short videos of context-specific social behaviors on a mobile digital device can provide concrete options for the person to use when they are distressed or confused in a social context.

Performance skill patterns are best learned in natural contexts and embedded into habits and routines. It is often more effective to teach a "morning routine" than to teach the several isolated tasks common to morning routines. Teaching the use of visual schedules and visual cues in the performance setting can offer support for the development of mastery and self-determination, while having the same effect of enhancing performance skills that direct instruction of the specific skills would have.

Extrinsic Supports for Learning

Context is defined in the *OTPF-4* (AOTA, 2020, pp. 36-37) as "the environmental and personal factors specific to each client (person, group, population) that influence engagement and participation in occupations." The *OTPF-4* definition includes both extrinsic (environmental) and intrinsic (personal) factors as contexts for occupational engagement. An IDD often creates a situation where the capabilities of the individual do not "fit" the demands of extrinsic environments in which the person must function. Recognizing this lack of fit leads occupational therapy professionals to focus their efforts on modifying the context within which the child with IDD must perform daily occupations. Environmental accommodation can be achieved either through changing the physical environment, such as is accomplished through user-centered design, or through introducing personalized supports, such as assistive devices. Gallimore and colleagues (1989) studied stress and quality of life in families of children with disabilities. They found that the families with the highest sense of well-being had constructed a personalized "ecocultural niche" of daily routines as an external context "that sustain[s] coherent and satisfying daily activities" (p. 216). The authors reported that for this personalized performance context to be sustainable, the emergent "niche" must have (1) ecological fit, (2) congruence, and (3) meaningfulness (Weisner et al., 2005). In occupational therapy terms, *ecological fit* is the balance between available resources and constraints in the performance environment. Supporting ecological fit includes identifying the best contexts for occupational engagement. *Congruence* refers to a balance between individual needs and abilities within the whole family system. Meaningfulness, in this instance, refers to the routine as supportive of parental values and goals. Occupational therapists, through the use of activity analysis, can collaborate with families in the selection or construction of an environmental "niche" that is an ecological fit for the family and has both congruence and meaningfulness. Case Study 4-1 illustrates the result of a challenge to adaptation caused by the extrinsic environment. In this case, Marina was unable to adapt her learned strategy for dressing or to develop a new approach. The result of this was that she was unable to participate in a desired occupation: not because of IDD, but because of a disruption in her routine and poor adaptation.

Adaptive Capacity

Many children with IDD are challenged to engage in activities that are valued by both the child and the persons in the child's daily life. Engagement in occupations is often restricted for children and youth with IDD because the supports for engagement and skill acquisition that are common in early childhood are not adequate for their learning needs. The failure to succeed in desired activities results in a pattern of learned

> ## Case Study 4-1
>
> Marina, a third-grade girl with Williams syndrome, was excited about the opportunity to go to the swimming pool with her Girl Scout troop. Because Marina had experience in swimming pools, and was independent in both dressing and functional mobility, none of the adults involved had concerns about her ability to participate in this activity. Everyone was surprised, then, when they found Marina in the pool locker room crying loudly. Although she knew how to change into her swimsuit, Marina did not know how to ask for help to solve her dilemma in the locker room.
>
> The dilemma was that Marina had a routine for dressing. She always sat in a chair and placed the clothing she wanted to put on to her right. She dressed/undressed her lower body first, and then her upper body. The pool locker room had no chairs or benches. Although lockers were available, there was no flat surface on which to organize her clothing. Marina's dressing independence was "cue bound," meaning that her performance was tied to a familiar environmental set-up. When the environment was changed, motivation to achieve was not enough to overcome her lack of adaptive capacity (i.e., the ability to choose, use, and revise strategies to overcome a challenge; Grajo, 2019).

helplessness that further limits occupational engagement. To build adaptive capacity, the individual needs to be actively engaged in occupation and must persist in the face of challenges. Unfortunately, as reported by Floyd and Olsen (2017), children with IDD have difficulty actively engaging in the problem-solving discussions used by parents to teach children social-emotional and behavioral regulation. In response to this, the parents adapt to the children's needs by being more directive than other parents. This adaptive strategy used by parents can be effective in supporting positive family interactions, but it leads the child with IDD to engage in less-active problem solving. These authors noted that the children with IDD were less engaged in interpersonal interactions in general and that mothers' positive problem solving and active listening strategies resulted in more active problem solving by the children; when mothers were highly directive, the children engaged in less problem solving.

Executive function abilities involving attention, working memory, mental storage of information, and mental retrieval of information, all supportive of adaptive capacity, are learned throughout childhood through active engagement in participation and with the guidance of parents and teachers. Providing support and coaching for the adults who support children with IDD in facilitating discovery learning that is graded to build on the child's current abilities will support the development of adaptive capacity in the child.

Coping and Self-Regulation

Coping can be conceptualized as the result of a developmental process grounded in self-regulation (Compas et al., 2017) and executive function skills (Erdmann & Hertel, 2019). Children and youth with IDD may lack the executive function skills to success-fully regulate their emotions and their behaviors to respond productively to stressful experiences. In typically developing children, both executive function and emotional self-regulation abilities emerge as a result of parental modeling and feedback. Through this process, the parents offer extrinsic emotional support to the child in the form of gen-eral responsiveness and behavior modeling, as well as verbal "emotion coaching" (Baker et al., 2019). This developmental process, through which children receive external sup-port from caring adults to help them regulate their emotions and behaviors, is called co-regulation (Erdmann & Hertel, 2019). Children and youth with IDD benefit from an integration of emotion coaching with explicit didactic teaching of strategies for prob-lem solving, behavioral persistence, and attentional refocusing (Baker et al., 2019). In Marina's case (Case 4-1), an inability to adapt to the change in routine and cope with the emotions she felt as a result led to distress, a breakdown of performance patterns, and a reduction in her sense of mastery. Teaching Marina specific help-seeking behaviors that she could use in times of distress could have diverted Marina from her negative trajectory in the locker room.

Unlike Marina, Jeffrey (Case Study 4-2) has learned help-seeking behaviors and has learned to rely on trusted others to help him evaluate and manage his own emo-tions. Jeffrey has a sense of mastery, a belief that his actions will make a difference. He has confidence that his friend and his teacher will support him. Finally, Jeffrey demon-strates basic coping skills. He is distressed, but he understands the need to get out of the

---

Case Study 4-2

Jeffrey, a ninth-grade boy with Down syndrome, had just started high school. He was in a special education classroom but was mainstreamed for many classes. Jeffrey had strong family support and had friends from middle school who were also in the high school. The first day of school, Jeffrey went into the bathroom and found that there were urinals rather than toilets. He watched his classmates use the urinals and tried to copy what he saw.

Because Jeffrey had poor fine motor coordination, and could not manage clothing fasteners well, his mother had provided him with elastic-waist blue jeans so that he could fit in with the other boys. That day at the urinals, there was much laughing and teasing as Jeffrey pulled his pants down and exposed his buttocks to the group. Jeffrey was upset, pulled up his pants, and quickly left the bath-room. He found a friend in the hall and tearfully reported what had happened. Jeffrey's friend smiled and told him he could help. Jeffrey's friend went with him to find a teacher to explain the problem. The teacher reassured Jeffrey and told him that she would call his school occupational therapist to help him come up with a solution. The addition of a Velcro front closure to all of his pants solved Jeffrey's problem and Jeffrey continued to enjoy his interactions with age peers.

situation and ask for help. Jeffrey's prior successes with learning and his confidence that he is supported serve as protective factors for him in the face of challenges.

The two case stories presented here offer simple challenges with manageable solutions. Young adults with Williams syndrome and with Down syndrome are often successful in the community. Jeffrey, who has a sense of mastery and coping skills, has a far greater chance of succeeding in this adult setting than Marina does. The difference between the two is not in their adaptive capacity, but rather in the specific skills that they have learned and their sense of mastery. Returning to the occupational profile of Victoria at the start of this chapter, Victoria's early experiences and social support network helped her face the trials and traumas of her cancer treatment. Her mother commented on her "can do" attitude: when expressing her own concern about starting another round of chemotherapy, Victoria told her: "Mom, we got this. We did it already." Victoria was able to hold on to the idea that once something had been achieved, it could be done again.

Victoria, Jeffrey, and Marina have extrinsic supports for coping with trusted friends and family. As these young people become more engaged in the community, nonhuman supports such as assistive devices can be an excellent extrinsic resource for coping (Gentry et al., 2015; Golisz et al., 2018). Marina could have a smartphone or other device that she learns to use when distressed. The phone could have a stored "to do" list of things to try, such as "find an adult to ask for help," "call mom," "tell a friend what the problem is." Martina may not be able to remember the strategies, but she would be able to remember that there is a list on her phone.

Resilience

Resilience is the ability to produce a positive, adaptive response in the face of significant adversity (National Scientific Council on the Developing Child, 2015). Resilience is a dynamic concept that is context specific, meaning that a person may be resilient in some aspects of daily life but not in others. A child who has persevered through many serious challenges may have greater resilience than an adult who has not been seriously challenged (ten Hove & Rosenbaum, 2018). Victoria, in her ongoing battle with cancer, has demonstrated a robust level of resilience, which greatly exceeds that seen in many other persons undergoing cancer treatments. Victoria has the three main sources of support reported to foster resilient behavior in children and youth with IDD when faced with adversity: external social supports, including family; an internalized sense of mastery; and intrinsic feelings, attitudes, or beliefs within the individual that enable them to build internal supports for themselves (ten Hove & Rosenbaum, 2018).

Authors ten Hove and Rosenbaum (2018) describe three main sources of support drawn upon in the face of adversity. The first of these are *"I have"* factors that are extrinsic, drawn from the social and environmental contexts of the child. "I have" factors exist as contextual factors and provide supports when the child needs to overcome a challenge or adversity. An "I have" factor could be family financial resources that make private therapy possible. A second source of resilience is *"I can"* factors that focus on things in which the child has achieved some degree of mastery. Earlier in this chapter, emotional co-regulation was described as the process through which young children regulate their emotions and behaviors with guidance and other external supports provided by caring adults (Erdmann & Hertel, 2019). This process of emotional co-regulation also provides a sense of mastery supporting the sense that "I can," making the child more likely to be able to demonstrate resilience. The third source of resilience is the *"I am"* factors, reflecting the person's identity and beliefs (ten Hove & Rosenbaum, 2018). According to Barrett et al. (2012), parents report that they rarely see mastery-oriented behaviors from their children with IDD. She noted that in her studies of children with IDD, she was able to see mastery motivation in controlled situations. Barrett proposes that parents may seldom see their children in optimally challenging situations. Occupational therapy interventions to support mastery, including those that involve any combination of accommodation, activity modification, and parent coaching, will help build the child's capacity for resilience.

THE ROLE OF OCCUPATIONAL THERAPY: BEST AND EVIDENCE-BASED PRACTICES FOR ASSESSMENT

Best practice in assessments is the use of functional strength-based measures that reflect performance in natural environments. Here, I outline several methods to facilitate a strength-based approach.

1. Developmental Assessment

In young children, performance is often evaluated relative to typical patterns of development. The utilization of a developmental systems frame of reference (Cronin & Graebe, 2018) informs the assessment process; when used in combination with social learning theories, this frame of reference guides valid and evidence-informed clinical reasoning to support intervention decisions for children and youth with IDD. Many developmental assessment tools can be effectively used with this population to measure performance in natural environments. The *Battelle Developmental Inventory, Third Edition [BDI-3]* (Newborg, 2020), is an especially appropriate tool as it includes a subsample of children with IDD up through age 7 in its normative sample, making interpretation of scores more valid. This assessment measures areas of age-normative occupational performance and adaptation. The *BDI-3* also contains an Early Academic Survey, with two subdomains specifically designed to measure foundational literacy and mathematics skills. Although developmental assessments are typically used to qualify children for therapy services in early childhood, a function-based assessment is recommended from the primary grades on.

2. Collaborative Goal-Setting Assessments

Assessments that consider family needs and concerns are vital in retaining a family-centered focus on the occupational therapy process. The *Routines Based Interview (RBI)* is a collaborative goal-setting tool that is widely used in early childhood practice because it is family-centered and offers insight into the occupational performance of both the parent and the child, as well as into coping strategies used by the parents in managing challenging situations or performance demands. The RBI is a semi-structured interview designed to develop functional outcome goals that address child and family priorities (McWilliam et al., 2009). This interview focuses on daily routines, asking parents to report their day from the beginning to the end of the day. This collaborative tool helps when planning for an individual with IDD, especially for those in the severe and profound ranges, whose routines and performance patterns have the oversight of a supervising adult. Through the use of this tool in planning interventions that support family functioning, the occupational therapist can support the development of resilience within the entire family.

The *Canadian Occupational Performance Measure (COPM*; Law et al., 2005) is a client-centered functional outcome measure that identifies participants' priorities for improving the performance of everyday tasks. Through a client-centered interview process, the respondent(s) (which could be a child, a parent, or both) identifies up to five priorities for intervention with an emphasis on change in self-care, productivity, and leisure activities. The COPM is often used as a basis to guide occupational performance coaching and other collaborative intervention processes (An et al., 2019). Like the RBI, the COPM can be used in planning interventions that support child and family functioning in a manner that also enhances resilience within the family.

3. Assessments of Functional Performance in Natural Environments

The *Pediatric Evaluation of Disability Inventory-Computer Adaptive Test [PEDI-CAT]* (Haley et al., 2012) is a standardized assessment that is administered in natural performance settings. The assessment includes the three functional skill domains of daily activities, mobility, and social/cognitive. Also, the PEDI-CAT assesses a "responsibility" domain that has a Responsibility Scale with responses that give insight into performance autonomy and self-regulation. Unlike the developmental sequence format of the BDI-3, the PEDI-CAT is criterion focused. This test is especially useful for children and youth with uneven developmental progressions. The PEDI-CAT normed up to age 20 years can be used into adulthood.

The *Communication Matrix* is an assessment designed to measure early communication behavior (Rowland, 2011). This tool is a behavior inventory that focuses on communication behaviors used before the child develops language. This tool is widely used as an assessment to support decisions about communication strategies in children with IDD who have complex communication needs. The occupational therapist can use this tool of communication behaviors as a means of distinguishing and reinforcing intentional behaviors in persons with severe and profound IDD. The communication matrix offers insight into functional cognition in persons with limited adaptive capacity that is not available from other standardized tests.

Table 4-5

Standardized Functional Assessment Tools		
Tool and Author	Age Group Intended	Assessment Focus
Goal-Oriented Assessment of Lifeskills (GOAL; Miller et al., 2013)	7 to 17 years	Uses structured task performance to evaluate the functional motor abilities needed for daily living.
Do-Eat Assessment (Josman et al., 2010)	Chronological or behavioral age of 5 to 8 years	Evaluation of areas of strength and difficulty in IADL/ADL. Can serve as a measure of executive function in this age group.
School Function Assessment (SFA; Coster, Deeney, et al., 1998)	K to sixth grade	Identifies a student's level of participation; assesses the need for task supports within the school environment.
Participation and Environment Measure–Children and Youth (PEM-CY; Coster, Law, et al., 2014)	5 years to 17 years	Evaluates participation in the home, at school, and in the community, and environmental factors within each of these settings.

4. Functional Performance in a Learning Context

Occupational therapists work collaboratively with other members of the school Individualized Education Plan (IEP) team in the areas of screening, assessment, program planning, designing, and implementing interventions. School-based occupational therapists focus on removing barriers from students' ability to learn and helping students develop skills that increase their independence in the school environment.

Data used to determine the educational need for occupational therapy may be obtained through a variety of assessment methods, including the following: skilled observations of the student's engagement in typical school environments and activities, assessment of environmental barriers and supports for participation and learning in the school environment, review of student work samples, and non-standardized functional performance assessments. Relatively few standardized assessment tools are valid for students with IDD. Table 4-5 includes some commonly used tests of functional performance supportive of goal setting in school-based practice for students with mild IDD.

THE ROLE OF OCCUPATIONAL THERAPY: BEST AND EVIDENCE-BASED PRACTICES FOR INTERVENTION

The most strongly evidence-based interventions for children and youth with IDD are grounded in the behavioral sciences and integrate attention, motivation, and reward for performance utilizing a teaching-learning process (Condillac & Baker, 2017). This category of interventions includes occupation-based coaching, an intervention combining the principles of coaching with occupation-centered reasoning that focuses on "increasing positive child-caregiver interactions and child-learning opportunities in everyday routines and contexts" (Little et al., 2018, p. 2).

In an occupation-based coaching model, there is active collaboration between the occupational therapist and the parent. Coaching is a therapeutic strategy that utilizes the strengths of both the parent and the child. Ogourtsova and colleagues (2019) describe five elements as essential to coaching intervention in childhood disability: joint planning, observation of the new strategy, real-life opportunity to practice the strategy, self-assessment of performance, and feedback that includes information on the intervention, the child's development, supportive resources, and additional strategies. This type of occupation-based coaching is built upon natural observation of the child/youth's adaptive capacity and ability to respond to challenges in occupational performance. This provides the insight needed to set challenges for the child that are achievable, while pushing the child to build new skills. As a coach, the occupational therapist leverages the strengths of the parent and the child to increase occupational engagement and provide opportunities for mastery. With mastery and the act of "doing," the child/youth will encounter challenges. Coaching can provide guidance for discovery learning and build the child's ability to dynamically adapt while engaging in occupations. This will offer a foundation for the development of coping and resilience, and can provide a strategy through supporting the child in acquiring these more complex skills.

Engagement in Occupation

The main approaches to support mastery are to identify goals and rewards that are meaningful to the child. For example, handwriting probably has no meaning for the child who does not read. The task may seem arbitrary and abstract to the child, and the child may not be motivated to engage. Play-based interventions are effective with young children because they are intrinsically motivating and can support both engagement and the development of mastery motivation (Fabrizi & Hubbell, 2017; Blanche et al., 2016). These interventions are characterized by playful interactions in a sensory-rich environment that offers enough challenge to elicit an adaptive response.

For older children, the ability to use free time appropriately is a crucial skill in both the community and the school setting. Collaborating to build a socially supportive environment by incorporating the preferred activities of the student with IDD into social clubs can improve social engagement and support the development of mastery motivation (Koegel et al., 2012). When the activity itself is not intrinsically motivating (for example, sitting quietly at a desk), the therapist can add extrinsic reinforcers to support engagement. Children and youth with IDD may need tangible rewards to support motivation. In these cases, a systematic choice assessment process can help identify motivating rewards. Systematic choice assessment requires the occupational therapist to collect several things that the child may like: things like fidgets, sensory toys, or candy. Two (of several) possible rewards are placed in front of the child. The child chooses one, and that one remains, while the object that was not chosen is removed and replaced with another option. Repeat this process until the child's preferences can be ranked in terms of level of motivation. When using behavioral strategies to support occupational engagement, the occupational therapy practitioner should collaborate with the behavioral specialist on the child's interprofessional team.

Skill Scaffolding

As children transition from home to primary school and expanded community contexts, occupational therapy interventions should include the use of multiple strategies that allow application and practice of skills across settings, to facilitate the generalization of learned skills into everyday life situations. The use of behavioral teaching methods supports the introduction of required skills in small increments to accommodate the limited adaptive capacity of children with IDD (Condillac & Baker, 2017). *Scaffolding* is breaking up the performance of the desired task into segments, like links on a chain. Then one uses those links to build a complex occupational performance pattern.

Chaining is a behavioral intervention to teach a multistep or complex task. Chaining is most effective when the child has the motor ability to perform some steps in the chain already. Using the example of self-feeding, if the child cannot already hold the spoon, none of the other steps in the chain can be introduced. In this case, the occupational therapist must determine how important the skill of self-feeding is to the child and family. If this is a high-priority goal, then the use of a task modification, such as a cuff to keep the spoon in hand, could be introduced. This strength-based modification would let the child focus on the transportation of the spoon to the mouth and compensate for an inconsistent grasp. If self-feeding is a lower priority, then a deficit-based intervention approach to build functional grasp patterns could be introduced.

There are two main types of chaining used with children and youth with IDD: backward chaining and forward chaining. In backward chaining, you teach the behavioral chain beginning with the last step. Backward chaining is often the best chaining approach to use with persons with IDD because they see the successful result immediately. For example, in teaching self-feeding with a spoon, you would provide physical prompts to hold the spoon, to scoop, to transport the loaded spoon near the mouth. When the loaded spoon is very near the mouth, you would stop the physical prompts and verbally encourage the person to take a bite. The food rewards the behavior, supporting learning. Backward chaining teaches the link between performance and the reinforcer. This link to the reinforcer motivates occupational engagement as well as building a skill. Once the last step of a backward chain is mastered at an independent level, then move to the last two steps, then the last three steps, and so on.

Forward chaining teaches a behavioral chain beginning with the first step. In this approach, you would have the child complete the first step independently and then prompt all remaining steps. Using the self-feeding example, the child would independently pick up and hold the spoon, and then all remaining steps are prompted. In forward chaining, the sequence looks like the sequence used by others, but requires that the child understand the purpose of the activity. In a forward-chaining approach, the use of tangible rewards can support motivation. As noted earlier, when using behavioral strategies to enhance skill development, the occupational therapy practitioner should collaborate with the behavioral specialist on the child's interprofessional team.

A GLOBAL PERSPECTIVE

IDD is viewed differently in different cultures. The cultural views may support or hinder the occupational therapist who wants to encourage inclusion in the community or who values personal independence as a therapy outcome. Collaboration remains an essential part of the assessment and intervention process, but people coming from different backgrounds may not fully understand the contexts or values of others on the team. Everyday tasks are performed differently in different geographical areas. For example, independence in toileting in the United States will require a very different skill set than independent toileting using a pit toilet in rural Sri Lanka.

ESSENTIAL CONSIDERATIONS FOR OCCUPATIONAL THERAPISTS WORKING WITH CHILDREN AND YOUTH WITH INTELLECTUAL DISABILITIES

Table 4-6 outlines some of the essential things occupational therapists should consider to promote adaptation, coping, and resilience in children and youth with intellectual disabilities.

Table 4-6

The Essential Things Occupational Therapists Need to Consider
1. **Use a strength-based perspective**. Children and youth with IDD have impairments in intellectual function that are chronic. The impairments may not improve with therapy, but functional performance does change.
2. **Environments matter**. Assessment in natural environments will give a truer perspective on the person's abilities. Interventions in natural environments support situated learning and can help the individual gain context-specific skills. Environmental modifications can make occupational performance possible and can support the family as well as the individual with IDD.
3. **Collaborate to build a social convoy**. Collaboration is essential in all aspects of the occupational therapy process. Putting child and family values front and center helps build strong relationships and creates the confidence to set higher goals. Siblings, neighbors, teachers, and classmates can all make the team stronger and build a convoy of social relationship that can move with the child through life. Multiple professionals will be involved in supporting both the child and the family. Linking the professionals and the social convoy can create an emotional safety net for times of need.
4. **Build adaptive capacity**. Using a collaborative coaching approach with families in meaningful occupations within optimized environments, occupational therapists can facilitate collaborative building of strategies to overcome performance challenges.
5. **Keep a future perspective**. When developing goals with the team, look at what is likely to be most useful in the long run, rather than focusing on the short term. For the child who does not read, successful navigation of communication apps on a smartphone will have a much greater impact into adulthood than practicing writing the alphabet.

REFERENCES

Adair, B., Ullenhag, A., Keen, D., Granlund, M., & Imms, C. (2015). The effect of interventions aimed at improving participation outcomes for children with disabilities: A systematic review. *Developmental Medicine & Child Neurology, 57*(12), 1093-1104. https://doi.org/10.1111/dmcn.12809

American Association on Intellectual Developmental Disabilities. (2010). *Intellectual disability: Definition, classification, and systems of supports.* AAIDD. https://doi.org/10.1002/9781118660584.ese2604

American Occupational Therapy Association. (2020). Occupational therapy practice framework: Domain and process (4th ed.). *American Journal of Occupational Therapy, 74*(Suppl. 2), 7412410010. https://doi.org/10.5014/ajot.2020.74S2001

American Psychological Association. (2013). *Diagnostic and statistical manual of mental disorders* (5th ed.). Author.

An, M., Palisano, R., Chiarello, L., Yi, C., Dunst, C., & Gracely, E. (2019). Effects of a collaborative intervention process on parent empowerment and child performance: A randomized controlled trial. *Physical & Occupational Therapy in Pediatrics, 39*(1), 1-15. https://doi.org/10.1080/01942638.2017.1365324

Baker, J., Fenning, R., & Moffitt, J. (2019). A cross-sectional examination of the internalization of emotion co-regulatory support in children with ASD. *Journal of Autism & Developmental Disorders, 49*(10), 4332-4338. https://doi.org/10.1007/s10803-019-04091-0

Barrett, K. C., Fox, N. A., Morgan, G. A., Fidler, D. J., & Daunhauer, L. A. (2012). *Handbook of self-regulatory processes in development: New directions and international perspectives.* https://doi.org/10.4324/9780203080719

Blanche, E., Chang, M., Gutierrez, J., & Gunter, J. S. (2016). Effectiveness of a sensory-enriched early intervention group program for children with developmental disabilities. *American Journal of Occupational Therapy, 70*(5), 7005220010. http://dx.doi.org/10.5014/ajot.2016.018481

Boat, T., & Wu, J. (2015). Clinical characteristics of intellectual disabilities. In T. Boat & J. Wu (Eds.), *Mental disorders and disabilities among low-income children* (pp. 169-178). National Academies Press.

Bremer, C., Kachgal, M., & Schoeller, K. (2003). Self-determination: Supporting successful transition. *Research to Practice Brief: Improving Secondary Education and Transition Services through Research, 2*(1). http://www.ncset.org/publications/viewdesc.asp?id=962

Case-Smith, J. (2013). Systematic review of interventions to promote social-emotional development in young children with or at risk for disability. *American Journal of Occupational Therapy, 67*(4), 395-404. http://dx.doi.org/10.5014/ajot.2013.004713

Compas, B., Jaser, S., Bettis, A., Watson, K., Gruhn, M., Dunbar, J., Williams, E., & Thigpen, J. (2017). Coping, emotion regulation, and psychopathology in childhood and adolescence: A meta-analysis and narrative review. *Psychological Bulletin, 143*(9), 939-991. https://doi.org/10.1037/bul0000110

Condillac, R., & Baker, D. (2017). Chapter 28 Behavioral intervention. In M. Wehmeyer, I. Brown, M. Percy, K. Shogren, & W. L. A. Fung (Eds.), *A comprehensive guide to intellectual and developmental disabilities* (2nd ed., pp. 401-411). Brooks Publishing.

Coster, W., Deeney, T., Haltiwanger, J., & Haley, S. (1998). *School Function Assessment (SFA)*. Pearson Assessments..

Coster, W., Law, M., Bedell, G., Anaby, D., Khetani, M., & Teplicky, R. (2014). *Participation and Environment Measure-Children and Youth (PEM-CY)*. CanChild.

Cronin, A., & Graebe, G. (2018). *Clinical reasoning in occupational therapy*. AOTA Press.

Eismann, M., Weisshaar, R., Capretta, C., Cleary, D., Kirby, A., & Persch, A. (2017). Characteristics of students receiving occupational therapy services in transition and factors related to postsecondary success. *The American Journal of Occupational Therapy, 71*(3), 7103100010p1-7103100010p8. https://doi.org/10.5014/ajot.2017.024927

Eklund, M., & Bejerholm, U. (2017). Staff ratings of occupational engagement among people with severe mental illness—psychometric properties of a screening tool in the day center context. *BMC Health Services Research, 17*, 1-11. https://doi.org/10.1186/s12913-017-2283-3

Erdmann, K. A., & Hertel, S. (2019). Self-regulation and co-regulation in early childhood—Development, assessment and supporting factors. *Metacognition and Learning, 14*, 229-238. https://doi.org/10.1007/s11409-019-09211-w

Fabrizi, S., & Hubbell, K. (2017). Promoting play participation and parent competence in early intervention: A program effectiveness study. *American Journal of Occupational Therapy, 71*(4, Suppl. 1), 7111520312p1. https://doi.org/10.5014/ajot.2017.71S1-PO6090

Faria, S., Esgalhado, G., & Pereira, C. (2019). Efficacy of a socioemotional learning programme in a sample of children with intellectual disability. *Journal of Applied Research in Intellectual Disabilities, 32*(2), 457-470. https://doi.org/10.1111/jar.12547

Floyd, F., & Olsen, D. (2017). Family-peer linkages for children with intellectual disability and children with learning disabilities. *Journal of Applied Developmental Psychology, 52*, 203-211. https://doi.org/10.1016/j.appdev.2017.08.001

Gallimore, R., Weisner, T., Kaufman, S., & Bernheimer, L. (1989). The social construction of ecocultural niches: Family accommodation of developmentally delayed children. *American Journal on Mental Retardation, 94*(3), 216-230.

Gentry, T., Kriner, R., Sima, A., McDonough, J., & Wehman, P. (2015). Reducing the need for personal supports among workers with autism using an iPod Touch as an assistive technology: Delayed randomized control trial. *Journal of Autism and Developmental Disorders, 45*(3), 669-684. https://doi.org/10.1007/s10803-014-2221-8

Giles, G., Edwards, D., Baum, C., Furniss, J., Skidmore, E., Wolf, T., & Leland, N. (2020). Making functional cognition a professional priority. *American Journal of Occupational Therapy, 74*(1), 1-6. https://doi.org/10.5014/ajot.2020.741002

Gilmore, L., & Cuskelly, M. (2017). Associations of child and adolescent mastery motivation and self-regulation with adult outcomes: A longitudinal study of individuals with Down syndrome. *American Journal on Intellectual & Developmental Disabilities, 122*(3), 235-246. https://doi.org/10.1352/1944-7558-122.3.235

Golisz, K., Waldman-Levi, A., Swierat, R., & Toglia, J. (2018). Adults with intellectual disabilities: Case studies using everyday technology to support daily living skills. *British Journal of Occupational Therapy, 81*(9), 514-524. https://doi.org/10.1177/0308022618764781

Grajo, L. (2019). Occupational adaptation as a normative and intervention process: Schkade and Schultz's legacy. In L. C. Grajo & A. Boisselle (Eds.), *Adaptation through occupation: Multidimensional perspectives* (pp. 83-104). SLACK Incorporated.

Haley, S. M., Coster, W. J., Dumas, H. M., Fragala-Pinkham, M. A., Ni, P. S., Kramer, J., Feng, T., Kao, Y. C., Moed, R., & Ludlow, L. H. (2012). *PEDI-CAT: Development, standardization and administration manual.* CRECare LLC.

Houwen, S., Visser, L., van der Putten, A., & Vlaskamp, C. (2016). The interrelationships between motor, cognitive, and language development in children with and without intellectual and developmental disabilities. *Research in Developmental Disabilities, 53-54,* 19-31. https://doi.org/10.1016/j.ridd.2016.01.012

Howe, T., Kramer, P., & Hinojosa, J. (2020). Developmental perspective: Fundamentals of developmental theory. In P. Kramer, J. Hinojosa, & T. Howe (Eds.), *Frames of reference for pediatric occupational therapy (4th ed.,* pp. 20-66). Wolters Kluwer.

Josman, N., Goffer, A., & Rosenblum, S. (2010). *Do-Eat assessment.* Therapro.

Kim, H., Carlson, A., Curby, T., & Winsler, A. (2016). Relations among motor, social, and cognitive skills in pre-kindergarten children with developmental disabilities. *Research in Developmental Disabilities* (June-July), 53-54, 43-60. https://doi.org/10.1016/j.ridd.2016.01.016

Koegel, L., Vernon, T., Koegel, R., Koegel, B., & Paullin, A. (2012). Improving social engagement and initiations between children with autism spectrum disorder and their peers in inclusive settings. *Journal of Positive Behavior Interventions, 14*(4), 220. https://doi.org/10.1177/1098300712437042

Law, M., Baptiste, S., Carswell, A., McColl, M., Polatajko, H., & Pollock, N. (2005). *Canadian Occupational Performance Measure* (4th ed.). CAOT Publications.

Little, L., Pope, E., Wallisch, A., & Dunn, W. (2018). Occupation-based coaching by means of telehealth for families of young children with autism spectrum disorder. *American Journal of Occupational Therapy, 72*(2), 1-7. https://doi.org/10.5014/ajot.2018.024786

Mahoney, W. (2020). Intellectual disability and occupational therapy. In K. Bryze (Ed.), *Occupational therapy for adults with developmental disability* (pp. 1-9). SLACK Incorporated.

Mancini, D. F., & Greco, C. M. (2012). *Intellectual disability: Management, causes and social perceptions.* Nova Biomedical/Nova Science Publishers.

McWilliam, R. A., Casey, A., & Sims, J. (2009). The routines-based interview: A method for gathering information and assessing needs. *Infants & Young Children, 22*(3), 224-233. https://doi.org/10.1097/IYC.0b013e3181abe1ddMiller, L., Oakland, T., & Herzberg, D. (2013). *Goal-Oriented Assessment of Lifeskills (GOAL™).* Western Psychological Services.

Morgan, C., Novak, I., Dale, R. C., & Badawi, N. (2015). Optimising motor learning in infants at high risk of cerebral palsy: A pilot study. *BMC Pediatrics, 15,* 30. https://doi.org/10.1186/s12887-015-0347-2

Mumbardó-Adam, C., Guàrdia-Olmos, J., Adam-Alcocer, A. L., Carbó-Carreté, M., Balcells-Balcells, A., Giné, C., & Shogren, K. A. (2017). Self-determination, intellectual disability, and context: A meta-analytic study. *Intellectual & Developmental Disabilities, 55*(5), 303-314. https://doi.org/10.1352/1934-9556-55.5.303

National Scientific Council on the Developing Child. (2015). *Supportive relationships and active skill-building strengthen the foundations of resilience (Working Paper 13).* http://www.developingchild.harvard.edu

Newborg, J. (2020.) *Battelle Developmental Inventory, Third Edition [BDI-3].* Riverside Assessments.

Ogourtsova, T., O'Donnell, M., & Majnemer, A. (2019). Coach, care coordinator, navigator or keyworker? Review of emergent terms in childhood disability. *Physical & Occupational Therapy in Pediatrics, 39*(2), 119-123. https://doi.org/10.1080/01942638.2018.1521891

Percy, M., Brown, I., & Fung, W. L. A. (2017). Factors causing or contributing to intellectual and developmental disabilities. In M. Wehmeyer, I. Brown, M. Percy, K. Shogren, and W. L. A. Fung (Eds.), *A comprehensive guide to intellectual and developmental disabilities* (2nd ed., pp. 175-194). Brooks Publishing.

Rosner, T., Grasso, A., Scott-Cole, L., Villalobos, A., & Mulcahey, M. J. (2020). Scoping review of school-to-work transition for youth with intellectual disabilities: A practice gap. *American Journal of Occupational Therapy, 74*(2), 7402205020p1-7402205020p23. https://doi.org/10.5014/ajot.2019.035220

Rowland, C. (2011). Using the Communication Matrix to assess expressive skills in early communicators. *Communication Disorders Quarterly, 32*(3), 190-201. https://doi.org/10.1177/1525740110394651

Sattler, J. (2002). *Assessment of children: Behavioral and clinical applications.* Sattler Press.

Selanikyo, E., Yalon-Chamovitz, S., & Weintraub, N. (2017). Enhancing classroom participation of students with intellectual and developmental disabilities. *Canadian Journal of Occupational Therapy, 84*(2), 76-76. https://doi.org/10.1177/0008417416661346

Shaw, S., & Jankowska, A. (2018). *Pediatric intellectual disabilities at school: Translating research into practice.* Springer Nature.

Shogren, K., Wehmeyer, M., & Singh, N. (Eds.). (2017). *Handbook of positive psychology in intellectual and developmental disabilities: Translating research into practice.* Springer. https://doi.org/10.1007/978-3-319-59066-0

Sulkes, B. (2018). Intellectual disability. https://www.merckmanuals.com/professional/pediatrics/learning-and-developmental-disorders/intellectual-disability

ten Hove, J., & Rosenbaum, P. (2018). The concept of resilience in childhood disability: Does the International Classification of Functioning, Disability and Health help us? *Child: Care, Health & Development, 44*(5), 730-735. https://doi.org/10.1111/cch.12590

Waldman-Levi, A., & Erez, A. B.-H. (2015). Will environmental interventions affect the level of mastery motivation among children with disabilities? A preliminary study. *Occupational Therapy International, 22*(1), 19-27. https://doi.org/10.1002/oti.1380

Waldman-Levi, L. A., Golisz, K., Swierat, R. P., & Toglia, J. (2019). Scoping review: Interventions that promote functional performance for adolescents and adults with intellectual and developmental disabilities. *Australian Occupational Therapy Journal, 66*(4), 458-468. https://doi.org/10.1111/1440-1630.12577

Weisner, T., Matheson, C., Coots, J., & Bernheimer, L. (2005). Sustainability of daily routines as a family outcome. In A. Maynard & M. Martini (Eds.), *Learning in cultural context* (pp. 41-73). Springer.

Wilder, J., & Granlund, M. (2015). Stability and change in sustainability of daily routines and social networks in families of children with profound intellectual and multiple disabilities. *Journal of Applied Research in Intellectual Disabilities, 28*(2), 133-144. https://doi.org/10.1111/jar.12111

Zablotsky, B., Black, L. I., & Blumberg, S. J. (2017). Estimated prevalence of children with diagnosed developmental disabilities in the United States, 2014-2016. *NCHS Data Brief No. 291.* National Center for Health Statistics. https://www.cdc.gov/nchs/data/databriefs/db291.pdf

5

Children and Youth With Behavioral and Mental Health Disorders

Catherine Candler, OTR, PhD, BCP and
Rebecca Crossland, OTR, MOT

CHAPTER OBJECTIVES By the end of this chapter, the reader will be able to:

- Describe the diagnostic categories of mental health disorders common in children and youth.
- Explain the occupational challenges faced by children and youth with identified mental health disorders and the impact of those challenges on adaptation, coping and resilience.
- Select among interventions that promote adaptation, coping, and resilience in children and youth with identified mental health disorders.
- Discuss the opportunities and challenges for occupational therapy practice in mental health in family-centered care, collaboration with professionals, and global contexts.

OVERVIEW OF THE POPULATION

This chapter focuses on children and youth with identified mental health and behavioral disorders. There are different ways to identify conditions atypical of the general population. From a societal perspective, children and youth with identified mental disorders are placed in tier three of the multitiered public health framework used today in school, community, and health care settings. Tier three is the category where the

Grajo L. C., & Boisselle, A. K. (Eds.). *Adaptation, Coping, and Resilience in Children and Youth: A Comprehensive Occupational Therapy Approach* (pp. 103-132). © 2022 Taylor & Francis Group.

risk of dysfunction and disability is high (Bazyk & Arbesman, 2013). Unlike the general population-based approaches of tier one, or the group-focused interventions of tier two, tier three includes the most individualized and customized approaches to treatment. In legal terms, identified mental disorder among children is defined through the Individuals with Disabilities Education Act (2004) eligibility of emotional disturbance (§ 300.8(c)(4)). Emotional disturbance includes any one of five characteristics that occur to a marked degree over a long period of time and adversely affect educational performance. Those characteristics are:

1. An inability to learn that cannot be explained by intellectual, sensory, or health factors;
2. An inability to build or maintain satisfactory interpersonal relationships with peers and teachers;
3. Inappropriate types of behavior or feelings under normal circumstances;
4. A general pervasive mood of unhappiness or depression; or
5. A tendency to develop physical symptoms or fears associated with personal or school problems.

Etiology is another method frequently used for the identification of conditions, but the etiology of identified mental disorder in children and youth remains an unanswered blend between physical and psychosocial factors. Neurological differences between those with and without mental disorder are confirmed by research and this has led to a call to remove the distinction between neurological and psychiatric disorders (David & Nicholson, 2015). However, the exact nature of these differences and their relationship to the symptoms experienced remain elusive. Genetics plays a role, as research also confirms that mental disorder occurs in families, yet no direct links have been made between specific genetic makeup and the categorized symptoms and signs of mental disorder predominantly used today (Smoller et al., 2019). It is known that environmental factors are related to prevalence of mental disorder. These include poverty, stressful life events, parental psychopathology, maltreatment, and family dysfunction (Shanahan et al., 2011). Yet, because not all individuals exposed to these develop mental disorders, they may be more accurately considered risk factors or contributors rather than direct sources of mental disorder.

Because direct etiology has not been established, ultimately mental health conditions atypical of the general population are identified through descriptions of behavior and function. Currently the features described by the *Diagnostic and Statistical Manual of Mental Disorders, Fifth Edition* (*DSM-5*; American Psychiatric Association, 2013) are the primary criteria used to delineate between mental health issues in the general population and identified mental disorders. Behavioral and mental health issues have a different prevalence among children vs. adults (Ghandour et al., 2019). Most identified disorders are less frequent in younger children and appear more often in adolescence. This chapter addresses the conditions more predominant among children and youth according to the Centers for Disease Control and Prevention (CDC; 2019) and are listed in Table 5-1. These are disorders of anxiety, mood, and oppositional defiant and conduct disorders. Severe mental disorder, schizophrenia, also occurs but rarely.

Table 5-1

Types of Identified Mental Illnesses

Anxiety Disorders

Condition	Prevalence		Gender	Description
	Childhood	Adolescence		
Separation anxiety	4%	1.6%	Both	Developmentally inappropriate fear/anxiety of separation from an attachment figure.
Selective mutism	0.03% to 1%	Rare	Both	Failure to speak.
Specific phobia	5%	16%	Girls	Fear/anxiety about a specific object or situation.
Social anxiety	3% to 6.8%, with higher percentage ranges for adolescents		Girls	Fear/anxiety/avoidance of situations of perceived social scrutiny.
Panic	0.4%	2% to 3%	Girls	Recurrent unexpected abrupt surges of intense fear or discomfort.
Agoraphobia	Uncommon	1.7%	Girls	Fear/anxiety about transportation, open or enclosed spaces, being alone or in a crowd.
Generalized	May be overdiagnosed	0.9%	Girls	Excessive, persistent, and pervasive worries about a number of events or activities.

(continued)

Table 5-1 (continued)

Types of Identified Mental Illnesses

Depressive Disorders

Condition	Prevalence		Gender	Description
	Childhood	Adolescence		
Disruptive mood dysregulation disorder	2% to 5%	Higher in school age than in adolescence	Boys	Chronic severe persistent irritability with frequent temper outbursts and angry mood.
Major depressive disorder	2%	4% to 8%	Both in childhood / Girls in adolescence	Depressed mood nearly every day and loss of interest or pleasure in nearly all activities; includes five symptoms: appetite changes, sleep disturbance, agitation or slowness of activity, decreased energy, sense of worthlessness or guilt, impaired ability to think and make decisions, recurrent thoughts of death.
Persistent depressive disorder (dysthymia)	0.5% for adults DSM-5 combines category of chronic major depressive disorder	When studied in combination with major depressive disorder, 11.2%		Depressed mood that occurs for most of the day for more days than not and includes two or more symptoms: appetite changes, sleep disturbance, decreased energy, low self-esteem, impaired ability to think and make decisions, feelings of hopelessness.

Disruptive, Impulse-Control, and Conduct Disorders

Condition	Prevalence		Gender	Description
	Childhood	Adolescence		
Oppositional defiant disorder	3.3%	12.6% lifetime prevalence	Boys more than girls prior to adolescence	Frequent persistent patterns of angry/irritable mood and argumentative/defiant behavior or vindictiveness.
Conduct disorder	2% to 10%	Prevalence rises from childhood to adolescence Lifetime prevalence 6.8%	Boys	A pattern of behavior where the rights of others or major social norms or rules are violated.

Psychotic Disorder

Condition	Prevalence		Gender	Description
	Childhood	Adolescence		
Schizophrenia	Rare	less than 0.04%	Both	Loss of contact with reality for a significant portion of time over 6 months, with accompanying impairment in interpersonal, academic, or daily life functioning and is generally considered a lifetime condition.

Synthesized from Centers for Disease Control and Prevention. (2019, April 19). *Data and statistics on children's mental health*. CDC. https://www.cdc.gov/childrensmentalhealth/data.html

Anxiety Disorders

> Jill didn't know why she got those feelings in her middle. They just seemed to well up, making her shaky and afraid. When they happened, her heart beat fast and it was hard to talk and she just wants to hide, hide, hide. They got worse when it was time to go to school; and if she didn't go to school, then they went away. She started having tummy aches in the morning and Mommy allowed her to stay home more often but usually she still had to go to school. Some days it was okay, but it was hard to do all the things a girl has to do at school with that scary feeling always hovering, waiting to jump out.

Anxiety disorders are typified by excessive fear and anxiety in situations that are non-threatening for most individuals. *Fear* refers to a response to a perceived present threat. *Anxiety* occurs in anticipation of a future threat (American Psychiatric Association, 2013). Recent evidence suggests anxiety disorders are identified in 7.1% or approximately 4.4 million children aged 3 to 17 years (Ghandour et al., 2019). Many anxiety disorders present among adults developed in childhood (Copeland et al., 2015), and prevalence of anxiety disorders among children has been increasing (Bitsko et al., 2018; Hitchcock et al., 2009). Prevalence data and descriptions of types of anxiety disorders according to the *DSM-5* are displayed in Table 5-1.

Occupational Implications

Anxiety consumes mental and physical energy; thus, children with anxiety disorders are impaired in their ability to do things efficiently, such as being able to focus on educational tasks amid the distraction of worry. Children with anxiety disorders often feel stressed, tired, and irritable, which may impede completion of daily routines. Avoidance or withdrawal from occupations most children enjoy may also occur, particularly occupations involving social participation. Occupational therapy practitioners often address these concerns using cognitive behavioral approaches to create self-established occupational routines and habits. These may include the design of enjoyable activities that promote optimal levels of arousal or relaxation, as well as assisting the child in developing strategies for managing symptoms (American Occupational Therapy Association [AOTA], 2016; Schwartz et al., 2019).

Depressive Disorders

> The boys were playing with the blocks and construction toys again. Donna had retreated to the building center because it was in a corner and she could sit screened from the classroom. She built a house with thick walls for the scared people inside. Donna saw Fred come closer to her with the dump truck. Donna felt irritation at the interruption. Fred filled the truck with the unused blocks lying next to her. Truck full, Fred drove the truck away across the carpet and Donna didn't pursue the interaction . . . it just didn't seem worthwhile.

The identifying features of depressive disorders are sad, empty, or irritable moods (American Psychiatric Association, 2013). An estimated 3.2% of children experience depression, and of these, the majority will have another accompanying disorder. It has been estimated that 78% of children with depression also experience anxiety and 48% exhibit behavioral problems (Ghandour et al., 2019). Two types, major and persistent depressive disorder (as identified by *DSM-5*), present with a combination of depressed mood and loss of interest in activities. Of the two, individuals with major depressive disorder demonstrate more symptoms with greater severity (including suicide risk).

Disruptive mood dysregulation disorder was introduced by the American Psychiatric Association in 2013 and does not appear in previous editions of the *DSM*. Diagnoses of this condition are restricted to children under the age of 18 with onset before the age of 10. An impetus to this addition was the emergence of an increase in the diagnosis rates of bipolar disorder, a condition historically occurring in less than 1% of children. Disruptive mood dysregulation disorder is typified by temper outbursts of strength and frequency outside of age norms with a chronic, severe irritability most of the day for most days. The chronicity of irritable mood differentiates disruptive mood dysregulation disorder from bipolar disorder, as individuals with bipolar disorder show wide swings in mood, often with stability in between. The long-term significance of this discriminating factor remains under study (Fristad et al., 2016).

Occupational Implications

Depression is most frequently treated with a combination of pharmacotherapy and psychotherapy and is organized along three phases (Patra, 2019). The target in the acute phase is a 50% reduction in symptoms. Subsequent to the acute phase (2 weeks to 2 months), intervention is focused on maintaining gains in emotional well-being followed by a recovery phase of relapse prevention. Shifts in occupational performance occur along this continuum. For the acute phase, onset of a depressive episode may be signaled by an unexplained disinterest in activities the child formerly found enjoyable. Disengagement from schoolwork may occur, as well as irritable responses to invitations or demands for engagement. Education of parents and educators regarding these signs of depression is critical. As the child moves toward recovery, modifications in school demands and schedule may be required to reduce stress (AOTA, 2009). Opportunities to engage in favored occupations should remain present as symptoms decrease and interest returns.

Disruptive, Impulse-Control, and Conduct Disorders

> She just didn't want to do what the teacher said and it was easier to just not do it; and so she didn't do it even though the teacher was looking hard at her again. Josephine looked hard right back. As she did, she felt in control, though ultimately she wasn't in control, and now she wasn't allowed to go to recess, which bothered her. She liked recess and needed recess because she felt in control there, in a world where teachers didn't make demands. Josephine's grades were terrible, and she didn't like that. But maybe she didn't care. In any case, she just wasn't going to do it.

Disruptive, impulse-control, and conduct disorders concern problems in emotional and behavioral self-regulation that evidence themselves in behaviors that violate the rights of others and/or set the individual in direct conflict with societal norms or authority figures. The prevalence of behavior/conduct problems is 7.4% of children aged 3 to 17 years, which equates to approximately 4.5 million within the United States (Ghandour et al., 2019). Within the *DSM-5*, two types of disorders are predominant for children: oppositional defiant and conduct disorders. These disorders emerge in childhood or adolescence and only rarely in adulthood.

Oppositional defiant disorder is characterized by frequent persistent patterns of angry/irritable mood and argumentative/defiant behavior or vindictiveness. The addition of these behaviors and the severity of symptoms differentiates the condition from the persistent irritability of disruptive mood dysregulation disorder (Ghosh et al., 2017). *Conduct disorder* is a pattern of behavior where the rights of others or major social norms or rules are violated. These include aggression to people and animals, destruction of property, theft, running away, and truancy. Comorbidity with attention deficit hyperactivity disorder is high (American Psychiatric Association, 2013; see Chapter 6 on attention deficit/hyperactivity disorders). Onset may occur in childhood before the age of 10. Oppositional defiant disorders often precede later identification of conduct disorder. Childhood onset is associated with persistence of the disorder into adulthood. Adolescent onset signals a better—though still difficult—prognosis, although this premise has been questioned (Fairchild, 2018).

Occupational Implications

Oppositional defiant and conduct disorders signal dysfunction in occupations linked with societal expectations. Issues of disobedience, disregard of rules, and flaunting social conventions arise with school and community life. Interventions as listed by Ghosh et al. (2017) include parental management training, school-based training, functional family therapy/brief strategic family therapy, and cognitive behavioral therapy. Intervention must be multimodal and long term (Sagar et al., 2019). Activity-based training and social skills programs are evidence-based approaches implemented by occupational therapists (Arbesman et al., 2013).

Psychotic Disorders

The whispers were scary and hard to understand. Sometimes they called her name, other times they just chattered. She couldn't pay attention to them and couldn't not pay attention to them and the people around her didn't seem to be a part of what was going on. When the shadows started walking and flitting around her, she knew it was time to hide and she screamed before she ran. They found her in the bathroom stall and she collapsed crying in her teacher's arms.

Psychosis refers to a loss of contact with reality (National Institute of Mental Health, 2015). Psychotic symptoms are key features in psychotic disorders, but may also occur as episodes in other conditions such as a depressive or bipolar disorder (American Psychiatric Association, 2013). Psychotic breaks with reality occur in five ways:

1. Delusions (i.e., beliefs that persist in spite of evidence to the contrary;
2. Hallucinations (i.e., perceptions that occur without an environmental stimulus);
3. Disorganized thinking, typically expressed through speech where the individual's communication is significantly impaired by abrupt switches of topic, responses unrelated to topic, or total incoherence;
4. Grossly disorganized motor behavior such as agitation, silliness, or catatonia, a shutdown of reactivity to the environment; and
5. Negative signs associated with psychosis, lack of emotional expression and motivation for activity.

Although psychotic diagnoses in the general population are uncommon, the mean prevalence of experiences of hallucination or delusion is relatively high at a worldwide estimate of 5.8%, with hallucination experiences (5.2%) more predominant than delusions (1.3%; McGrath et al., 2015). Approximately 20% of those reporting psychotic experiences continue to do so, while 80% do not (Linscott & van Os, 2013). A recent meta-analysis concerning these experiences found a higher (9.9%) prevalence among children and youth (Healy et al., 2019). Systematic reviews suggest a relationship between psychotic experiences and subsequent development of a mental disorder, although this topic of study is still in development (Healy et al., 2019; Linscott & van Os, 2013; Maijer et al., 2018).

Childhood schizophrenia is a rare diagnosis, with a prevalence of less than 0.04% (Driver et al., 2013). Making the diagnosis involves a meticulous process of ruling out other etiology. Children with schizophrenia demonstrate psychotic symptoms for a significant portion of time over 6 months with accompanying impairment in interpersonal, academic, or daily life functioning. This is generally considered a lifetime condition.

Occupational Implications

Schizophrenia is a severe mental disorder, and intervention involves both pharmacologic and psychiatric approaches. Though a chronic condition, treatment must be timely and involve multiple modalities and disciplines (Abidi, 2013). Support systems are essential. Occupational therapy can be instrumental in the development or re-establishment of essential routines to maintain quality rhythms for daily life. These include individualized adaptations and strategies for self and community support.

Defining Adaptation, Coping, and Resilience for Children and Youth With Behavioral and Mental Health Disorders

Although mental health and quality of life are achieved by individuals with mental disorders, these conditions frequently carry lifetime challenges. The Great Smoky Mountains Study (Copeland et al., 2015) followed 1,420 persons from age 9 to 26 with and without mental health issues. Participants with an identified childhood psychiatric disorder had six times higher odds of at least one adverse outcome in adulthood even if the children as adults no longer had psychiatric problems. Higher odds—three times that of those without childhood mental health issues—were also detected for the children who did not meet psychiatric diagnosis criteria but exhibited subclinical symptoms.

Inability to successfully direct one's behavior within a community of others has significant implications for quality of life. Individuals with mental disorder often take blame for their disabilities and induce a paradox of confusion among their associates. Friends and family members who are motivated to provide support also need affirmation, which the individual with mental disorder may provide only intermittently. Mentally ill behaviors are by definition socially destructive, cutting those with mental disorder off from the very community they need to function optimally. This is exacerbated by the chronicity of mental disorder, which extends these challenges over a lifetime.

The significance of these challenges is illustrated clearly with today's concept of the term *recovery* in relation to severe mental disorder (Davidson et al., 2005). As recently as 2005, the standard professional response to severe mental disorders such as schizophrenia was that these conditions could not be functionally addressed and amelioration of symptoms through medication was the only meaningful intervention that could be offered. Recovery today goes beyond psychotic symptoms into concepts associated with resilience in the personal process of living with mental disorder, a holistic approach consistent with the tenets of occupational therapy.

Early research that takes a deeper look into the lives of individuals with severe mental disorder reveals life patterns that do improve over time (Harding et al., 1987). Key to positive changes is an increase in coping and adaptive skills, which results in self-generated strategies to live optimally with the condition. Initially proposed from a narrative review of the literature in 2011 (Leamy et al., 2011), and more recently affirmed by a scoping review conducted by van Weeghel et al. (2019), areas key to recovery include connectedness, hope and optimism about the future, identity, meaning in life, and empowerment.

Case Study 5-1

Harry

Harry could remember how messed up going to school was in the fifth grade. Things always got out of control when he was with the regular class, so he spent most of his day in a special classroom with other "messed-up" kids. He was the youngest of four and lived with his mom and stepdad and his stepdad's three kids. It made for a chaotic household and things got physical sometimes. Some might call it abuse but he wasn't so sure. He would comment that that's the way his family did things. His birth dad has bipolar disorder and he had a great uncle who was schizophrenic, after all. Harry did know it was rough. He was a tough kid to teach. Most of the time he didn't care much about doing schoolwork and he liked to do things his own way. Sometimes he got a bit impulsive and when they changed things, well, it took time to get used to it. Memorizing to know things just didn't work for him, writing was a struggle, and socializing with other kids? Let's just say that friendship was a day-to-day thing. Some days he got along good, other days not so much. Now that he was grown and starting out at the community college, things weren't that much different. Managing his life remained a struggle. But at least he knew how to do it, even though actually doing it didn't always happen. He remembered the occupational therapist who showed up back then. She had gathered the class together and taught him something she called Goal-Plan-Do-Check (Polatajko & Mandich, 2004). He still used it today. When things got to be too much, he knew that what worked best was to just stop doing and think about it. If he could boil down the chaos to one goal, one thing he wanted, then he could make a plan. If he focused just on his plan and checked on how he was doing, usually he could work his way out. What a difference such a simple little thing could make for a graduate from self-contained classrooms for children with an emotionally disturbed eligibility!

Functional mechanisms for adaptation and coping are essential for quality of life throughout the lifespan of individuals with mental health challenges. Building these skills early, as a foundation for lifetime support, is critical to optimal outcomes for children. Success in occupations of scholastic achievement or work are good predictors of adult success in these areas. More importantly, occupations that emphasize adaptation and coping in social function tend to have a more generalized positive benefit for multiple life tasks (Henry & Coster, 1996). Case Study 5-1 paints a picture of life in a youth with behavioral disorder.

The Role of Occupational Therapy for Children With Behavioral and Mental Disorders: Best and Evidence-Based Practices for Assessment and Intervention

Assessment

An occupation-focused approach to effective intervention for children with identified mental health disorders relies on evaluation that is holistic and, thus, includes a variety of information sources based on the child's age and developmental level. The evaluation, therefore, should also include caregivers and families, as children's developing patterns of behavior are typically learned from the home environment. Depending on the practice setting, effective occupational therapy evaluation may occur as a multidisciplinary effort, which may include a team of providers such as nurses, case managers, recreational therapists, psychiatrists, and social workers. To ensure an occupational perspective, the evaluation includes the development of an occupational profile and an analysis of occupational performance as outlined in the *Occupational Therapy Practice Framework, Fourth Edition* (AOTA, 2020).

Due to the variability and severity of symptoms seen across practice areas, the evaluation may be performed across multiple sessions to provide a comprehensive view of the client. Standardized evaluations as well as parent/caregiver report, teacher report, and observation of play in structured and unstructured tasks will be necessary. Important areas to consider include cognitive abilities, sensory needs, social interactions, and difficulties with self-management, as these influence engagement in childhood occupations of education, play, and activities of daily living. Targeted assessment of occupations is critical, because a component-based perspective does not encompass the child's ability to perform the complex tasks of daily life (Rogers & Holm, 2016). Table 5-2 includes a list of potential assessments that may be used to develop a holistic and multidimensional evaluation.

Intervention

Adaptive capacity is the ability to plan, execute, and revise ways or strategies, as needed, to overcome an occupational challenge (Grajo, 2019). Development of explicit skills requiring flexibility, goal setting, and problem solving improves adaptive capacity (Grajo et al., 2018). The coping process involves information processing, emotions, and behavioral response that occurs repeatedly throughout life (Lazarus & Folkman, 1987). Coping includes purposeful responses that are either problem focused, which serves to eliminate the negative stressor; or emotion focused, which reduces negative emotions due to stress and, thus, improves the ability to cope. Thus, in order to develop adaptive capacity and coping skills, children need strong executive function and self-regulation skills to manage their own behavior.

Table 5-2

Some Assessments for Children and Youth With Mental Disorders

Assessment of Occupational Performance

Child Occupational Self Assessment (COSA; Kramer et al., 2014)

Self-report questionnaire for children under 12 years concerning their self-perception of occupational competence.

Available from https://www.moho.uic.edu/default.aspx

Canadian Occupational Performance Measure (COPM; Law, 2019)

Self-report questionnaire and evidence-based outcome measure concerning self-perception of performance in everyday living. Ages 6 to 17.

Available from http://www.thecopm.ca

Young Children's Participation and Environment Measure (YC-PEM; Khetani et al., 2013)

Parent-completed measure of the child's participation in home, daycare/preschool, and community settings and the impact of each setting's environment on that participation. Ages 0 to 5 years.

Available from https://www.canchild.ca/en/shop

Vineland Adaptive Behavior Scales, Third Edition (Sparrow et al., 2016)

Semi-structured interview or questionnaire to assess personal and social skills for daily activities. Ages 0 to 90 years.

Available from https://www.pearsonassessments.com

Assessment of School Participation

Occupational Therapy Psychosocial Assessment of Learning (OT PAL) Version 2.0 (Townsend, 1999)

Structured observation-based rating scale inclusive of parent, teacher, child interviews concerning social competence in school children. School-aged children.

Available from https://www.moho.uic.edu/default.aspx

Devereux Student Strengths Assessment (DESSA; K-8 and High School Editions; LeBuffe et al., 2014)

Likert-scale assessment of eight social and emotional competencies to assist educators in planning, documenting, and monitoring progress in social-emotional learning.

Available from https://apertureed.com/dessa-overview

Assessment of Social Skills

Evaluation of Social Interaction (ESI; Fisher & Griswold, 2008)

Observational tool that measures quality of social interaction in natural contexts. Test administration training required. Age 2.5 and up.

Available from https://www.innovativeotsolutions.com

(continued)

Table 5-2 (continued)

Some Assessments for Children and Youth With Mental Disorders

Social Profile: Assessment of Social Participation in Children, Adolescents and Adults (Donohue, 2013)

Observational measure of social participation in groups or individuals in social settings.

Available from https://www.maryvdonohue.com

Social Skills Rating System (SSRS; Gresham & Elliott, 1990)

Teacher, parent, and student rating forms for social skills, problem behaviors, and academic competence. Ages 3 to 18 years.

Available from https://pearsonclinical.in

Assessment of Interests and Play Behavior

Children's Assessment of Participation and Enjoyment (CAPE) and Preferences for Activities with Children (PAC; Law et al., 2004)

Picture-based questionnaire and rating scale. Children report their level of participation, enjoyment, and preferences among a wide variety of play activities. Ages 6 to 21 years.

Available from https://www.pearsonassessments.com

Pediatric Activity Card Sort (PACS; Mandich et al., 2004)

Utilizes a card-sorting task to help to determine the child's level of occupational performance and engagement in typical childhood occupations. Ages 6 to 12 years.

Available from https://www.caot.ca

Test of Playfulness (Skard & Bundy, 2008)

Assess a child's playfulness during free play. Ages 6 months to 18 years.

Available in Parham, L. D. & Fazio, L. S. (2008). *Play in occupational therapy for children* (2nd ed.). Mosby Elsevier.

Assessment of Coping

Children's Coping Strategies Checklist (CCSC; Program for Prevention Research at Arizona State University,1999)

Self-report inventory of 52 items where children describe their coping efforts. Ages 9 to 13 years.

Available from http://www.ravansanji.ir/?9311011032

Adolescent Coping Scale, Second Edition (ACS; Frydenburg & Lewis, 2012)

A 60-item, self-report inventory that describes an individual's degree of usage of 20 coping strategies and an evaluation of their perceived helpfulness. Ages 12 to 18 years.

Available from https://shop.acer.edu.au

(continued)

Table 5-2 (continued)

Some Assessments for Children and Youth With Mental Disorders

Coping Inventories (Zietlin, 1985)

Assessment of the behavior patterns and skills used to meet personal needs and adapt to the demands of the environment.

Coping Inventory Observational Form: Ages 3 to 16 years

Coping Inventory Self-Report Form: Age 15 to adult

Early Coping Inventory: A Measure of Adaptive Behavior: Ages 4 to 36 months.

Available from https://ststesting.com/COPI.html

Parent and Caregiver Assessments

Parenting Stress Index, Fourth Edition (Abidin, 2012)

Questionnaire that evaluates the parenting system and identifies issues that may lead to problems in the child's or parent's behavior. Ages 0 to 12 years.

Available from https://www.parinc.com/Products/Pkey/335

Promoting Adaptive Capacity: Occupational Engagement

Meaningful Activities. The use of occupation to improve health, well-being, and adaptation forms the distinct value of occupational therapy and should be present in all occupational therapy intervention (AOTA, 2017). Occupational therapy involves directly engaging clients in occupation and thus, by nature, is a holistic approach incorporating understanding of personal and environmental factors, rather than focus on impairment and symptoms (Krupa et al., 2009). An occupational approach allows individuals to learn and experience the effects of adaptation and coping within the context of activities important to them, thus contributing to resilience in the face of personal challenges. The Occupational Therapy Training Program (https://www.ottp.org) in California illustrates the occupational approach well. Adaptive behaviors are facilitated in the context of engagement in occupations from across the spectrum of self-care, work, and play/leisure.

In a systematic review of occupations used to engage children with mental health disorders, Cahill et al. (2020) identified moderate-strength evidence supporting the use of yoga, sports, play, and creative arts as occupation-based interventions. Adaptive capacities such as problem solving, self-regulation, and social skills are examples of areas that can be targeted using occupation-based intervention. Another systematic review sponsored by the American Occupational Therapy Association probed the literature for occupation- and activity-based approaches for mental health intervention and confirmed their effectiveness (Arbesman et al., 2013). Among tier three interventions specific to children and youth with diagnosed mental disorder, Arbesman et al. found strong evidence of efficacy for social skills training. Occupations that emphasize adaptation and coping in social function tend to have a generalized positive benefit to multiple life tasks (Henry & Coster, 1996). Figure 5-1 shows an example of providing opportunities for meaningful therapeutic activities.

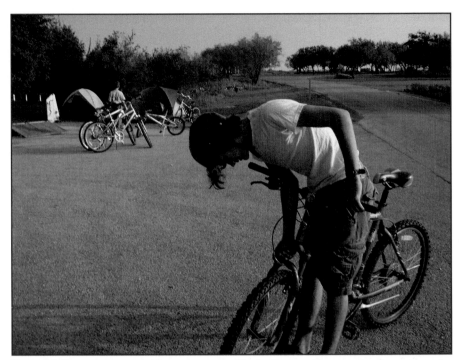

Figure 5-1. Summer camps provide many opportunities for therapeutic occupational engagement.

Life Balance and Coaching. Functional routines and balance in occupational engagement form a base for resilience for children and youth with identified mental disorders. Analysis of the nature and frequency of daily occupations and task analysis of the routines associated with them is an overarching occupational approach. This analysis becomes a good tool for adaptation when combined with the collaborative intervention approach of coaching (Graham et al., 2009). In coaching, the therapist takes a facilitating role with the client, who may be the child, adolescent, teacher, and/or caregiver. Using techniques of questioning rather than direct provision of advice or instruction, the client is asked to identify their challenges and then prompted to reflect on possible strategies. The occupational therapist adds information about occupational balance and functional routines as needed by the client to facilitate the client's choices of strategies for improvement. Coaching continues beyond problem identification and strategies into strategy implementation. As coach, the therapist provides feedback and encouragement, prompting the child or adolescent to respond to the results experienced in the implementation by either revising or adopting the new way of adapting.

Social Skills Training. An occupation-based approach to social skills includes addressing them within a social context of occupation, and may also include explicit teaching of specific behaviors that lie within that context. *Social skills* are behaviors that have been accepted by others as typical and appropriate. They enable an individual to interact in positive ways and avoid rejection or negative responses (Elliott et al., 1995). Some examples are how to greet a peer, effective ways to disconnect from a conversation, appropriate table manners, and how to thank or apologize. More involved skills may include how to say no or language to use to avoid confrontation. Video modeling has emerged as an evidence-based approach to this type of instruction (Arbesman et al., 2013). Children view a video of the appropriate behavior in order to learn it. Other approaches are social stories and short illustrations of social interactions, as well as role play and other teaching techniques.

Problem-Focused Coping

Problem solving involves the ability to objectively consider a situation, analyze it, form a plan for addressing it, and integrate feedback from the plan's intervention. Effective problem solving requires the use of feedback from the situation and metacognition, which is the awareness and understanding of one's own thought processes. Metacognitive interventions use guided teaching approaches of self-discovery in which the client is coached into an understanding and reflection on their own thinking in order to make changes that address the client's personal needs.

Behavior Therapy. Behavior therapy concerns the explicit address of observable behavior using targeted outcomes. It is implemented by structuring the events that occur before and immediately after the targeted behavior in order to shape or change that behavior (Benjamin et al., 2011). Behavior therapy includes explicitly stated expectations, ready feedback on performance, reward, and contingencies. These strategies are used routinely in occupational therapy practice within the context of instruction and behavior management. Behavior therapy as an exclusive focus of intervention is particularly applicable for children with externalizing disorders such as oppositional defiance and for children whose level of functioning is low.

A critique of behavior therapy from the perspective of adaptation is that when used exclusively it relies heavily on externally imposed rewards and expectations, thus placing the child in a passive position in an artificially constructed environment (Knestrict, 2019). Intervention exclusively based on behavior therapy has been operationalized in formats of applied behavior analysis (Cooper et al., 2020). These range from stringent approaches such as discrete trial training, where small pieces of behavior are shaped through rituals of prompt and reward, and pivotal response training, a more naturalistic form that incorporates the child's internal motivations. Occupational therapy practitioners also may encounter and participate in positive behavioral support programs (Koegel et al., 1996). Positive behavioral support programs are frequently implemented within schools, and use a team approach. The team works to understand the child's unique motivation for a challenging behavior and to intervene collaboratively using strategies to prevent, change, or remove the reward from the behavior.

Cognitive-Behavioral Therapy. Cognitive-behavioral therapy (CBT) is based on a combination of behavioral and cognitive theories of human function (Benjamin et al., 2011) that consider the effect of maladaptive assumptions and thinking patterns on behavior. CBT seeks to make changes in the client's internal perspectives in order to influence behavioral health. The efficacy of CBT approaches is strongest with internalizing disorders such as anxiety and depression; they are less effective with externalizing disorders such as disruptive and conduct disorders.

Bazyk and Arbesman (2013) identify five strategies rooted in CBT that can be applied within occupational therapy practice:

1. *Psychoeducation.* Here the therapist works with the child and family to demystify the diagnosis and empower their involvement in finding solutions.
2. *Affective education* involves the child's understanding of their own emotions.
3. *Cognitive restructuring* employs self-talk as a tool to assist the child in reflecting on and changing their own emotions or actions.
4. *Relaxation training* is used to reduce feelings of anxiety.
5. *Graded exposure to fears and contingency management,* which refers to rewarding favored activity, is used to address avoidance and unwanted behaviors.

Cognitive Orientation to daily Occupational Performance (CO-OP). The CO-OP was developed by occupational therapists as a performance-based treatment for teaching clients how to learn new skills (Dawson et al., 2017). The intervention was originally developed to serve children with motor planning difficulties, and since then has been expanded for use in multiple populations. CO-OP involves explicitly teaching the client an overarching global strategy called Goal-Plan-Do-Check. The children learn to verbalize this strategy and apply it to skills they wish to learn. Adaptive capacity is increased, as the child is encouraged to apply the strategy across any problem-solving situation.

Emotion-Focused Coping

Social-Emotional Learning. Social-Emotional Learning (SEL) refers to an initiative that advocates for inclusion of social emotional targets in curriculum standards and seeks to provide explicit direction to teachers in how to address social-emotional development of the children in their classrooms (Shriver & Weissberg, 2020). The focus of SEL is to teach children and youth to understand emotions, set and achieve positive goals, feel and show empathy for others, establish and maintain positive relationships, and make responsible decisions. SEL can be presented in multiple ways and is typically integrated in a school system. Research has been positive for tier one school-wide implementation (Durlak et al., 2011). Tier 3 interventions, which can be utilized by occupational therapists for children with identified mental disorder, include teaching explicit SEL skills, such as self-awareness, self-management, social awareness, relationship skills, and responsible decision making.

Sensory and Metacognitive Applications to Self-Regulation. Individuals with identified mental disorder may also exhibit sensory differences (Fraser et al., 2017). Sensory differences can negatively affect a child's behavior, emotional regulation, maintenance of optimal levels of arousal, and development of positive social interactions (Schaaf et al., 2017). Sensory techniques involving sensory processing and sensory modulation can assist with self-regulation in order to further develop the skills necessary to build adaptive capacity and coping skills. Sensory techniques may include activities that are calming/alerting, sensory diets to maintain a level of arousal, a sensory room that children can turn to, or environmental sensory strategies to use in the classroom, hospital, or home environment. Sensory techniques are frequently used by occupational therapists for children with behavioral disorders. Use of more targeted sensory integration interventions, such as Ayres Sensory Integration, for some behavioral populations such as children with autism has been encouraging (Schaaf et al., 2017). However, studies specifically examining this approach for children with identified mental disorder are lacking. Thus, sensory-based approaches should be viewed as potentially helpful as adjuncts to rather than a replacement for multimodal psychosocial interventions (Tzang et al., 2019).

The Alert Program. Also known by the title *How Does Your Engine Run?* (Williams & Shellenberger, 1996), the Alert Program is a metacognitive approach for behavior that calls on the immediate influence of sensory input to self-regulate arousal level. In this program, children are taught to recognize behavioral cues that signal high arousal (engines running in high), low arousal, and optimal arousal levels. Concurrently, children are guided in exploring how various sensory inputs affect their feelings of arousal. For example, does the child experience jumping up and down as arousing or calming? Based on this knowledge, children are facilitated in designing their own sensory-based strategies to bring their arousal levels to optimum (just right engines). The program can be used at a classroom or individual level. A randomized controlled trial of the Alert Program for children with sensory reactive issues related to fetal alcohol syndrome found moderate support for effectiveness (Wells et al., 2012). Two other interventions, Zones of Regulation and The Incredible 5-Point Scale, are similar programs. More research on these programs utilizing different populations remains to be done.

Zones of Regulation. The Zones of Regulation curriculum (Kuypers & Winner, 2011) teaches self-regulation skills using cognitive behavioral strategies incorporating executive functions, emotional regulation, and sensory processing. Participants learn to understand their current arousal state by identifying specific colors: blue (low state of alertness), green (optimal state of alertness), yellow (increasing arousal, less emotional control), and red (high arousal, very little emotional control). Designed to be delivered as a tier 1 intervention, the curriculum consists of 18 lessons through which participants are introduced to an array of concrete cognitive, sensory, and calming tools and strategies to regulate their behavior in a variety of contexts.

The Incredible 5-Point Scale. The Incredible 5-Point Scale program is focused toward managing anxiety. The program breaks down social and emotional concepts into a number system to organize the child's emotions or behavior (Buron & Curtis, 2003). Using the scale, the child better understands what activities produce stress and improves self-awareness and understanding of emotions.

Yoga, Physical Exercise, and Techniques for Relaxation. Yoga, physical exercise, mindfulness, and relaxation strategies are promising activities that can improve coping abilities and reduce anxiety in children (Figure 5-2). In a systematic review, Cahill et al. (2020) found moderate-strength evidence that yoga could improve mental health, positive behavior, and social participation. Physical exercise has been shown to reduce psychiatric and depressive symptoms (Stubbs et al., 2018). Mindfulness is a form of meditation and includes focus on the breath, attending to what is occurring in one's own mind and body, and taking note of the experience (Rempel, 2012). The use of mindfulness has been advocated for use in school settings and as a means to address anxiety and stress.

Figure 5-2. Even young children can benefit from the practice of yoga.

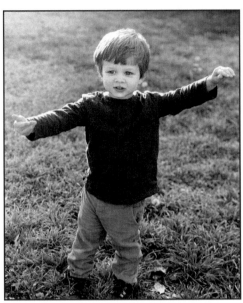

Creative Self-Expression. Participation in play and creative self-expression are important components of planning interventions with children with mental disorder. These can include free-form types of art, such as watercolor or finger painting. The ability to create can allow children to express underlying emotions. Based on Brooks and Goldstein (2008), children's self-esteem affects personal resilience and their ability to cope. Activities that can improve self-efficacy include self-reflection activities such as reflecting on the child's performance of activities rather than therapist or parent reactions to that performance. The activities should be chosen by the child in order to facilitate meaningful participation.

Accommodations and Supports. Children with identified mental disorders experience many challenges. Developing a supportive context is an important aspect of developing adaptive capacity and coping skills (Compas et al., 2001). Adapting the environment to scale challenges closer to current capabilities provides opportunity for adaptive growth. Examples of accommodations and supports to consider are listed in Table 5-3.

COLLABORATIVE APPROACH WITH FAMILIES AND THE SOCIAL ENVIRONMENT

Family-centered care is based on the recognition that the family forms the primary foundation of strength and support for developing children. Thus, information and the perspectives of the family in intervention are essential. A review of family-centered care over the past 20 years found that it is practiced widely and perceived as valuable by both families and practitioners (Cunningham & Rosenbaum, 2014). Family-centered care

Table 5-3

Accommodations and Supports
• Reduce demands for decision making
• Encourage development of daily routines
• Reduce length of the school day
• Modify classroom expectations
• Educate others concerning signs of mental disorder
• Invite, do not push participation
• Keep conversations short and simple
• Increase opportunity for and encourage physical exercise
• Post a daily schedule
• Encourage writing things down or journaling
• Ensure a calming bedtime routine
• Minimize environmental distractions
• Provide time, demonstration, and repetition when introducing novel tasks
• Create routine or rituals for transitions
• Organize work spaces

has additional meaning for occupational therapy practitioners in that occupation-based intervention includes not only a family perspective but also the occupations of the family as a unit. This calls on occupational therapy practitioners to incorporate the meaning family members ascribe to their daily occupations and routines (DeGrace, 2003). In addition, occupational therapy practitioners need to take into consideration the readiness of the caregivers themselves to participate in intervention (Sepulveda et al., 2020). This can be accomplished through careful questioning on how intervention strategies affect the family unit. Family readiness can also be accomplished through screening caregivers for mental health risks. The Parenting Stress Index (Abidin, 2012) can provide insight into caregiver coping. From an occupational therapy perspective, the assessment tool called Life Participation for Parents (Fingerhut, 2013) assesses caregivers' ability to engage in life occupations while caring for their child.

BUILDING INTERPROFESSIONAL COLLABORATIONS

Individuals coping with mental disorder require the services of multiple disciplines. Multidisciplinary intervention is a hallmark of mental health practice, as most identified mental health disorders are chronic conditions that affect occupational engagement across settings, situations, and lifetimes. Disciplines involved with mental health are many and include psychiatrists, psychologists, counselors, specialized mental health nurses, social workers, and teachers, as well as family and community members. Competence in working in interprofessional teams is measured in four areas: (1) respect for the contribution of other disciplines, (2) using knowledge of one's own professional role and that of others to appropriately address client needs, (3) communicating in a responsive and responsible manner, and (4) applying relationship building and team dynamics for effective performance (Interprofessional Education Collaborative, 2016).

Over time, occupational therapists have become less frequent contributors to mental health teams. A current challenge for those in this area of practice is a solid understanding of occupational therapy's role by other team members as well as the occupational therapy practitioners themselves (Miles & Morely, 2013; Wimpenny & Lewis, 2015). For example, in a qualitative study of occupational therapy practitioners in mental health, participants reported challenges in maintaining their focus on occupation and pressure to instead adopt psychiatric frames of reference (Ashby et al., 2017). Thus, the first step toward effective collaboration with other professionals may involve strengthening the practitioner's own occupational therapy identity. The American Occupational Therapy Association provides many resources for this, both informational (AOTA, n.d.) and through access to peers, such as the listserv CommunOT or communities of practice (Bazyk et al., 2015). A practitioner equipped in this way can communicate the distinct value of occupational therapy in mental health. Krupa et al. (2009) outlined the basic tenets of the profession with emphasis on the meaning of occupation and how it is used to enable participation in personally and socially meaningful ways.

A GLOBAL PERSPECTIVE

Behavioral and mental health disorders are a human condition and challenge individuals worldwide. Overall, the prevalence of mental health disorders is estimated at 10% of the world's population (James et al., 2018). In addition, persons with mental disorders constitute 14% of those living with disability, and this number has remained stable since 1990. The World Health Organization (WHO) carries this estimate forward for children, indicating that 10% to 20% of the world's children experience mental disorders, with half of these manifesting before the age of 14 (WHO, n.d.). The dispersion of specific mental health disorders worldwide is primarily uniform, though there are some exceptions. Conflict-affected countries show higher prevalence of mental disorder overall (22.1%; Charlson et al., 2019). Outside of conflict areas, paradoxically, anxiety disorders are more prevalent in the United States and European countries (American Psychiatric Association, 2013).

In response to the high impact of mental disorder on populations, WHO initiated the Mental Health Action Plan 2013-2020 (Saxena et al., 2014) with proposed actions and targets for member states to address globally pervasive challenges, including the macro effects of national policies, social protection, living standards, working conditions, and community social supports. Individuals with mental disorders also face stigmatization and marginalization and mental disorders often lead to poverty, which releases its own cascade of negative consequences.

Table 5-4

Essential Considerations for Occupational Therapists

- Identified mental disorders tend to be chronic, with implications across occupations and the lifespan; thus, it is essential that strength in adaptation, coping, and resilience be fostered early for lifetime benefit.
- Occupational therapists contribute to this development by offering challenging experiences within the context of occupation.
- An occupational approach allows individuals to learn and experience the effects of adaptation and coping within the context of activities important to them, thus contributing to resilience in the face of personal challenges.
- Although occupational therapy is well positioned to provide meaningful contributions toward adaptation, coping, and resilience by children and youth with identified mental disorders, these services are underrepresented in mental health practice settings and occupational therapy practitioners themselves may be uncertain concerning their role.
- Advocacy for occupational therapy services to these populations must be built on the distinct value of occupational therapy. Namely, the facilitation of participation and engagement in occupations, the meaningful, necessary, and familiar activities of everyday life.

The World Federation of Occupational Therapists (WFOT) supports the Mental Health Action Plan. The Federation's position statement embraces recovery-oriented approaches that emphasize building capacities in adaptation, coping, and resilience (WFOT, 2019). However, challenges exist throughout the profession in meeting these goals. Although occupational therapy emerged from the field of mental health, practice over the last decades has focused on medical models of disorder. Global directions toward social determinants of health have caught the profession by surprise, leaving questions of preparedness for meeting mental health needs and insufficient advocacy for occupational therapy's role (Gutman & Raphael-Greenfield, 2014; Miles & Morley, 2013; Wimpenny & Lewis, 2015). Yet, occupational therapists worldwide are suited well for the work at hand (WFOT, 2019). Occupational therapy's holistic, bio-psychosocial, and person-centered approach to building capacities in individuals to use their strengths through meaningful activities that motivate recovery is a perfect match for the global issues concerning mental health today.

ESSENTIAL CONSIDERATIONS FOR OCCUPATIONAL THERAPISTS WORKING WITH CLIENTS WITH MENTAL DISORDERS

Five essential considerations for occupational therapists working with clients with mental disorders are specified in Table 5-4.

Case Study 5-2

Beth

Beth is a 4-year-old girl who is diagnosed with disruptive mood dysregulation disorder. Beth currently demonstrates symptoms of anxiety and depression, including poor self-regulation and limited initiation of play and socialization with peers. Beth's mother and a developmental pediatrician have asked for an occupational therapy evaluation due to behavioral concerns in the home and limited interest in gross motor play.

Beth currently is at home with her mother and siblings during the day. She was previously expelled from daycare due to inappropriate, aggressive behavior, including screaming when presented with non-preferred tasks and hitting and kicking peers and teachers. Her mother provides structure to the day, much like preschool with routines and structure of play. Beth enjoys sedentary activities such as reading books, playing puzzles, crafts, and coloring, and prefers to perform these activities to the extent that she refuses to participate in gross motor activities.

Cognitively, Beth demonstrates developmentally appropriate skills, such as the ability to perform two- to four-step commands, identify and sort colors and shapes, count up to 10 well and is initiating counting to 20. She demonstrates sustained attention to preferred tasks for 20 to 45 minutes at a time. Beth shows developmentally appropriate self-care skills and her motor skills are also appropriate to her age with fine motor strengths.

Beth's executive functioning skills are delayed and limit her ability to participate in developmentally appropriate play at times. She demonstrates limited mental flexibility, which affects cooperative and imaginative play with peers and siblings. She does demonstrate interest in other children and will observe them playing; however, she will not engage with them when provided opportunities to do so. She demonstrates deficits in inhibition and self-regulation. When Beth is confronted with a change in routine or expectations, she demonstrates poor impulse control and self-regulation and will throw tantrums or refuse to participate in tasks. These limit the family's participation in outings, including going to the park. Her mother reports that Beth rarely demonstrates positive emotions at home but will demonstrate negative emotions such as sadness, worry, and anger.

The possibility of challenges with sensory modulation were assessed using the Sensory Profile-2 Caregiver Report. The sensory profile revealed that Beth has a low threshold for sensory stimulation and is sensory avoidant. She demonstrated a definite difference in her emotional and social responses through modulation of sensory information that affects her emotional responses and behavior. She also demonstrated poor coping behavior, as indicated by the Early Coping Inventory, with rigid and limited range of self-management strategies.

At her visit to the clinic, Beth wore plastic gloves for the duration of the session. Beth's mother explained that Beth is biting her fingernails, causing bleeding at times. Beth demonstrated avoidance of activities that involve sensory

(continued)

Case Study 5-2 (continued)

stimulation or gross motor movements, including various swings or gym equipment. She would become anxious, as evidenced by biting her gloves, turning away from the therapist, and refusing to participate in novel tasks presented by the therapist. She was observed to have a flat affect for the duration of the session.

Goals for Beth include expression and identification of positive and negative emotions, prosocial adaptation to novel and non-preferred activities, improved sensory processing and modulation in order to participate in leisure tasks, and socialization with peers in order to participate in cooperative play. Planned intervention strategies include the following:

Strategies for Adaptation	Strategies for Social-Emotional Learning	Sensory Strategies
• Transition between novel activities • Visual schedule for awareness of change; plan, do, review technique • Explore activity prior to completing and follow client's readiness to participate • Stop to discuss anxiety or unwillingness to participate	• Structured opportunities to engage with peers in small group • Identify emotions in others through watching videos and discussion • Identify stressors using The Incredible 5-Point Scale or Zones of Regulation • Identify how activities make her feel • Therapist models and provides examples	• Vestibular input for alerting, including slide into crash pad, bounce on large therapy ball, swing in circular motion • Tactile defensiveness: Incremental exposure using the hierarchy sequence of touch • Home program for mother to expose to sensations

Beth has participated in occupational therapy for 3 months and has shown progress, including not having to wear gloves and not biting fingernails. She can identify emotions of others with good accuracy; will report feeling happy, sad, and mad with fair accuracy; will attempt novel activities with minimal assistance; transitions between preferred and non-preferred activities with verbal cues; has limited tantrums at home; and participates in cooperative play during games and structured play with siblings, with limited use of imaginative play.

REFERENCES

Abidi, S. (2013). Psychosis in children and youth: Focus on early-onset schizophrenia. *Pediatrics in Review, 34*(7), 296-306. https://doi.org/10.1542/pir.34-7-296

Abidin, R. R. (2012). *Parenting Stress Index* (4th ed.). Psychological Assessment Resources.

American Occupational Therapy Association. (n.d.). Mental health. https://www.aota.org/Practice/Mental-Health.aspx

American Occupational Therapy Association. (2009). Occupational therapy and school mental health. https://www.aota.org/-/media/corporate/files/practice/children/browse/school/mental-health/ot%20%20school%20mental%20health%20fact%20sheet%20for%20web%20posting%20102109.pdf

American Occupational Therapy Association. (2016). Occupational therapy's role in mental health in children and youth. https://www.aota.org/-/media/Corporate/Files/AboutOT/Professionals/WhatIsOT/MH/Facts/MH%20in%20Children%20and%20Youth%20fact%20sheet.pdf

American Occupational Therapy Association. (2017). Philosophical base of occupational therapy. *American Journal of Occupational Therapy, 71*(Suppl. 2), 7112410045. https://doi.org/10.5014/ajot.2017.716S06

American Occupational Therapy Association. (2020). Occupational therapy practice framework: Domain and process (4th ed.). *American Journal of Occupational Therapy, 74*(Suppl. 2), 7412410010. https://doi.org/10.5014/ajot.2020.74S2001

American Psychiatric Association. (2013). *Diagnostic and statistical manual of mental disorders* (5th ed.). Author. https://doi.org/10.1176/appi.books.9780890425596

Arbesman, M., Bazyk, S., & Nochajski, S. M. (2013). Systematic review of occupational therapy and mental health promotion, prevention, and intervention for children and youth. *American Journal of Occupational Therapy, 67*(6), e120-e130. https://doi.org/10.5014/ajot.2013.008359

Ashby, S., Gray, M., Ryan, S., & James, C. (2017, February 1). An exploratory study into the application of psychological theories and therapies in Australian mental health occupational therapy practice: Challenges to occupation-based practice. *Australian Occupational Therapy Journal, 64*(1), 24-32. https://doi.org/10.1111/1440-1630.12302

Bazyk, S., & Arbesman, M. (2013). *Occupational therapy practice guidelines for mental health promotion, prevention, and intervention for children and youth.* American Occupational Therapy Association.

Bazyk, S., Demirjian, L., LaGuardia, T., Thompson-Repas, K., Conway, C., & Michaud, P. (2015). Building capacity of occupational therapy practitioners to address the mental health needs of children and youth: A mixed-methods study of knowledge translation. *American Journal of Occupational Therapy, 69*(6), 6906180060p1-6906180060p10. https://doi.org/10.5014/ajot.2015.019182

Benjamin, C. L., Puleo, C. M., Settipani, C. A., Brodman, D. M., Edmunds, J. M., Cummings, C. M., & Kendall, P. C. (2011). History of cognitive-behavioral therapy (CBT) in youth. *Child and Adolescent Psychiatric Clinics of North America, 20*(2), 179-189. https://doi.org/10.1016/j.chc.2011.01.011

Bitsko, R. H., Holbrook, J. R., Ghandour, R. M., Blumberg, S. J., Visser, S. N., Perou, R., & Walkup, J. T. (2018). Epidemiology and impact of health care provider-diagnosed anxiety and depression among US children. *Journal of Developmental and Behavioral Pediatrics: JDBP, 39*(5), 395-403. https://doi.org/10.1097/DBP.0000000000000571

Brooks, R., & Goldstein, S. (2008). The mindset of teachers capable of fostering resilience in students. *Canadian Journal of School Psychology, 23*(1). https://doi.org/10.1177/0829573508316597

Buron, K. D., & Curtis, M. (2003). *The incredible 5-point scale: The significantly improved and expanded second edition.* AAPC Publishing.

Cahill, S. M., Egan, B. E., & Seber, J. (2020). Activity- and occupation-based interventions to support mental health, positive behavior, and social participation for children and youth: A systematic review. *American Journal of Occupational Therapy, 74*(2), 7402180020p1-7402180020p28. https://doi.org/10.5014/ajot.2020.038687

Centers for Disease Control and Prevention. (2019, April 19). *Data and statistics on children's mental health | CDC.* https://www.cdc.gov/childrensmentalhealth/data.html

Charlson, F., van Ommeren, M., Flaxman, A., Cornett, J., Whiteford, H., & Saxena, S. (2019). New WHO prevalence estimates of mental disorders in conflict settings: A systematic review and meta-analysis. *The Lancet, 394*(10194), 240-248. https://doi.org/10.1016/S0140-6736(19)30934-1

Compas, B. E., Connor-Smith, J. K., Saltzman, H., Thomsen, A. H., & Wadsworth, M. E. (2001). Coping with stress during childhood and adolescence: Problems, progress, and potential in theory and research. *Psychological Bulletin, 127*(1), 87-127. https://doi.org/10.1037//0033-2909.127.1.87

Cooper, J. O., Heron, T. E., & Heward, W. L. (2020). *Applied behavior analysis* (3rd ed.). Pearson.

Copeland, W. E., Wolke, D., Shanahan, L., & Costello, E. J. (2015). Adult functional outcomes of common childhood psychiatric problems: A prospective, longitudinal study. *JAMA Psychiatry, 72*(9), 892-899. https://doi.org/10.1001/jamapsychiatry.2015.0730

Cunningham, B. J., & Rosenbaum, P. L. (2014). Measure of processes of care: A review of 20 years of research. *Developmental Medicine & Child Neurology, 56*(5), 445-452. https://doi.org/10.1111/dmcn.12347

David, A. S., & Nicholson, T. (2015). Are neurological and psychiatric disorders different? *The British Journal of Psychiatry, 207*(5), 373-374. https://doi.org/10.1192/bjp.bp.114.158550

Davidson, L., Harding, C., & Spaniol, L. (2005). *Recovery from severe mental illnesses: Research evidence and implications for practice* (Vol. 1). Center for Psychiatric Rehabilitation, Boston University.

Dawson D., McEwen, S. E., & Polatajko, H. J. (2017). *Cognitive orientation to daily occupational performance in occupational therapy: Using the CO-OP approach™ to enable participation across the lifespan.* AOTA Press.

DeGrace, B. W. (2003). Occupation-based and family-centered care: A challenge for current practice. *American Journal of Occupational Therapy, 57*(3), 347-350. https://doi.org/10.5014/ajot.57.3.347

Donohue, M. (2013). *Social profile: Assessment of social participation in children, adolescents and adults.* AOTA Press.

Driver, D. I., Gogtay, N., & Rapoport, J. L. (2013). Childhood onset schizophrenia and early onset schizophrenia spectrum disorders. *Child and Adolescent Psychiatric Clinics of North America, 22*(4), 539-555. https://doi.org/10.1016/j.chc.2013.04.001

Durlak, J. A., Weissberg, R. P., Dymnicki, A. B., Taylor, R. D., & Schellinger, K. B. (2011). The impact of enhancing students' social and emotional learning: A meta-analysis of school-based universal interventions: Social and emotional learning. *Child Development, 82*(1), 405-432. https://doi.org/10.1111/j.1467-8624.2010.01564.x

Elliott, S. N., Racine, C. N., & Busse, R. T. (1995). Best practices in preschool social skills training. In A. Thomas & J. Grimes (Eds.), *Best practices in school psychology-III* (pp. 1009-1020). National Association of School Psychologists.

Fairchild, G. (2018). Adult outcomes of conduct problems in childhood or adolescence: Further evidence of the societal burden of conduct problems. *European Child & Adolescent Psychiatry, 27*(10), 1235-1237. https://doi.org/10.1007/s00787-018-1221-1

Fingerhut, P. E. (2013). Life participation for parents: A tool for family-centered occupational therapy. *American Journal of Occupational Therapy, 67*(1), 37-44. https://doi.org/10.5014/ajot.2013.005082

Fisher, A. G., & Griswold, L. A. (2008). *Evaluation of social interaction research* (4th ed.). Three Star Press.

Fraser, K., MacKenzie, D., & Versnel, J. (2017). Complex trauma in children and youth: A scoping review of sensory-based interventions. *Occupational Therapy in Mental Health, 33*(3), 199-216. https://doi.org/10.1080/0164212X.2016.1265475

Fristad, M. A., Wolfson, H., Algorta, G. P., Youngstrom, E. A., Arnold, L. E., Birmaher, B., Horwitz, S., Axelson, D., Kowatch, R. A., & Findling, R. L. (2016). Disruptive mood dysregulation disorder and bipolar disorder not otherwise specified: Fraternal or identical twins? *Journal of Child and Adolescent Psychopharmacology, 26*(2), 138-146. https://doi.org/10.1089/cap.2015.0062

Frydenburg, E., & Lewis, R. (2012). *Adolescent coping scale* (2nd ed.). ACER Press.

Ghandour, R. M., Sherman, L. J., Vladutiu, C. J., Ali, M. M., Lynch, S. E., Bitsko, R. H., & Blumberg, S. J. (2019). Prevalence and treatment of depression, anxiety, and conduct problems in US children. *The Journal of Pediatrics, 206*, 256-267.e3. https://doi.org/10.1016/j.jpeds.2018.09.021

Ghosh, A., Ray, A., & Basu, A. (2017). Oppositional defiant disorder: Current insight. *Psychology Research and Behavior Management, 10*, 353-367. https://doi.org/10.2147/PRBM.S120582

Graham, F., Rodger, S., & Ziviani, J. (2009). Coaching parents to enable children's participation: An approach for working with parents and their children. *Australian Occupational Therapy Journal, 56*(1), 16-23. https://doi.org/10.1111/j.1440-1630.2008.00736.x

Grajo, L. (2019). Occupational adaptation as a normative and intervention process: Schkade and Schultz's legacy. In L. C. Grajo & A. Boisselle (Eds.), *Adaptation through occupation: Multidimensional perspectives*. SLACK Incorporated.

Grajo, L., Boisselle, A., & DaLomba, E. (2018). Occupational adaptation as a construct: A scoping review of literature. *The Open Journal of Occupational Therapy, 6*(1). https://doi.org/10.15453/2168-6408.1400

Gresham, F. M., & Elliott, S. N. (1990). *Social skills rating system (SSRS)*. American Guidance Services.

Gutman, S. A., & Raphael-Greenfield, E. I. (2014). Five years of mental health research in the *American Journal of Occupational Therapy*, 2009-2013. *American Journal of Occupational Therapy, 68*(1), e21-e36. https://doi.org/10.5014/ajot.2014.010249

Harding, C. M., Brooks, G. W., Ashikaga, T., Strauss, J. S., & Breier, A. (1987). The Vermont longitudinal study of persons with severe mental illness, II: Long-term outcome of subjects who retrospectively met DSM-III criteria for schizophrenia. *The American Journal of Psychiatry, 144*(6), 727-735. https://doi.org/10.1176/ajp.144.6.727

Healy, C., Dooley, N., Coughlan, H., Kelleher, I., Brannigan, R., Clarke, M., & Cannon, M. (2019). Childhood and adolescent psychotic experiences and risk of mental disorder: A systematic review and meta-analysis. *Psychological Medicine, 49*(10), 1589-1599. https://doi.org/10.1017/S0033291719000485

Henry, A. D., & Coster, W. J. (1996). Predictors of functional outcome among adolescents and young adults with psychotic disorders. *American Journal of Occupational Therapy, 50*(3), 171-181. https://doi.org/10.5014/ajot.50.3.171

Hitchcock, C. A., Chavira, D. A., & Stein, M. B. (2009). Recent findings in social phobia among children and adolescents. *The Israel Journal of Psychiatry and Related Sciences, 46*(1), 34-44.

Individuals with Disabilities Education Act, 20 U.S.C. § 1400 (2004).

Interprofessional Education Collaborative. (2016). *Core competencies for interprofessional collaborative practice: 2016 update*. Author.

James, S. L., Abate, D., Abate, K. H., Abay, S. M., Abbafati, C., Abbasi, N., Abbastabar, H., Abd-Allah, F., Abdela, J., Abdelalim, A., Abdollahpour, I., Abdulkader, R. S., Abebe, Z., Abera, S. F., Abil, O. Z., Abraha, H. N., Abu-Raddad, L. J., Abu-Rmeileh, N. M. E., Accrombessi, M. M. K., . . . Murray, C. J. L. (2018). Global, regional, and national incidence, prevalence, and years lived with disability for 354 diseases and injuries for 195 countries and territories, 1990-2017: A systematic analysis for the Global Burden of Disease Study 2017. *The Lancet, 392*(10159), 1789-1858. https://doi.org/10.1016/S0140-6736(18)32279-7

Khetani, M. A., Coster, W., Law, M., & Bedell, G. M. (2013). *Young children's participation and environment measure (YC-PEM)* [review copy]. Colorado State University.

Knestrict, T. D. (2019). *Controlling our children: Hegemony and deconstructing the positive behavioral intervention support model*. Peter Lang.

Koegel, L. K., Koegel, R. L., & Dunlap, G. (Eds.). (1996). *Positive behavioral support: Including people with difficult behavior in the community*. Paul H. Brookes Publishing.

Kramer, J., ten Velden, M., Kafkes, A., Semonti, B., Federico, J., & Kielhofner, G. (2014). *Child occupational self assessment (COSA) version 2.2*. The University of Illinois at Chicago.

Krupa, T., Fossey, E., Anthony, W. A., Brown, C., & Pitts, D. B. (2009). Doing daily life: How occupational therapy can inform psychiatric rehabilitation practice. *Psychiatric Rehabilitation Journal, 32*(3), 155-161. https://doi.org/10.2975/32.3.2009.155.161

Kuypers, L. M., & Winner, M. G. (2011). *The zones of regulation: A curriculum designed to foster self-regulation and emotional control*. Think Social Publishing.

Law, M. (2019). *COPM manual: Canadian occupational performance measure*. COPM, Inc.

Law, M., King, G., King, S., Hurley, P., Rosenbaum, P., Hanna, S., . . . Young, N. (2004). *Children's assessment of participation and enjoyment and preferences for activities of children*. Psychological Corporation.

Lazarus, R. S., & Folkman, S. (1987). Transactional theory and research on emotions and coping. *European Journal of Personality, 1*(3), 141-169. https://doi.org/10.1002/per.2410010304

Leamy, M., Bird, V., Boutillier, C. L., Williams, J., & Slade, M. (2011). Conceptual framework for personal recovery in mental health: Systematic review and narrative synthesis. *British Journal of Psychiatry, 199*(6), 445-452. https://doi.org/10.1192/bjp.bp.110.083733

LeBuffe, P. A., Shapiro, V. B., & Naglieri, J. A. (2014). *The Devereaux student strengths assessment (DESSA): Assessment, technical manual, and user's guide*. Apperson, Inc.

Linscott, R. J., & van Os, J. (2013). An updated and conservative systematic review and meta-analysis of epidemiological evidence on psychotic experiences in children and adults: On the pathway from proneness to persistence to dimensional expression across mental disorders. *Psychological Medicine, 43*(6), 1133-1149. https://doi.org/10.1017/S0033291712001626

Maijer, K., Begemann, M. J. H., Palmen, S. J. M. C., Leucht, S., & Sommer, I. E. C. (2018). Auditory hallucinations across the lifespan: A systematic review and meta-analysis. *Psychological Medicine, 48*(6), 879-888. https://doi.org/10.1017/S0033291717002367

Mandich, A. D., Polatajko, H. J., Miller, L. T., & Baum, C. (2004). *Paediatric activity card sort.* CAOT Publications ACE.

McGrath, J. J., Saha, S., Al-Hamzawi, A., Alonso, J., Bromet, E. J., Bruffaerts, R., Caldas-de-Almeida, J. M., Chiu, W. T., de Jonge, P., Fayyad, J., Florescu, S., Gureje, O., Haro, J. M., Hu, C., Kovess-Masfety, V., Lepine, J. P., Lim, C. W., Mora, M. E. M., Navarro-Mateu, F., . . . Kessler, R. C. (2015). Psychotic experiences in the general population: A cross-national analysis based on 31,261 respondents from 18 countries. *JAMA Psychiatry, 72*(7), 697-705. https://doi.org/10.1001/jamapsychiatry.2015.0575

Miles, H., & Morley, M. (2013). Developing mental health occupational therapy practice to meet the needs of people with mental health problems and physical disability. *British Journal of Occupational Therapy, 76*(12), 556-559. https://doi.org/10.4276/030802213X13861576675321

National Institute of Mental Health. (2015). Fact sheet: First episode psychosis: Facts about psychosis. https://www.nimh.nih.gov/health/topics/schizophrenia/raise/fact-sheet-first-episode-psychosis.shtml

Occupational Therapy Training Program. (n.d.). About us. http://www.ottp.org/about-3

Patra, S. (2019). Assessment and management of pediatric depression. *Indian Journal of Psychiatry, 61*(3), 300-306. https://doi.org/10.4103/psychiatry.IndianJPsychiatry_446_18

Polatajko, H. J., & Mandich, A. (2004). *Enabling occupation in children: The Cognitive Orientation to Daily Occupational Performance (CO-OP) approach.* CAOT.

Program for Prevention Research at Arizona State University. (1999). *Children's Coping Strategies Checklist and the How I Coped under Pressure Scale (CCSC).* Arizona State University.

Rempel, K. D. (2012). Mindfulness for children and youth: A review of the literature with an argument for school-based implementation. *Canadian Journal of Counseling and Psychotherapy, 46*(3), 201-220.

Rogers, J. C., & Holm, M. B. (2016). Functional assessment in mental health: Lessons from occupational therapy. *Dialogues in Clinical Neuroscience, 18*(2), 145-154.

Sagar, R., Patra, B. N., & Patil, V. (2019). Clinical Practice Guidelines for the management of conduct disorder. *Indian Journal of Psychiatry, 61*(Suppl. 2), 270-276. https://doi.org/10.4103/psychiatry.IndianJPsychiatry_539_18

Saxena, S., Funk, M., & Chisholm, D. (2014). WHO's Mental Health Action Plan 2013-2020: What can psychiatrists do to facilitate its implementation? *World Psychiatry, 13*(2), 107-109. https://doi.org/10.1002/wps.20141

Schaaf, R. C., Dumont, R. L., Arbesman, M., & May-Benson, T. A. (2017). Efficacy of occupational therapy using Ayres Sensory Integration®: A systematic review. *American Journal of Occupational Therapy, 72*(1), 7201190010p1-7201190010p10. https://doi.org/10.5014/ajot.2018.028431

Schwartz, C., Barican, J. L., Yung, D., Zheng, Y., & Waddell, C. (2019). Six decades of preventing and treating childhood anxiety disorders: A systematic review and meta-analysis to inform policy and practice. *Evidence Based Mental Health, 22*(3), 103-110. https://doi.org/10.1136/ebmental-2019-300096

Sepulveda, A., Barlow, K., Benen Donichick, B., & Flanagan, J. E. (2020). Children's mental health: Promoting mental health through early screening and detection. *OT Practice, 25*(4), 10-14. https://www.aota.org/publications-news/otp/archive/2020/children-mental-health

Shanahan, L., Copeland, W. E., Costello, E. J., & Angold, A. (2011). Child-, adolescent-, and young adult-onset depressions: Differential risk factors in development? *Psychological Medicine, 41*(11), 2265-2274. https://doi.org/10.1017/S0033291711000675

Shriver, T. P., & Weissberg, R. P. (2020). A response to constructive criticism of social and emotional learning. *Phi Delta Kappan, 101*(7), 52. https://doi.org/10.1177/0031721720917543

Skard, G., & Bundy, A. (2008). Test of playfulness. In L. D. Parham & L. S. Fazio (Eds.), *Play in occupational therapy for children* (pp. 71-93). Mosby Elsevier.

Smoller, J. W., Andreassen, O. A., Edenberg, H. J., Faraone, S. V., Glatt, S. J., & Kendler, K. S. (2019). Psychiatric genetics and the structure of psychopathology. *Molecular Psychiatry, 24*(3), 409-420. https://doi.org/10.1038/s41380-017-0010-4

Sparrow, S. S., Cicchetti, D. V., & Saulnier, C. A. (2016). *Vineland adaptive behavior scale* (3rd ed.). Pearson.

Stubbs, B., Vancampfort, D., Hallgren, M., Firth, J., Veronese, N., Solmi, M., Brand, S., Cordes, J., Malchow, B., Gerber, M., Schmitt, A., Correll, C. U., De Hert, M., Gaughran, F., Schneider, F., Kinnafick, F., Falkai, P., Möller, H.-J., & Kahl, K. G. (2018). EPA guidance on physical activity as a treatment for severe mental illness: A meta-review of the evidence and position statement from the European Psychiatric Association (EPA), supported by the International Organization of Physical Therapists in Mental Health (IOPTMH). *European Psychiatry, 54*, 124-144. https://doi.org/10.1016/j.eurpsy.2018.07.004

Townsend, S. (1999). *Occupational therapy psychosocial assessment of learning (OT PAL) Version 2.0.* University of Illinois at Chicago.

Tzang, R.-F., Chang, Y.-C., Kao, K.-L., Huang, Y.-H., Huang, H.-C., Wang, Y.-C., Muo, C.-H., Wu, S.-I., Sung, F.-C., & Stewart, R. (2019). Increased risk of developing psychiatric disorders in children with attention deficit and hyperactivity disorder (ADHD) receiving sensory integration therapy: A population-based cohort study. *European Child & Adolescent Psychiatry, 28*(2), 247-255. https://doi.org/10.1007/s00787-018-1171-7

van Weeghel, J., van Zelst, C., Boertien, D., & Hasson-Ohayon, I. (2019). Conceptualizations, assessments, and implications of personal recovery in mental illness: A scoping review of systematic reviews and meta-analyses. *Psychiatric Rehabilitation Journal, 42*(2), 169-181. https://doi.org/10.1037/prj0000356

Wells, A. M., Chasnoff, I. J., Schmidt, C. A., Telford, E., & Schwartz, L. D. (2012). Neurocognitive habilitation therapy for children with fetal alcohol spectrum disorders: An adaptation of the Alert Program. *American Journal of Occupational Therapy, 66*, 24-34. https://doi.org/10.5014/ajot.2012.002691

Williams, M. S., & Shellenberger, S. (1996). *How does your engine run? A leader's guide to the Alert Program for self regulation.* TherapyWorks Inc.

Wimpenny, K., & Lewis, L. (2015). Preparation for an uncertain world: Professional agency and durability in the practice preparation of mental health in occupational therapy. *South African Journal of Occupational Therapy, 45*(2), 22-28. https://doi.org/10.17159/2310-3833/2015/v45n2a5

World Federation of Occupational Therapists. (2019). Position statement: Occupational therapy and mental health. https://wfot.org/resources/occupational-therapy-and-mental-health

World Health Organization. (n.d.). Improving the mental and brain health of children and adolescents. http://www.who.int/mental_health/maternal-child/child_adolescent/en

Zietlin, S. (1985). Coping inventory: A measure of adaptive behavior. Scholastic Testing Service.

6

Children and Youth With Attention Deficit/ Hyperactivity Disorders

*Elaina DaLomba, PhD, OTR/L, MSW and
Lisa Griggs-Stapleton, PhD, OTR/L*

CHAPTER OBJECTIVES By the end of this chapter the reader will be able to:
- Define attention deficit/hyperactivity disorder and its implications for occupational participation of children.
- Describe the adaptation, coping, and resilience of children and youth with attention deficit/hyperactivity disorder.
- Apply an occupational adaptation perspective in the assessment of and intervention for children and youth with attention deficit/hyperactivity disorder.

OVERVIEW OF THE POPULATION

Attention deficit/hyperactivity disorder (ADHD) is a neurodevelopmental disorder that has the potential to affect every aspect of occupational participation. Individuals with ADHD experience an inability to attend to tasks, hyperactivity, and/or impulsivity (American Psychiatric Association [APA], 2013). There are three subtypes of ADHD: inattentive, hyperactive, and combined types. People with *inattentive type* are often seen as daydreamers; they have difficulty focusing on tasks and are often seen staring out the window in class instead of taking notes. Those with *hyperactive type* are often diagnosed quickly as children because they have difficulty sitting still and are in seemingly constant motion. Individuals with *combined type* present with both hyperactive and inattentive symptoms. Compounding these symptoms are often other clinical issues, such as

2022 Taylor & Francis Group.

- 133 -

Table 6-1

Perceived Strengths and Challenges for People With ADHD	
Strengths	**Challenges**
<ul><li>Ability to hyperfocus (flow)</li><li>High psychological and physical energy level</li><li>Creativity (divergent thinking)</li><li>Social intelligence as adults</li><li>Humor</li><li>Self-acceptance and acceptance of others</li><li>Recognition of feelings</li><li>Resilience</li><li>Curiosity</li><li>Non-conformist</li><li>Self-regulation</li><li>Persistence</li><li>Adventurous</li></ul>	<ul><li>Social challenges</li><li>Hyperactivity</li><li>Sensory processing differences</li><li>Visual perception</li><li>Gross motor coordination issues</li><li>Fine motor coordination Issues</li><li>Executive functioning issues, including:<ul><li>Attending to task</li><li>Planning</li><li>Prioritizing</li><li>Organizing</li><li>Working memory</li><li>Impulsivity</li></ul></li><li>Language processing disorders. including:<ul><li>Dysgraphia</li><li>Dyslexia</li><li>Dyscalculia</li></ul></li><li>Common mental health comorbidities:<ul><li>Anxiety</li><li>Depression</li><li>Conduct disorder</li><li>Oppositional defiant disorder</li></ul></li><li>Unpredictability of medication effects and side effects</li><li>Emotional regulation</li><li>Sleep disorders</li><li>At risk for substance abuse, aggressive behavior, and delinquency</li></ul>
Sources: APA (2013), Dvorsky and Langberg (2016), Hupfeld et al. (2019), Muris et al. (2018), and Sedgwick et al. (2019).	

dysgraphia, sensory processing issues, visual perception challenges, and gross and fine motor coordination deficits (Table 6-1). ADHD is typically diagnosed in childhood, and although people find ways to cope with its effects, they do not outgrow it.

The specific cause of ADHD is not yet known, but much progress has been made in understanding the mechanisms of the disorder. For example, a strong genetic link has been demonstrated through sibling studies (Chen et al., 2017). Once assumed to be controllable behaviors, more recent findings in functional magnetic resonance imaging studies demonstrate widespread dysfunction in regions of the brain associated with ADHD symptoms such as inattention and impulsivity (Schneider et al., 2010). Additionally, people with ADHD demonstrate differences in neuropsychological functioning correlated with dopaminergic system differences compared to typical peers (Levy & Swanson, 2001). Dopamine is a neurotransmitter that underlies one's ability to regulate emotional responses and is part of the reward system that motivates action to pursue and experience pleasure from rewards (Bressan & Crippa, 2005). Thus, the individual with ADHD may be at increased risk for poor emotional regulation.

Although much is still unknown about ADHD, it is one of the most common and controversial childhood disorders (Wolraich et al., 2019). Changes in treatment and diagnosis criteria have led to an increase in the number of children diagnosed, as well as the perception by the public that too many children are diagnosed with the disorder (Schwarz & Cohen, 2013). Prevalence estimates of children with ADHD increased by 33% between 1997 and 2008 (Boyle et al., 2011). In 2016, it was estimated that there were 6.1 million children (9.4% of the population) between the ages of 2 and 17 years diagnosed with ADHD in the United States (Danielson et al., 2018). More recent research places the rate of incidence between 7% and 11% (Thomas et al., 2015; Visser et al., 2015). Minority children, however, are less likely to receive the diagnosis, for reasons that are not well explored in literature; lack of proper diagnosis leaves children unable to access the critical services described in this chapter (Morgan et al., 2013). This creates a compelling need for clinicians to better understand ADHD and its potential impact on occupational functioning.

Treatment recommendations for ADHD vary by age. Parent training in behavior management (PTBM) and behavioral classroom interventions (BCIs) are the first lines of treatment for children between 4 and 6 years of age (Wolraich et al., 2019). If these interventions are not successful, stimulant medication may be indicated. Initial treatment recommendations for children over 6 years of age include PTBM, BCI, and medication. In a national study of children aged 4 to 17 years, based on parent report, 78.2% of non-Hispanic white children with ADHD received medication for their condition (Visser et al., 2015). Poignantly, studies reveal disparities in the rate of treatment of ADHD in non-white children. Visser et al. (2015) noted that only 69.5% of Hispanic children in their study received medication in the past week, and even fewer (66.8%) of non-Hispanic Black children received medication. Families of children with ADHD also rely on behavioral therapy, with 44% reporting its use within the past year. In spite of the available research on the efficacy of medication and behavioral interventions, almost a quarter of children with ADHD (21%) were found to be receiving neither.

Complicating diagnosis and treatment, the majority of children with ADHD have comorbid disorders (Centers for Disease Control, 2017). Almost half (45%) are also diagnosed with a specific learning disorder such as a reading disorder (see Chapter 3 on children with learning disabilities). Additionally, almost two-thirds (64%) were found to have a comorbid mental health diagnosis, with behavioral and conduct challenges being most common in 52% of the children (Danielson et al., 2018; see Chapter 5 on children with behavioral and mental health disorders). Anxiety (33%) and depression (17%) are also common in this population. The American Academy of Pediatrics recommends that all patients with ADHD be screened for comorbid conditions so as to pay proper attention to these conditions (Wolraich et al., 2019). The complexity of their health profiles has potential to result in numerous coping challenges to those with ADHD and their families.

People with ADHD face many challenges as a result of their symptomology. These are listed in Table 6-1. Social challenges, emotional regulation, and sensory processing differences are well documented, as are motor coordination issues (Gol & Jarus, 2005). Visual processing challenges and even color perception differences are common for people with ADHD (Soyeon et al., 2014). However, executive functioning tasks remain some of the most challenging for people with ADHD, especially tasks requiring attention, planning, or memory (Ahmann et al., 2018; Muris et al., 2018). Impulsivity is another area of concern for most people with ADHD, as it affects every occupation, especially the ability to form social connections and participate in (and benefit from) traditional educational settings.

While there are many challenges to face in ADHD, there are lesser-known strengths that come from growing up with ADHD. Some people with ADHD acknowledge their hyperactivity but also recognize the usefulness of their boundless energy (Hupfeld et al., 2019; Sedgwick et al., 2019). They also identify curiosity, creative thinking, persistence, and an adventurous spirit as assets. Additionally, the ability of people with ADHD to hyperfocus on tasks they enjoy is recognized as a trait that can often yield an advantage over peers.

Research into how occupational therapists support children and youth with ADHD remain underexplored. In the United Kingdom, researchers found that sensory-based intervention was the most popular approach, followed by perceptual motor training, and therapeutic recreation activities such as active play (Spiliotopoulou, 2009). Some evidence indicates that sensory integration by using weighted vests improves cognitive processing speed and the ability to attend to task (Lin et al., 2014). However, the evidence for sensory-based interventions is considered weak and this area requires much more extensive research (Cahill & Beisbier, 2020).

Occupational therapists in the United States often address dysgraphia issues as well. Interventions can enhance speed and accuracy in letter formation in handwriting (Case-Smith et al., 2011). There are continued calls for additional research into occupational therapy interventions to continue to develop new ways to meet these needs (Nielsen et al., 2017). There are many occupational challenges for children with ADHD, but there are also untapped strengths in these individuals that warrant further research and focus.

DEFINING ADAPTATION, COPING, AND RESILIENCE FOR CHILDREN WITH ATTENTION DEFICIT/HYPERACTIVITY DISORDER

The adage "Nothing succeeds like success, nothing fails like failure," may help to frame the occupational challenges of the child with ADHD perhaps more accurately than any other. As noted earlier, research into ADHD has been deficit-focused. It is easy

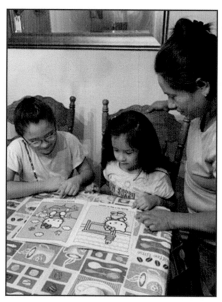

Figure 6-1. Parent facilitates play to promote successful social engagement.

to see why children with ADHD, who are often unable to attend to developmentally enhancing experiences and interactions, are at risk for inaccurate processing of these environmental transactions. These inaccurately assessed experiences may then be stored in memory, which can result in the use of ineffective approaches to future life challenges (Barkley & Murphy, 2010). Children with ADHD can be aware of their lack of success in many situations, often attributing the blame to their own behaviors and lacking insight into the breakdown between what they intended to do vs. what they actually did (Gallichan & Curle, 2008; Levanon-Erez et al., 2017). This can lead to diminished self-esteem, depression, and anxiety (Biederman, 2005). Because successfully facing life challenges leads to increases in adaptive capacity (i.e., the ability to use a variety of responses to overcome a challenge) and identity formation (Schkade & Schultz, 1992; Gallichan & Curle, 2008), it becomes critically important for the child with ADHD to have successful experiences.

Seminally, Folkman and Lazarus (1984) describe this normative process of learning to appraise challenging life situations, with the aim of resolving problems and reducing social tensions, as *coping*. This process unfolds in all areas of life; therefore, the child with ADHD is likely to struggle to succeed in family, academic, and social environments (Aduen et al., 2018; Barkley & Murphy, 2010; Daley & Birchwood, 2010). The inattentive and impulsive child is at risk for developing inadequate coping skills. It is also easy to see how children who are impulsive, emotionally reactive, and have difficulty learning from experiences might place unusually high levels of demand on those who care for them. Yet, having supportive family, adults, and peers in their lives is known to be a protective feature, or buffer, for children with ADHD (Dvorsky & Langberg, 2016). See Figure 6-1 for an example of a family supportive of social engagement. Children with ADHD can also have remarkable success in social and academic environments because of their energetic, creative, and curious style, or when offered various forms of individualized support that focus on successful resolution of environmental challenges (Barkley, 2020). These buffer areas provide inlets of possible change into the faulty adaptive cycle. The case story at the end of this section highlights how these particular challenges often result in occupational dysadaptation but nevertheless offer windows of opportunity.

Occupational Adaptation

Like all humans, children require opportunities for engagement in occupation to develop and grow throughout their lives (Hooper & Wood, 2014). *Active engagement* in occupations is thought to be central to the process whereby individuals learn to overcome challenges in life and develop their sense of self (Grajo et al., 2018). As the primary occupations of children are education and play (American Occupational Therapy Association [AOTA], 2020), concerns about inattentive, impulsive behaviors, sensory processing issues, and decreased fine and gross motor skills would often be identified and felt by teachers, as children spend a large portion of their days in school environments. In fact, behavioral concerns, particularly the excessive physical activity associated with ADHD, can be seen in children as young as 3 years old (Gleason & Humphreys, 2016), when they often experience social demands and (pre)academic instruction for the first time without parental support. Traditional elementary, middle-, and high-school settings require students to sit for long periods of time, engage in active listening (often combined with note-taking), organize their work, keep track of classwork, and engage in planning for projects due in the future. The very nature of the formal school environment presupposes an increasing level of development in executive functioning, including working and long-term memory, problem solving, organization, and planning to successfully engage in school activities. The child with ADHD likely has deficits in a few, if not all, of these areas, leaving them vulnerable to disengagement from the educational process.

Typical life transitions demand individual adaptation, change, and mastery of all children. These normative demands, however, may be magnified for children with ADHD if their social-emotional, cognitive, and self-regulation skills are mismatched (Ringer, 2019) with the unique expectations of successive environments. These changes may include new physical surroundings, new peer groups, and new teachers with differing teaching styles and levels of understanding of children with ADHD. Periods of transition are noted to be catalysts in occupational adaptation (Grajo et al., 2018). Therefore, successive underperformance, or not mastering adaptive challenges during these times, may have a cascading negative effect on the developing child with ADHD. This in turn can affect the family (problems with stress and relationship dysfunction), school (decreased academic performance), and society (increased risk-taking behaviors, missed work days, and poor job performance in adulthood), as summarized by Barkley (2020) and Becker et al. (2012).

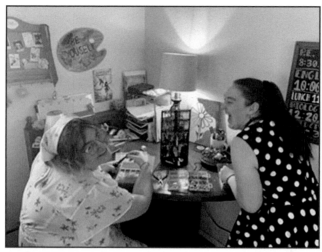

Figure 6-2. Teens crafting jewelry to express creativity and identity.

Coping and Resilience

Coping has been described as a fluid process of recognizing the results of one's efforts when interacting with the environment and changing one's behavior to achieve desired results (Compas et al., 2001). However, if a child's appraisals are inaccurate (such as routinely blaming others, or not seeing their own contribution to the results), as they are noted to be in children with ADHD, they cannot benefit from life experiences and develop healthy coping mechanisms as effectively as other children (Graziano & Garcia, 2016). Perhaps it is unsurprising that much of the literature on coping in ADHD describes how others cope *with* the child with ADHD (e.g., López-Liria et al., 2020; Ringer, 2019) rather than how the child with ADHD copes. The varied, multifaceted, and consistent emotional and even physical energy demands placed on parents and teachers by children with ADHD justifies the need for focused research and intervention into the coping process of others (Barkley, 2020; Lee et al., 2016). More recent data on coping show that children with ADHD have limited coping flexibility in response to stressful situations, with blame for perceived failures often being attributed to external factors and tendencies to use domineering attitudes to control a situation, which results in sparse coping skills repertoires (Babb et al., 2010). Children may default to aggression or verbal outbursts out of frustration and lack of insight into stressful situations (Becker et al., 2012). These externalized behaviors—ones that are outwardly visible—can cause stigma and social isolation (Mikami & Normand, 2015). This can further deprive the child of opportunities to develop healthy skills of appraisal and social negotiation, which are central to the development of a desired sense of self-identity (Figure 6-2).

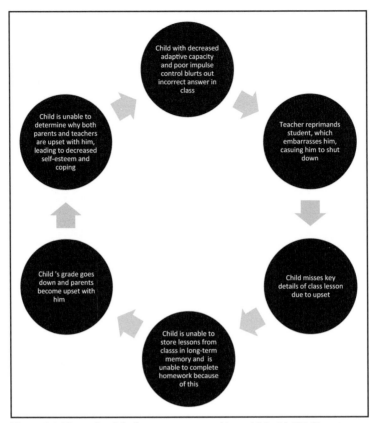

Figure 6-3. The cycle of challenges encountered by a child with ADHD.

Resilience represents the outcome or evidence of successful, accumulated, and routinely utilized coping strategies (Compas et al., 2001). Children with ADHD who have limited coping skills therefore appear to be less resilient than typically developing children, due to having more negative outcomes in managing increasingly complex social and academic situations in life (Regalla et al., 2015). If children lack insight into the results of their behaviors and cannot employ positive behavioral changes to effectively meet personal goals, then adaptive capacity does not increase and resilience remains static. Figure 6-3 shows how the challenges of a child with ADHD might result in difficulties in occupational adaptation, coping, and resilience. Case Study 6-1 illustrates an example of how this cycle of poor adaptation, coping, and resilience may manifest in a child.

Case Study 6-1

Mandy is a 13-year-old female who lives with her mother, father, and older brothers. She was recently diagnosed with ADHD, inattentive type. At age 7 years, she was diagnosed with specific learning disability (SLD) and decreased auditory processing skills, for which she has an Individualized Education Program (IEP). She receives special education through an inclusion/co-teaching model, 2 hours each week for English and math. When first diagnosed with SLD, she received occupational therapy for 1 year to address handwriting, and met her goals. She continues to use a wrapped thumb grasp, but complains of hand, eye, and mental fatigue after 20 minutes of any academic task. Now in seventh grade, she must independently organize her work and turn assignments in on time, but struggles with organization and memory challenges that make meeting these expectations difficult. Mandy failed pre-Algebra because she neglected to turn in three major assignments; she hid this dereliction from her parents. Now her teachers, the school psychologist, and her parents all remind her about homework and assignments and the impact poor performance may have on her future. They also remind her that her frequent "zoning out" is problematic. As a result of the perceived negative focus, her self-esteem has suffered. Mandy was referred to occupational therapy to develop her organizational skills, review keyboarding skills, and recommend possible adaptations to how she completes work so that she can be more successful in class. When asked what her goals would be in working with the occupational therapist, Mandy stated that she did not really know, but she wants to stop making everyone mad at her. Her teachers and parents would like assistance in determining how to help Mandy succeed in school and life.

THE ROLE OF OCCUPATIONAL THERAPY: BEST AND EVIDENCE-BASED PRACTICES FOR ASSESSMENT AND INTERVENTION OF CHILDREN WITH ADHD

Occupational therapy interventions for ADHD focus primarily on sensory processing challenges, motor skills, and handwriting development, as previously discussed. However, there are many other areas that occupational therapy can successfully address, including developing coping skills, metacognition, executive functioning, and behavioral regulation.

Assessing Needs of the Child With ADHD

Many standardized assessments are available to help identify issues in children and youth with ADHD once the therapist completes a comprehensive occupational profile. A summary of the assessments most commonly used appears in Table 6-2.

Table 6-2

Common Assessments Used With Children With ADHD			
Assessment and Authors	Purpose	Description/Tasks	Score Reporting and Interpretation
Pediatric Evaluation of Disability Inventory (PEDI) (Haley, 1992)	Assess key functional abilities (and levels of assistance) in children 6 months to 7 years old in self-care, mobility, and social function.	Caregiver/parent questionnaire that guides tracking of all areas.	Raw scores are converted to normative standard and scaled scores, with a mean standard scale score of 30 to 70 equaling performance with 95% of normative sample.
Conners' Continuous Performance Test—III (Conners, 2008)	Assess cognitive, emotional, and behavior problems in children aged 6 to 18.	Parent and self-assessment questionnaire for children and adolescents aged 8 to 18; can provide information on ADHD-related behaviors, as well as academic issues and mental health concerns.	Scores are reported in scales including the following behaviors: • Sustained attention • Hyperactivity-impulsivity • Vigilance
The Behavior Rating Inventory of Executive Function (BRIEF) (Gioia et al., 2000)	Assesses eight areas of behavioral regulation and metacognition in children 5 to 18 years old, including working memory, planning, and impulse control.	Individually administered rating scale completed by client and/or caregivers/parents.	Scores are given as indexes, including Behavioral Regulation Index, Emotional Regulation, and Metacognition Index. These are combined to create a Global Executive Composite.

(continued)

Table 6-2 (continued)

Common Assessments Used With Children With ADHD			
Assessment and Authors	Purpose	Description/Tasks	Score Reporting and Interpretation
The Barkley Deficits in Executive Functioning Scale (BDEFS) and Barkley Deficits in Executive Functioning Scale—Children and Adolescents (BDEFS-CA; Barkley, 2012)	Assesses clinically significant executive functioning of individuals aged 6 to 17 (BDEFS-CA), and adults over age 18 (BDEFS).	The BDEFS has "self" and "other" forms that address self-awareness, inhibition, working memory, emotion regulation, and plan/problem solving. The BDEFS-CA has short and long parent forms that look at child's/adolescent's capacities in time management, organization and problem solving, self-restraint, self-motivation, and self-regulation of emotions.	Scores reported in scales for self-management to time, self-organization (planning/problem solving), self-restraint (inhibition), self-motivation (executive actions), and self-regulation of emotion (behavioral inhibition and working memory).
The Learning and Study Strategies Inventory (LASSI) (Cano, 2006)	Assesses 10 areas that support 3 component areas: skill, will, and self-regulation. Adaptation in the classroom is measured by information processing, attitude, motivation, concentration, and time management.	Self-report assessing learning strategies (cognitive, general, and strategic learning).	Results reported on scales for Information Processing, Selecting Main Ideas, Test Strategies, Attitude, Anxiety, Motivation, Self-Testing, Concentration, Time Management, and Study Aids.

(continued)

Table 6-2 (continued)

Common Assessments Used With Children With ADHD			
Assessment and Authors	Purpose	Description/Tasks	Score Reporting and Interpretation
School Function Assessment (SFA) (Coster et al., 1998)	Criterion-referenced observational assessment with 320 items; measures skills that affect academic and social performance of children in kindergarten to sixth grade.	Questionnaires completed by one or more school professionals in three parts, including: student's level of participation in different settings; task supports, or the extent of assistance provided to the student to enable engagement in school-related tasks; and activity performance, assessing the student's physical and cognitive performance in specific activities.	Raw scores are converted to criterion scores for each section. Criterion cut-off scores are given for each setting, task, or activity.
Sensory Profile 2 (Dunn, 2014)	Assesses children from birth to 14 years 11 months in sensory processing patterns in the context of home, school, and community-based activities.	Parent questionnaires for infant, toddler, and child formats; short forms; and a school companion completed by teachers if desired.	Scores are reported for sensory systems, sensory patterns, and behavior.

Interventions Focusing on Adaptation, Coping, and Resilience

Occupational therapy has a significant role in the treatment of children with ADHD and their families. Evidence shows the efficacy of occupational therapy interventions and education in developing coping skills, metacognition, executive functioning, social skills, and behavioral regulation (Ahmann et al., 2018). A few of these are outlined in this section.

Interventions Focused on Skill Building

Direct skill building can be a focus of occupational therapy interventions. For example, coaching is a technique that involves goal setting, planning for potential obstacles to goal completion, and use of organization and reminder systems. A coach also provides external accountability in addition to evaluating the client's progress and performance. This aligns with professional standards of occupational therapy process, noted in the *Occupational Therapy Practice Framework: Domain and Process, Fourth Edition* (*OTPF-4*; AOTA, 2020). Coaching offers improved coping, problem solving, and goal planning, which can lead to improved occupational adaptation (Ahmann et al., 2018). Coaching strategies have been used in distinct areas such as sleep hygiene and habit development. For example, Sciberras et al. (2011) found that occupational therapy coaching interventions for sleep hygiene resulted in improved sleep routines and hygiene, enhanced habits and routines, and improved quality of sleep. They also noted enhancements in daily functioning, which may be attributed to enhanced sleep.

Other skills-based interventions are seen in the STEER driving-skills interventions program for new adolescent drivers and their parents (Fabiano et al., 2011). These researchers found that a combination of driving-simulation activities, discussion, and behavioral strategies resulted in small improvements in braking, speed, and general driving skills. These skills comprise some of the foundations of driving and, therefore, may contribute to increased personal and community safety and enhanced engagement in other occupations where teens must transport themselves (e.g., school, work, visiting friends' homes).

There are other limited but emerging areas of evidence for skill-level interventions. One example is the Cognitive Functional (Cog-Fun) model that targets cognitive, emotional, and environmental factors that affect occupational engagement through training and practicing executive function skills in enjoyable environments and activities (Maeir et al., 2014). The program has shown evidence of skills enhancement in areas such as memory, emotional control, and impulse control. A more recent randomized controlled trial of the Cog-Fun program (Hahn-Markowitz et al., 2017) showed significant improvements on both the BRIEF and the Canadian Occupational Performance Measure (COPM). As noted earlier, the BRIEF measures individual skills, but the use of the COPM gives some promising insights into how these skills may contribute to occupational engagement and satisfaction.

Other skills-based interventions have garnered only weak or inconclusive evidence. For example, there is limited evidence to show that mindfulness interventions are effective in decreasing anxiety and improving impulse control in children and youth with ADHD (Gu et al., 2018). Lin et al. (2014) used weighted vests to determine their impact on attention, impulse control, and on-task behavior of children with ADHD. Their protocol resulted in decreased inattention, increased speed of processing and responding, and increases in on-task behaviors (i.e., less out-of-seat behavior).

Therapists should be cautious when using or recommending some of these skill-based interventions due to limited research rigor at this time. Moreover, skill-based interventions are sometimes considered to conflict with a top-down occupations-based approach, and, therefore, may be seen as inconsistent with occupational therapy foundations.

Interventions Focusing on Academic Participation

Studies exploring interventions on academic participation by children with ADHD are not as well represented in the literature, in spite of the widely noted academic issues seen in these children. One study by Fedewa and Erwin (2011) targeted the externalizing,

Figure 6-4. Child completes homework in a quiet environment.

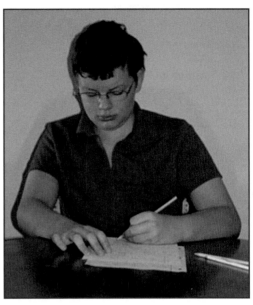

disruptive behaviors often associated with hyperactivity. The authors explored the use of stability balls on seated and on-task classroom behavior of eight children with ADHD and found significant increases in both. However, this sample size is small and there was no evidence of improved academic performance for the subject children; only an improvement in their ability to sit and focus, which may or may not translate into increased learning. Other small studies reveal only weak evidence of enhanced academic performance. However, some children with ADHD may be represented (although not identified) in other studies in areas such as handwriting or literacy. Figure 6-4 illustrates how selection of appropriate environments can support academic participation.

Interventions Focusing on Social Participation and Play

Social involvement and play are primary occupations of children and youth and thus, should be focus areas for the delivery of occupation-based interventions for occupational therapists. Evidence supporting the use of play is seen in Pfiffner et al. (2018), who used the Child Life and Attention Skills Treatment (CLAS) program that trains children to manage executive-function and social-skills deficits while engaging in daily activities. The program also developed behavioral programs for home and classroom that support the child's skill development in multiple environments. Significant improvements in attention, organizational skills, social skills, and global functioning were noted. Likewise, Wilkes-Gillan et al. (2017) used play-based interventions that included parents and peers that showed significant improvements on the Test of Playfulness ([TOP]; Bundy, 2010) such as motivation, control, suspension of reality, and framing. Another study that included video-recorded free-play sessions, video feed-forward/feedback from an occupational therapist, and peer modeling was found to significantly improve scores on the TOP for children with ADHD (Wilkes et al., 2011). The somewhat controversial

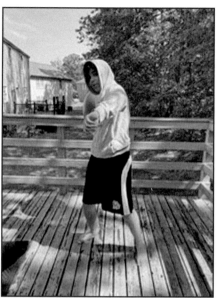

Figure 6-5. Teen practices ball throwing with appropriate force with peers.

area of video gaming is also emerging in the literature on ADHD. Video gaming-based interventions seem to affect specific areas of social function for children with ADHD, such as cooperation, as seen in Bul et al. (2016), where they used a computerized game with both play and serious components to it.

The overall evidence for play-based occupations' ability to enhance occupational participation for children and youth with ADHD is strong. Encouragingly, the evidence suggests that these interventions have even more impact when they include peers and parents, making treatment more contextually relevant, and perhaps enhancing the likelihood of increased participation and adaptation across environments. Ultimately, the play-based and some of the cognitive-based interventions (Figure 6-5, for example), with perceived success, seem to support the underlying components of coping, resilience, and adaptation, which enable individuals to face life challenges, learn to assess their choices, and use the outcomes of those choices to make better decisions, as described earlier.

COLLABORATIVE APPROACH WITH FAMILIES AND THE SOCIAL ENVIRONMENT

Families are systems, and the actions of one member have the potential to affect all the members. The literature suggests that raising a child with ADHD is uniquely challenging to parents and families. As noted earlier in this chapter, children with ADHD can display intense internalizing (e.g., poor self-efficacy) and externalizing behaviors (such as verbal and physical aggression). They may have unstable peer relationships and poor academic performance. All of these factors can challenge the well-being of the entire family unit and can negatively affect parental role competence and satisfaction (Barkley, 2020; Theule et al., 2013). Parenting styles and experiences can also reciprocally affect the child with ADHD: those who display warmth and acceptance of their child tend to experience improved child outcomes, and those displaying less warmth and acceptance tend to experience less favorable child outcomes (Heath et al., 2015). Just as with the child's experiences, successful mastery over life challenges promotes adaptation and resilience for facing future challenges as parents. The family context is, therefore, central to intervention with the child with ADHD, as parents are often the ones to implement the comprehensive strategies required for success outside of therapy and school times. Furthermore, family-centered intervention is best practice for children throughout childhood (Stoffel, 2016). Occupational therapy theory holds that children should be viewed within their individual contexts, with parents/caregivers typically representing primary members of a child's psychosocial context (AOTA, 2020). Parents are included in the evaluation process starting with the occupational profile, and tools commonly used by occupational therapists for comprehensive assessment of children with ADHD, such as the Sensory Profile, include parent questionnaires (Dunn, 2014). Establishing parent collaboration in the occupational therapy process is vital to the success of that process. Because evaluation results significantly rely on parent input, it follows that their collaboration in intervention is also fundamental to treatment planning and intervention.

When the occupational therapist facilitates positive change for one family member, that change has the potential to affect the health of the entire family. Parents may experience increased parental-role satisfaction and competence from being part of more successful interactions with their child when interventions are implemented in the home (Heath et al., 2015), and in turn, may parent with more warmth and understanding of their child's disability. As the occupational therapist determines the child's need, they can educate parents on the etiology of these (e.g., poor executive functions, sensory defensiveness) and advocate viewing the child as one with a neurodevelopmental disability rather than as simply willful or defiant. As suggested by Barkley (2014), keeping in mind that the child may not know how to control impulses, but can potentially learn skills to do so, can help parents maintain their perspective and avoid discouragement about parenting effectiveness. In fact, mutual problem solving and collaboration with parents have been shown to be effective in significantly reducing the symptoms associated with ADHD (Ollendick et al., 2016; Pfiffner et al., 2018), which benefits both the child and the family unit. Wilkes-Gillan et al. (2017) showed that a play-based pragmatic language intervention carried out in formal occupational therapy sessions, as well as by parents in the home, led to enhanced peer-to-peer social interactions of 6- to 11-year-old children with ADHD. Wilkes-Gillan et al. (2014) also found that play-based, social-skills interventions carried out with typical peers in the home were likewise effective at increasing the social interaction skills of young children with ADHD.

As noted earlier, children with ADHD are at risk for decreased social interaction and increased negative peer relationships. Because children often rely on their parents to access social and extracurricular events, the occupational therapist can collaborate with parents to consider the most effective plans for their child's engagement in these situations to promote positive peer interactions. For example, if the child wants to engage in community sports, the occupational therapist can assist parents in finding a league that has clear structure and rules, or a lower player-to-coach ratio, where the child can get more immediate feedback from the coach and more turns at practicing each skill. The therapist can make environmental suggestions, such as avoiding loud and crowded gymnasiums for a child with auditory sensitivity, or encouraging children to play faster-moving sports so they do not become distracted. Once parents begin to understand how to promote their child's successful interactions and behaviors at home, they may be able to facilitate positive friendships by structuring play dates with peers, monitoring for any decrease in their child's self-control (Barkley, 2020). If the child has success with this level of support, the parent and therapist can review how to upgrade the social challenge, reinforcing the use of strategies found to be helpful during these earlier experiences. Moreover, there is evidence that when the positive aspects of children with ADHD are emphasized to their peers, and children are encouraged and rewarded for working together regardless of their differences, social and behavioral improvements are even greater for the child with ADHD (Mikami et al., 2013). Not surprisingly, these areas of positive family and peer support are the strongest protective and mediating factors against poor academic performance and depressive symptoms in young people with ADHD (Dvorsky & Langberg, 2016), and give powerful evidence for therapeutic collaboration with both to promote coping and resilience in children with ADHD.

BUILDING INTERPROFESSIONAL COLLABORATIONS

The role of advocate may be the most impactful one the occupational therapist can play in the life of a child with ADHD. The inattentive or hyperactive child at home presents challenges for their family, but can present broader-reaching challenges and issues in the school and larger social settings. With an increase in the number of children per classroom and heightened focus on standardized testing, elementary-age children may spend 6 to 7 hours in the same crowded space, with much of this time spent in seated activities. The child who frequently disrupts the teaching process or quietly daydreams, missing important content, will likely decrease teaching effectiveness for their peers. Such children may also perform poorly academically and on standardized tests due to their not hearing information or not storing it in long-term memory for later use. Thus, it benefits everyone in the school context if all members can attend, participate, and succeed. Occupational therapists can reinforce the concept of ADHD as a neurodevelopmental disability to teachers and related services personnel as a starting point for understanding the underlying cause of the child's performance deficits. This can help adults to depersonalize the child's behaviors and anticipate potential individualized academic and social support needs. This also reinforces the importance of adults giving frequent and meaningful feedback so the child with ADHD understands when they have been successful, thereby promoting adaptive behavior (Pfiffner et al., 2018).

Occupational therapists can be an important link between home, school, and clinic performance for the individualized academic and social needs of the child with ADHD. Once effective strategies that address underlying process skills deficits are identified, the occupational therapist can work with teachers and professionals to ensure these strategies are carried over in school and other environments. For example, if the child is sensory seeking and frequently out of his seat during lessons, the occupational therapist can educate teachers about strategies that facilitate the child's ability to remain seated. Occupational therapists can likewise implement fine motor and visual motor strategies in the classroom to encourage engagement in typical classroom occupations. The ability to participate and complete academic work alongside their typical peers (which has both social and academic implications) can reinforce the child's sense of competence, break the cycle of dysadaptation discussed earlier in this chapter, and increase the child's resilience (Dvorsky & Langberg, 2016). With more consistency and predictability across contexts, there is evidence that children with ADHD can better understand what is expected of them, more effectively participate in normative experiences, and learn to adapt and cope to life challenges alongside neurotypical peers in multiple contexts.

Lastly, it is important to note that many children with ADHD and their families may need mental health services to help them develop effective coping skills and behavioral strategies. Social workers, counselors, and psychologists have specific training in areas such as cognitive-behavioral strategies, which have proven to be effective (Barkley, 2020). Speech therapists can focus on social communication and cognitive skills to facilitate more effective interactions (Hill, 2000). It also seems possible that the cycles of maladaptive coping noted earlier in this chapter might confer added risk for children with ADHD of developing comorbid mental health problems and diagnoses. The preponderance of evidence throughout this chapter supports the idea of building a team to support the child with ADHD; thus, referrals to other professionals may amplify therapeutic benefits.

A GLOBAL PERSPECTIVE

ADHD is a condition receiving attention all over the world. In the United Kingdom, researchers focused on the positive aspects of the condition (Sedgwick et al., 2019). Emerging treatments such as Cog-Fun and assessments for executive functioning are being produced in Israel (Maeir et al., 2014; Stern & Maeir, 2014). The Australian research community has also made significant contributions to ADHD research in the area of social skills (Barnes et al., 2017). Through a small randomized controlled trial of a play-based intervention, researchers found that treatment may yield a positive long-term impact on social play skills.

The international ADHD research community continues to grow and now supports multiple, yearly international conferences, such as the ADHD Congress, Children and Adults with Attention-Deficit/Hyperactivity Disorder (CHADD), European Network for Hyperkinetic Disorders (EUNETHYDIS), International Conference on ADHD (in the United Kingdom), and the Adult ADHD Network, to name a few. These are all valuable resources for therapists working with clients with ADHD and their families to facilitate the learning, coping, and adapting that allows for engagement in meaningful occupations. Also, with more of the world engaging in research and practice with individuals with ADHD, there seems even greater potential for finding more effective individual/family and societal-level ideas for enhancing occupational engagement, adaptation, coping, and resilience.

Essential Things Occupational Therapists Need to Consider to Build Adaptation, Coping, and Resilience in Children With ADHD

Table 6-3 lists essential considerations for occupational therapists working with children with ADHD.

Table 6-3

Essential Considerations for Occupational Therapists Working With Children With ADHD

- Children with ADHD face multiple occupational challenges that can affect their well-being, coping, resilience, and adaptation in many contexts.
- Comorbid diagnoses are common and may decrease opportunities to develop healthy coping and resilience.
- Strong evidence indicates that play-based occupational therapy interventions can improve occupational engagement, social skills, and global functioning for this population.
- Collaboration and incorporation of peers and family in treatment enhances the impact of many interventions for ADHD symptomology.
- Building a team of professional supports such as teachers and mental health providers can enrich occupational therapy interventions and enhance the child's capacity to adapt and cope with life situations.

Case Study 6-2

Trevor is a 7-year-old boy being raised by a single mother who works full-time while her son attends school. He was recently diagnosed with ADHD, combined type. Trevor has possible delays in fine motor and social-emotional skills development, as identified by his teacher. He loves outdoor activities and gross motor play and is extremely active. He also enjoys quiet play, such as with LEGOs and electronic games. When playing e-games, he is less active, and his mother can get housework done. However, if the game becomes too challenging, he becomes excessively angry and will slam his tablet down or bang it against his forehead. Trevor can dress himself, but needs constant verbal prompts or he gets distracted and stops dressing. In school, he excels in physical education and art (when the focus is hands-on activities such as working with clay, but

(continued)

Case Study 6-2 (continued)

he dislikes pencil sketching and listening to instructions). He has difficulty with handwriting and is often reprimanded for touching others and chewing on his pencil. He resists all tabletop activities and will often yell and spit at others if forced to sit and work for more than a few minutes. The school calls his mother several times each week to come pick him up because they cannot control his behavior. He was referred to occupational therapy services within the school district for evaluation of handwriting and possible sensory processing concerns. When asked what they hoped to achieve from occupational therapy services, the teacher stated that she would like Trevor to be able to write all numbers and letters and not disrupt the class; Trevor's mother stated that she would like him to be more independent and keep out of trouble; and Trevor noted that he would like to know how to make friends. The occupational therapy evaluation was completed, and scores were as follows.

Sensory Processing Measure (Teacher)

Definite dysfunction in Social Participation, Planning/Ideas, Touch, Body Awareness. Some problems in Hearing, Vision, Balance and Motion.

Berry Visual Motor Integration

Percentile score 6%: Definite visual motor challenges.

Behavior Rating Inventory of Executive Function (Teacher)

Clinically significant challenges in all areas, including Inhibit, Self-Monitor, Shift, Emotional Control, Initiate, Task Completion, Working Memory, Plan/Organize, Task-Monitor, Organization of Materials.

With the approval of his mother and school administration, Trevor started in occupational therapy group and individual sessions once a week in the therapy room. Group therapy focused on Trevor's need to improve the effectiveness of his social interactions with peers. Individual sessions addressed teacher concerns about his handwriting and his mother's desire that he become more independent.

Group Therapy Sessions

Trevor participated in occupational therapy groups with three other children. For his first session, he was chosen as the leader for a game activity. His peers stood at the opposite end of the room from Trevor. Each child would ask Trevor politely for a turn. Trevor would then roll the dice and ask them to "please" hop the number of spaces indicated on the dice. He completed the social interaction by thanking peers for participating. If someone hopped too many times, the group learned to tell that peer, "That's okay, just try again." The first child to reach Trevor was then the leader and the game started again.

(continued)

Case Study 6-2 (continued)

This activity addressed numerous areas of challenge for Trevor, but in a supported environment. Trevor had the opportunity to feel successful in a leadership role while learning to take turns in social interactions with other children, thus supporting adaptive social behavior for other settings. Additionally, Trevor learned coping strategies to support resilience when things did not work out as planned. Trevor's teacher reported hearing him tell himself, "That's okay, just try again" when he made a mistake at a tabletop task a few weeks later. Trevor was able to respond to demands of structured environment, assess his performance and responses received from his social environment, and add to his previously limited repertoire of responses for future use.

Individual Therapy Sessions

Goals for Trevor included increasing his willingness to participate in tabletop tasks and improving his handwriting. Knowing that Trevor enjoyed art, his occupational therapist began their tabletop sessions using clay to make letters. After two sessions using this activity, Trevor came into the third session and initiated the creation of clay letters without cueing. Trevor wrote his initials with encouragement to participate in the task. After writing his letters, he became upset, slammed down the marker, and said, "writing is stupid." His occupational therapist helped Trevor evaluate his performance and put words to his frustration that handwriting was difficult for him and made his hands tired. They discussed encouraging words he could use to tell himself when something is hard to do. Trevor wrote his full name and stopped several times due to frustration. Each time, the occupational therapist cued him to use his new coping strategies and then continue the task. The occupational therapist taped notecards with Trevor's new coping phrases on his desk, including "Keep trying" and "I can do it." The phrases taped to his desk helped compensate for Trevor's decreased working memory, allowing him to step out of dysadaptive habits and build new coping strategies until he reached relative mastery. Trevor's occupational therapist worked with Trevor's teacher and parent to teach them how to cue Trevor to use his new coping strategies across environments. As Trevor was able to transfer his successes to other settings, his confidence grew and he needed fewer cues to remember his coping phrases.

Now that Trevor is successful with new occupational responses in controlled settings, the next step will be to support Trevor in natural environments as he uses coping strategies in his roles as student, friend, and family member. His occupational therapist will continue to work with his teachers and parents to support Trevor as he develops adaptive responses to new occupational challenges.

REFERENCES

Aduen, P. A., Day, T. N., Kofler, M. J., Harmon, S. L., Wells, E. L., & Sarver, D. E. (2018). Social problems in ADHD: Is it a skills acquisition or performance problem? *Journal of Psychopathology and Behavioral Assessment, 40*, 440-451. https://doi.org/10.1007/s10862-018- 9649-7

Ahmann, E., Tuttle, L. J., Saviet, M., & Wright, S. D. (2018). A descriptive review of ADHD coaching research: Implications for college students. *Journal of Postsecondary Education and Disability, 31*(1), 17-39. https://files.eric.ed.gov/fulltext/EJ1182373.pdf

American Occupational Therapy Association. (2021). The Association—Improve your documentation and quality of care with AOTA's updated Occupational Profile Template. *American Journal of Occupational Therapy, 75*, 7502420010. https://doi.org/10.5014/ajot.2021.752001

American Occupational Therapy Association. (2020). Occupational therapy practice framework: Domain and process (4th ed.). *American Journal of Occupational Therapy, 74*(Suppl. 2), 7412410010. https://doi.org/10.5014/ajot.2020.74S2001

American Psychiatric Association. (2013). *Diagnostic and statistical manual of mental disorders* (5th ed.). Author. https://doi.org/10.1176/appi.books.9780890425596

Babb, K. A., Levine, L. J., & Arseneault, J. M. (2010). Shifting gears: Coping flexibility in children with and without ADHD. *International Journal of Behavioral Development, 34*(1), 10-23. https://doi.org/10.1177/0165025409345070

Barkley, R. A. (2012). Barkley deficits in executive functioning scale: Children and adolescents (BDEFS-CA). Guilford.

Barkley, R. A. (Ed.). (2014). *Attention-deficit hyperactivity disorder: A handbook for diagnosis and treatment.* Guilford.

Barkley, R. A. (2020). *Taking charge of ADHD: The complete, authoritative guide for parents.* Guilford Press.

Barkley, R. A., & Murphy, K. R. (2010). Impairment in occupational functioning and adult ADHD: The predictive utility of executive function (EF) ratings versus EF tests. *Archives of Clinical Neuropsychology, 25*(3), 157-173. https://doi.org/10.1093/arclin/acq014

Barnes, G., Wilkes-Gillan, S., Bundy, A., & Cordier, R. (2017). The social play, social skills and parent-child relationships of children with ADHD 12 months following a RCT of a play-based intervention. *Australian Occupational Therapy Journal, 64*(6), 457-465. https://doi.org/10.1111/1440-1630.12417

Becker, S. P., Luebbe, A., & Langberg, J. M. (2012). Co-occurring mental health problems and peer functioning among youth with ADHD: A review and recommendations for future research. *Clinical Child and Family Psychology Review, 15*, 279-302. https://doi.org/10.1007/s10567-012-0122-y

Biederman, J. (2005). Attention-deficit/hyperactivity disorder: A selective overview. *Biological Psychiatry, 57*(11), 1215-1220. https://doi.org/10.1016/j.biopsych.2004.10.020

Boyle, C. A., Boulet, S., Schieve, L. A., Cohen, R. A., Blumberg, S. J., Yeargin-Allsopp, M., . . . Kogan, M. D. (2011). Trends in the prevalence of developmental disabilities in US children, 1997-2008. *Pediatrics, 137*(6), 1034-1042. https://doi.org/10.1542/peds.2010-2989

Bressan, R. A., & Crippa, J. A. (2005). The role of dopamine in reward and pleasure behaviour-review of data from preclinical research. *Acta Psychiatrica Scandinavica, 111*(s427), 14-21. https://doi.org/10.1111/j.1600-0447.2005.00540.x

Bul, K. C., Kato, P. M., Van der Oord, S., Danckaerts, M., Vreeke, L. J., Willems, A., van Oers, H. J., Van Den Heuvel, R., Birnie, D., Van Amelsvoort, T. A., Franken, I. H., & Maras. A. (2016). Behavioral outcome effects of serious gaming as an adjunct to treatment for children with attention-deficit/hyperactivity disorder: A randomized controlled trial. *Journal of Medical Internet Research, 18*(2), e26. https://doi.org/10.2196/jmir.5173

Bundy, A. (2010). *Test of playfulness manual.* Colorado State University.

Cahill, S. M., & Beisbier, S. (2020). Occupational therapy practice guidelines for children and youth ages 5-21 years. *American Journal of Occupational Therapy, 74*(4), 7404397010p1-7404397010p48. https://doi.org/10.5014/ajot.2020.744001

Cano, F. (2006). An in-depth analysis of the Learning and Study Strategies Inventory (LASSI). *Educational and Psychological Measurement, 66*(6), 1023-1038. https://doi.org/10.1177/0013164406288167

Case-Smith, J., Holland, T., & Bishop, B. (2011). Effectiveness of an integrated handwriting program for first-grade students: A pilot study. *American Journal of Occupational Therapy, 65*(6), 670-678. https://doi.org/10.5014/ajot.2011.000984

Centers for Disease Control and Prevention. (2017). National survey of children's health. https://www.cdc.gov/nchs/slaits/nsch.htm

Chen, Q., Brikell, I., Lichtenstein, P., Serlachius, E., Kuja-Halkola, R., Sandin, S., & Larsson, H. (2017). Familial aggregation of attention-deficit/hyperactivity disorder. *Journal of Child Psychology and Psychiatry, 58*(3), 231-239. https://doi.org/10.1111/jcpp.12616

Compas, B. E., Connor-Smith, J. K., Saltzman, H., Thomsen, A. H., & Wadsworth, M. E. (2001). Coping with stress during childhood and adolescence: Problems, progress, and potential in theory and research. *Psychological Bulletin, 127*(1), 87. https://doi.org/10.1037/0033-2909.127.1.87

Conners, C. K. (2008). *Conners' continuous performance test* (3rd ed.). Pearson.

Coster, W., Deeney, T. A., Haley, S., & Haltiwanger, J. (1998). *School function assessment.* Psychological Corporation.

Daley, D., & Birchwood, J. (2010). ADHD and academic performance: Why does ADHD impact on academic performance and what can be done to support ADHD children in the classroom? *Childcare, Health & Development, 36*(4), 455-464. https://doi.org/10.1111/j.1365-2214.2009.01046.x

Danielson, M. L., Bitsko, R. H., Ghandour, R. M., Holbrook, J. R., Kogan, M. D., & Blumberg, S. J. (2018). Prevalence of parent-reported ADHD diagnosis and associated treatment among U.S. children and adolescents, 2016. *Journal of Clinical Child and Adolescent Psychology, 47*(2), 199-212. https://doi.org/10.1080/15374416.2017.1417860

Dunn, W. (2014). *Sensory profile 2.* Psych Corporation.

Dvorsky, M. R., & Langberg, J. M. (2016). A review of factors that promote resilience in youth with ADHD and ADHD symptoms. *Clinical Child and Family Psychology Review, 19*(4), 368-391. http://doi.org/10.1007/s10567-016-0216-z

Fabiano, G. A., Hulme, K., Linke, S., Nelson-Tuttle, C., Pariseau, M., Gangloff, B., . . . & Gormley, M. (2011). The Supporting a Teen's Effective Entry to the Roadway (STEER) program: Feasibility and preliminary support for a psychosocial intervention for teenage drivers with ADHD. *Cognitive and Behavioral Practice, 18*(2), 267-280. https://doi.org/10.1016/j.cbpra.2010.04.002

Fedewa, A. L., & Erwin, H. E. (2011). Stability balls and students with attention and hyperactivity concerns: Implications for on-task and in-seat behavior. *American Journal of Occupational Therapy, 65*(4), 393-399. https://doi.org/10.5014/ajot.2011.000554

Folkman, S., & Lazarus, R. S. (1984). *Stress, appraisal, and coping* (pp. 150-153). Springer.

Gallichan, D. J., & Curle, C. (2008). Fitting square pegs into round holes: The challenge of coping with attention-deficit hyperactivity disorder. *Clinical Child Psychology and Psychiatry, 13*(3), 343-363. https://doi.org/10.1177/1359104508090599

Gioia, G. A., Isquith, P. K., Guy, S. C., & Kenworthy, L. (2000). *Behavior rating inventory of executive function.* Psychological Assessment Resources.

Gleason, M. M., & Humphreys, K. L. (2016). Categorical diagnosis of extreme hyperactivity, impulsivity, and inattention in very young children. *Infant Mental Health Journal, 37*(5), 476-485. https://doi.org/10.1002/imhj.21592

Gol, D., & Jarus, T. (2005). Effect of a social skills training group on everyday activities of children with attention-deficit-hyperactivity disorder. *Developmental Medicine and Child Neurology, 47*(8), 539-545. http://doi.org/10.1017/S0012162205001052

Grajo, L., Boisselle, A., & DaLomba, E. (2018). Occupational adaptation as a construct: A scoping review of literature. *The Open Journal of Occupational Therapy, 6*(1), 2. https://doi.org/10.15453/2168-6408.1400

Graziano, P. A., & Garcia, A. (2016). Attention-deficit hyperactivity disorder and children's emotion dysregulation: A meta-analysis. *Clinical Psychology Review, 46,* 106-123. https://doi.org/10.1016/j.cpr.2016.04.011

Gu, Y., Xu, G., & Zhu, Y. (2018). A randomized controlled trial of mindfulness-based cognitive therapy for college students with ADHD. *Journal of Attention Disorders, 22*(4), 388-399. https://doi.org/10.1177/1087054716686183

Hahn-Markowitz, J., Berger, I., Manor, I., & Maeir, A. (2017). Impact of the Cognitive-Functional (Cog-Fun) intervention on executive functions and participation among children with attention deficit hyperactivity disorder: A randomized controlled trial. *American Journal of Occupational Therapy, 71*(5), 7105220010p1-7105220010p9. https://doi.org/10.5014/ajot.2017.022053

Haley, S. M. (1992). *Pediatric evaluation of disability inventory (PEDI): Development, standardization and administration manual.* Therapy Skill Builders.

Heath, C. L., Curtis, D. F., Fan, W., & McPherson, R. (2015). The association between parenting stress, parenting self-efficacy, and the clinical significance of child ADHD symptom change following behavior therapy. *Child Psychiatry and Human Development, 46*, 118-129. https://doi.org/10.1007/s10578-014-0458-2

Hill, G. P. (2000). A role for the speech-language pathologist in multidisciplinary assessment and treatment of attention-deficit/hyperactivity disorder. *Journal of Attention Disorders, 4*(2), 69-79. https://doi.org/10.1177/108705470000400201

Hooper, B., & Wood, W. (2014). The philosophy of occupational therapy: A framework for practice. In B. A. Boyt Schell, G. Gillen, & M. Scaffa (Eds.), *Willard and Spackman's occupational therapy* (12th ed., pp. 35-46). Lippincott Williams & Wilkins.

Hupfeld, K. E., Abagis, T. R., & Shah, P. (2019). Living "in the zone": Hyperfocus in adult ADHD. *ADHD Attention Deficit and Hyperactivity Disorder, 11*, 191-208. https://doi.org/10.1007/s12402-018-0272-y

Lee, S. S., Sibley, M. H., & Epstein, J. N. (2016). Attention-deficit/hyperactivity disorder across development: Predictors, resilience, and future directions. *Journal of Abnormal Psychology, 125*(2), 151. http://doi.org/10.1037/abn0000114

Levanon-Erez, N., Cohen, M., Traub Bar-Ilan, R., & Maeir, A. (2017). Occupational identity of adolescents with ADHD: A mixed methods study. *Scandinavian Journal of Occupational Therapy, 24*(1), 32-40. https://doi.org/10.1080/11038128.2016.1217927

Levy, F., & Swanson, J. M. (2001). Timing, space and ADHD: The dopamine theory revisited. *Australian & New Zealand Journal of Psychiatry, 35*(4), 504-511. https://doi.org/10.1046/j.1440-1614.2001.00923.x

Lin, H. Y., Lee, P., Chang, W. D., & Hong, F. Y. (2014). Effects of weighted vests on attention, impulse control, and on-task behavior in children with attention deficit hyperactivity disorder. *American Journal of Occupational Therapy, 68*(2), 149-58. https://doi.org/10.5014/ajot.2014.009365

López-Liria, R., Vargas-Muñoz, E., Aguilar-Parra, J. M., Padilla-Góngora, D., Mañas-Rodriguez, M. A., & Rocamora-Pérez, P. (2020). Effectiveness of a training program in the management of stress for parents of disabled children. *Journal of Child and Family Studies, 29*, 964-977.

Maeir, A., Fisher, O., Bar-Ilan, R. T., Boas, N., Berger, I., & Landau, Y. E. (2014). Effectiveness of cognitive-functional (Cog-Fun) occupational therapy intervention for young children with attention deficit hyperactivity disorder: A controlled study. *American Journal of Occupational Therapy, 68*(3), 260-267. https://doi.org/10.5014/ajot.2014.011700

Mikami, A. Y., Griggs, M. S., Lerner, M. D., Emeh, C. C., Reuland, M. M., Jack, A., & Anthony, M. R. (2013). A randomized trial of a classroom intervention to increase peers' social inclusion of children with attention-deficit/hyperactivity disorder. *Journal of Consulting and Clinical Psychology, 81*(1), 100-112. https://doi.org/10.1037/a0029654

Mikami, A. Y., & Normand, S. (2015). The importance of social contextual factors in peer relationships of children with ADHD. *Current Developmental Disorders Reports, 2*(1), 30-37. https://doi.org/10.1007/s40474-014-0036-0

Morgan, P. L., Staff, J., Hillemeier, M. M., Farkas, G., & Maczuga, S. (2013). Racial and ethnic disparities in ADHD diagnosis from kindergarten to eighth grade. *Pediatrics, 132*(1), 85-93. https://doi.org/10.1542/peds.2012-2390

Muris, P., Roodenrijs, D., Kelgtermans, L., Sliwinski, S., Berlage, U., Baillieux, H., & Deckers, A. (2018). No medication for my child! A naturalistic study on the treatment preferences for and effects of Cogmed working memory training versus psychostimulant medication in clinically referred youth with ADHD. *Child Psychiatry & Human Development, 49*(6), 974. https://doi.org/10.1007/s10578-018-0812-x

Nielsen, S. K., Kelsch, K., & Miller, K. (2017). Occupational therapy interventions for children with attention deficit hyperactivity disorder: A systematic review. *Occupational Therapy in Mental Health, 33*(1), 70-80. https://doi.org/10.1080/0164212X.2016.1211060

Ollendick, T. H., Greene, R. W., Austin, K. E., Fraire, M. G., Halldorsdottir, T., Allen, K. B., . . . & Noguchi, R. J. (2016). Parent management training and collaborative & proactive solutions: A randomized control trial for oppositional youth. *Journal of Clinical Child & Adolescent Psychology, 45*(5), 591-604. https://doi.org/10.1080/15374416.2015.1004681

Pfiffner, L. J., Rooney, M. E., Jiang, Y., Haack, L. M., Beaulieu, A., & McBurnett, K. (2018). Sustained effects of collaborative school-home intervention for attention-deficit/hyperactivity disorder symptoms and impairment. *Journal of the American Academy of Child & Adolescent Psychiatry, 57*(4), 245-251. https://doi.org/10.1016/j.jaac.2018.01.016

Regalla, M. A., Guilherme, P., Aguilera, P., Serra-Pinheiro, M. A., & Mattos, P. (2015). Attention deficit hyperactivity disorder is an independent risk factor for lower resilience in adolescents: A pilot study. *Trends in Psychiatry and Psychotherapy, 37*(3), 157-160. https://doi.org/10.1590/2237-6089-2015-0010

Ringer, N. (2019). Young people's perceptions of and coping with their ADHD symptoms: A qualitative study. *Cogent Psychology, 6*(1), 1608032. https://doi.org/10.1080/23311908.2019.1608032

Schkade, J. K., & Schultz, S. (1992). Occupational adaptation: Toward a holistic approach for contemporary practice, part 1. *American Journal of Occupational Therapy, 46*(9), 829-837. https://doi.org/10.5014/ajot.46.9.829

Schneider, M. F., Krick, C. M., Retz, W., Hengesch, G., Retz-Junginger, P., Reith, W., & Rösler, M. (2010). Impairment of fronto-striatal and parietal cerebral networks correlates with attention deficit hyperactivity disorder (ADHD) psychopathology in adults—a functional magnetic resonance imaging (fMRI) study. *Psychiatry Research: Neuroimaging, 183*, 75-84. https://pubmed.ncbi.nlm.nih.gov/20558047

Schwarz, A., & Cohen, S. (2013, March 31). ADHD seen in 11% of U.S. children as diagnoses rise. *The New York Times*. www.nytimes.com/2013/04/01/health/more-diagnoses-of-hyperactivity-causing-concern.html

Sciberras, E., Fulton, M., Efron, D., Oberklaid, F., & Hiscock, H. (2011). Managing sleep problems in school aged children with ADHD: A pilot randomized controlled trial. *Sleep Medicine, 12*(9), 932-935. https://doi.org/10.1016/j.sleep.2011.02.006

Sedgwick, J. A., Merwood, A., & Asherson, P. (2019). The positive aspects of attention deficit disorder: A qualitative investigation of successful adults with ADHD. *ADHD Attention Deficit and Hyperactivity Disorders, 11*, 241-253. https://doi.org/10.1007/s12402-018-0277-6

Soyeon, K., Chen, S., & Tannock, R. (2014). Visual function and color vision in adults with attention-deficit/hyperactivity disorder. *Journal of Optometry, 7*(1), 22-36. https://doi.org/10.1016/j.optom.2013.07.001

Spiliotopoulou, G. (2009). Management of children with attention deficit/hyperactivity disorder and learning disabilities: A survey of paediatric occupational therapists in the United Kingdom. *Mental Health and Learning Disabilities Research and Practice, 6*(1), 5-19. https://doi.org/10.5920/mhldrp.2009.615

Stern, A., & Maeir, A. (2014). Validating the measurement of executive functions in an occupational context for adults with attention deficit hyperactivity disorder. *American Journal of Occupational Therapy, 68*(6), 719-728. https://doi.org/10.5014/ajot.2014.012419

Stoffel, V. G. (2016). Coming home to family: Now is the time! *American Journal of Occupational Therapy, 70*(6), 700612010p1-7006120010p6. https://doi.org/10.5014/ajot.2016.706003

Theule, J., Wiener, J., Tannock, R., & Jenkins, J. M. (2013). Parenting stress in families of children with ADHD: A meta-analysis. *Journal of Emotional and Behavioural Disorders, 21*(1), 3-17. https://doi.org/10.1177/1063426610387433

Thomas, R., Sanders, S., Doust, J., Beller, E., & Glasziou, P. (2015). Prevalence of attention-deficit/hyperactivity disorder: A systematic review and meta-analysis. *Pediatrics, 135*(4), e994-e1001. https://doi.org/10.1542/peds.2014-3482

Visser, S. N., Bitsko, R. H., Danielson, M. L., Ghandour, R. M., Blumberg, S. J., Schieve, L. A., Holbrook, J. R., Wolraich, M. L., & Cuffe, S. P. (2015). Treatment of attention deficit/hyperactivity disorder among children with special health care needs. *The Journal of Pediatrics, 166*(6), 1423-1430. https://doi.org/10.1016/j.jpeds.2015.02.018

Wilkes, S., Cordier, R., Bundy, A., Docking, K., & Munro, N. (2011). A play-based intervention for children with ADHD: A pilot study. *Australian Occupational Therapy Journal, 58*(4), 231-240. https://doi.org/10.1111/j.1440-1630.2011.00928.x

Wilkes-Gillan, S., Bundy, A., Cordier, R., & Lincoln, M. (2014). Eighteen-month follow-up of a play-based intervention to improve the social play skills of children with attention deficit hyperactivity disorder. *Australian Occupational Therapy Journal, 61*(5), 299-307. https://doi.org/10.1111/1440-1630.12124

Wilkes-Gillan, S., Cantrill, A., Parsons, L., Smith, C., & Cordier, R. (2017). The pragmatic language, communication skills, parent-child relationships, and symptoms of children with ADHD and their playmates 18-months after a parent-delivered play-based intervention. *Developmental Neurorehabilitation, 20*(5), 317-322. https://doi.org/10.1080/17518423.2016.1188861

Wolraich, M., Hagan, J. F., Allan, C., Chan, E., Davison, D., Earls, M., . . . & Zurhellen, W. (2019). Clinical practice guideline for the diagnosis, evaluation, and treatment of attention-deficit/hyperactivity disorder in children and adolescents. *Pediatrics, 144*(4), 1-25. http://doi.org/10.1542/peds.2019-2528

Complex Medical and Other Multi-Systems Considerations

7

Children and Youth With Complex Medical Needs and Chronic Illnesses

Susan M. Cahill, PhD, OTR/L, FAOTA

CHAPTER OBJECTIVES By the end of this chapter, the reader will be able to:
- Identify the factors that influence adoption of the self-manager role by children and youth with chronic conditions.
- Understand the types of assessment tools that are useful for guiding interventions to promote self-management.
- Understand the intervention approaches used with children and youth with chronic conditions to support coping, adaptation, and resilience.

Children and youth with complex medical needs and chronic illnesses often require unique interventions to support the development of person systems and enhance occupational participation. Occupational therapy practitioners improve the health and well-being of children and youth by creating opportunities for them to meet role demands and expectations and balance the relative mastery of their health conditions with desired occupational pursuits (Grajo, 2019). Occupational therapy practitioners also create occupational contexts that encourage children and youth with complex medical needs and chronic illnesses to act as agents of change by collaborating with families during critical periods of transition.

Historically, medical care for children and youth with chronic illnesses was focused on symptom reduction and survival. Advancements in medical technology over the past several decades have resulted in the need for targeted services focused on transitioning to adulthood and independent health management (Goralski et al., 2017). Occupational

- 161 -

Grajo L. C., & Boisselle, A. K. (Eds.). *Adaptation, Coping, and Resilience in Children and Youth: A Comprehensive Occupational Therapy Approach* (pp. 161-182).
© 2022 Taylor & Francis Group.

therapy practitioners can play a critical role in supporting children with chronic health conditions by addressing adaption, coping, and resilience through health management interventions. *Health management* is defined as a series of activities related to managing and maintaining health through routines in order to more fully participate in other occupations (American Occupational Therapy Association [AOTA], 2020). Medication management, communication with health care providers, symptom management, and management of nutrition and activity routines are some examples of health management occupations (AOTA, 2020). Interventions focused on health management facilitate the continuation of care from pediatric to adult specialists, maximize independence, and support the transition to adulthood (Goralski et al., 2017). Occupational therapy practitioners support children and youth through the adaptive process by creating opportunities for the acquisition of knowledge and skills associated with chronic disease management, and partner with families to determine the best time to begin transitioning health management responsibilities from the parent to the child (Ödling et al., 2019). The child's developmental level is matched with health management expectations, so chronological age is not the primary determinant for beginning the transition of responsibilities (Ödling et al., 2019). The desired outcome of this transition of responsibilities is to maximize the child's adaptation, coping, and resilience in light of disease management and to minimize disruptions to health care and quality of life (Ödling et al., 2019).

Overview of the Population

Chronic illness is defined as a medical condition that, once developed, persists throughout the lifespan and affects all aspects of life. Some chronic conditions develop in adulthood; however, several conditions are prevalent in children and influence development. Such chronic conditions also create opportunities for children to acquire skills that support transition to adulthood, such as advance planning and scheduling, organization, prioritization.

The prevalence of chronic conditions in childhood has increased over the past 40 years (Miller et al., 2016). Chronic conditions may affect physical, cognitive, and psychological systems and generally involve some type of persistent medical management. Such medical management may cause children and youth to reconsider typical habits and routines (e.g., going out to eat with friends), affect engagement with peers, and potentially affect psychosocial well-being. Some examples of chronic conditions that are common in childhood include juvenile idiopathic arthritis, cystic fibrosis, and diabetes.

Juvenile Idiopathic Arthritis

Juvenile idiopathic arthritis (JIA) is a group of conditions that are identified in children prior to their turning 16 years old (Cron et al., 2019). Approximately 1 in every 1,000 children in the United States has a form of JIA (Cron et al., 2019). JIA is characterized by stiffness, swelling, and inflammation of few joints (oligoarticular) or many joints (polyarticular) for more than 6 weeks (Cron et al., 2019). Children with JIA typically experience flares of increased inflammation, which are associated with significant pain and decreased activity engagement (Stinson et al., 2012). Pain management is addressed through pharmacological interventions, cognitive behavioral therapy, sleep interventions, physical activity, and the application of orthoses (Stinson et al., 2012).

Cystic Fibrosis

Cystic fibrosis (CF) is caused by a genetic mutation that leads to thick mucus secretions, infections, and organ failure (Quittner et al., 2014). Children with CF experience chronic symptoms, including shortness of breath (dyspnea), cough, fatigue, sleep disturbances, malnutrition, and pain (Linnemann et al., 2016). CF is a condition with variable life expectancy based on symptom severity; early death caused by respiratory failure is not uncommon (Dellon et al., 2016). Medical interventions have led to increased survival rates for individuals with CF, but children and young adults with this condition have to balance symptom management, breathing treatments, and the demands of daily life activities (Linnemann et al., 2016).

Diabetes

Approximately 190 out of every 100,000 children in the United States have some form of diabetes (Centers for Disease Control, 2017). Type 1 diabetes is caused by the inability of the pancreas to create adequate amounts of insulin to control blood glucose levels (Chiang et al., 2014). Type 2 diabetes is associated with the body's inability to respond to insulin and control blood glucose levels (Pettitt et al., 2014). Children who are overweight or characterized as medically obese are at heightened risk for developing type 2 diabetes in childhood (Cameron & Wherrett, 2015). Glycemic control in type 1 and type 2 diabetes is managed through frequent monitoring of blood glucose levels, physical activity, medication, and healthy eating (Jackson et al., 2015).

Occupational Profile

The occupational history and experiences associated with complex medical management influence the occupational profile of children living with chronic conditions. Although children with chronic conditions and their families may seek occupational therapy for many reasons associated with general development and occupational participation and engagement, the primary focus of occupational therapy intervention associated with chronic illness is often focused on adaption, coping, and resilience leading to disease self-management (Cahill et al., 2016).

Chronic condition management is complex and requires children and youth to assume the life role of "self-manager" and develop performance patterns that promote optimal health (Cahill et al., 2016). The transition from having one's medical care and

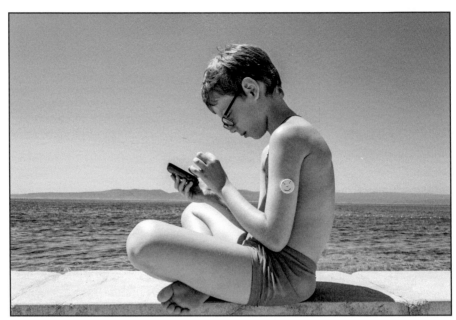

Figure 7-1. Child on vacation monitoring glucose level. (Kristina Kuptsevich/shutterstock.com.)

symptoms managed by a parent to becoming a self-manager, like other critical life transitions, causes a major disruption of the occupational adaptation process (Grajo, 2019). The child develops a new understanding of their occupational identity and the occupational therapist acts as a facilitator to assist the child in prioritizing this important role. This is accomplished by educating the child about the occupational demands associated with chronic disease self-management and providing opportunities to experience competence associated with self-management tasks (Figure 7-1). Table 7-1 includes examples of tasks associated with the self-manager role. These tasks can be used to explore the child's adaptive capacity: that is, the child's ability to perceive the need to change, modify, and/or refine a response to a role demand (Grajo, 2019). Understanding the child's adaptive capacity with regard to the self-manager role gives the occupational therapist a better understanding of the strategies the child uses to complete tasks that are challenging and how the child copes with frustration (Grajo, 2019). Competence experienced in the self-manager role may not only improve adherence to medical treatment plans, but also build the child's capacity to navigate challenging situations and solve problems in other areas of life.

Table 7-1

Tasks Associated With the Self-Manager Role	
Self-Management Focus	Tasks
General	Monitor and manage symptoms, prevent flares, avoid triggers, administer medication and treatments, cope with stress and functional impact of condition, manage condition-related equipment and technology, balance physical activity and rest, communicate with health care providers, implement an action plan when needed, and utilize social supports (Lozano & Houtrow, 2018).
JIA	Routinely use pain management strategies (e.g., muscle relaxation, guided imagery, mindfulness, calming breathing techniques), utilize joint-protection techniques, and monitor how pain affects sleep, mood, and concentration (Stinson et al., 2014).
Cystic fibrosis	Utilize energy-conservation techniques, monitor air quality and avoid environments with smoke and other pollutants, routinely use airway-clearing techniques, monitor diet for adequate nutrition and caloric intake (Bregnballe et al., 2017).
Diabetes	Plan time for blood glucose monitoring, manage and adjust diet, and navigate social situations that involve eating and drinking (Pyatak, 2011; Thompson, 2014).

DEFINING ADAPTATION, COPING, AND RESILIENCE FOR CHILDREN WITH COMPLEX MEDICAL NEEDS AND CHRONIC ILLNESS

The manner in which children and adolescents cope with stress influences their mental health and how they adjust to future stressors (Compas et al., 2001). The presence of a personal chronic illness may negatively affect a child or adolescent's ability to achieve developmental milestones associated with autonomy, self-acceptance, social relationships, and career readiness (Pinquart & Pfeiffer, 2015). Coping and adapting to stressors is an ongoing developmental process that changes based on personal resources (e.g., cognitive abilities, modulation of energy, initiation of actions, and regulation of emotions) and social resources (e.g., parental support, peer expectations; Compas et al., 2001).

Encountering stressful life events, such as receiving a diagnosis of a co-morbid condition or having a serious symptom exacerbation requiring hospitalization, influences the adaptation, coping, and resilience of children and youth with chronic conditions. The intensity and chronicity of stressful life events are important considerations, but so too are the child's appraisal of the stressful event, the lived experience of stress, their coping responses, and feelings of competence associated with overcoming the stressful situation (Zimmer-Gembeck & Skinner, 2016).

Challenges

Children and youth with chronic medical conditions often experience challenges related to adaptation, coping, and resilience in everyday life. Many of these challenges are associated with the unpredictable and fluctuating nature of chronic illness and the effect it has on daily life activities. Even when strictly adhering to medical recommendations, many children and youth are often uncertain when they will experience significant symptom fluctuations or an exacerbation resulting in temporary or permanent functional setbacks (Knudsen et al., 2018; Spencer et al., 2019). The transition to different life stages, such as the hormonal changes associated with the onset of puberty, may influence the disease process and lead to difficulty with coping or lack of a functional adaptive response (Heaton et al., 2016).

Many youth understand the complex nature of their illness, as well as the consequences associated with mismanagement and imprecise adherence to medical recommendations. Despite this, children and youth sometimes ignore symptoms that signal a medical setback and attend to other occupational demands, such as going out with friends or completing academic assignments (Spencer et al., 2019). The desire to have similar experiences as their peers can cause children and youth with chronic conditions to postpone or forego important critical health maintenance routines, which could have detrimental consequences for their health (Knudsen et al., 2018). Other children and youth choose to avoid and disengage from social activities and setting future goals, rather than decide between compromising their health and letting themselves and their friends down (Heaton et al., 2016; Knudsen et al., 2018; Spencer et al., 2019). Elijah, in Case Study 7-1, is an example of an adolescent with cystic fibrosis who is struggling to adapt to challenges associated with his chronic condition.

Adaptation

Children and youth who cope well with the stressors associated with their chronic condition adapt to different situations and develop resilience. One way that children and youth develop resilience is through accurate self-knowledge and a clear understanding of how their bodies will respond to delays and disruptions in their condition management routines. Self-knowledge is acquired through experimentation with symptom management and advice obtained from health providers (Spencer et al., 2019). For example, a teenager with JIA who usually rests after school may decide to attend a short club meeting to determine if adding an extracurricular activity at the end of the school day would overly tax their system or not. If the teenager does not experience increased pain after the meeting, they may consider joining the club on a regular basis. However, if the teenager does experience increased pain, they may decide to join an extracurricular activity that takes place on the weekend, rather than after a full day of school.

Case Study 7-1

Elijah is currently a junior in high school who lives with his grandma and is contemplating whether or not he should apply to universities away from home. It has always been his dream to go away for college; however, he is concerned that living on his own, managing his condition, and completing undergraduate coursework will be too much for him to handle. Elijah's grandma wants him to pursue his dreams and knows that universities provide accommodations (e.g., assignment to an air-conditioned room, opportunities to make up missed class-work, extended assignment deadlines) to students with cystic fibrosis and that these accommodations would support Elijah. Elijah's grandma tries to convince him to go on a campus visit and speak with a student-services representative. Elijah declines this invitation and explains to his grandma that he is concerned about the instability of his condition. He is worried that his symptoms will worsen when he is far from home and that regular treatments might not be effective. Even with accommodations, Elijah is concerned that he will not be able to meet his day-to-day responsibilities if he experiences a flare. Ultimately, Elijah decides to give up his dream of going away for college and applies to a local university that he can commute to on a daily basis.

Children and youth who have adapted to their chronic condition often demonstrate a strong sense of self-discipline (Knudsen et al., 2018). Health maintenance in the presence of a chronic condition requires diligence and sustained attention. Children and youth may adopt a proactive viewpoint and attempt to organize all aspects of their life (Spencer et al., 2019). In addition, they may plan ahead and attempt to anticipate challenges that may arise throughout the days or weeks, while carefully managing their schedules and routines (Knudsen et al., 2018). Planning ahead for assignments, balancing commitments, becoming health conscious, and engaging in more health-promoting activities are all examples of ways children and youth with chronic conditions can respond to the challenges associated with managing a chronic condition. Case Study 7-2 features Deja, a child with type 1 diabetes who is coping well with the demands associated with her chronic condition and adapting to different situations.

THE ROLE OF OCCUPATIONAL THERAPY: BEST AND EVIDENCE-BASED PRACTICES FOR ASSESSMENT AND INTERVENTION

The focus of occupational therapy assessment for children and youth with chronic conditions is on daily and lifelong medical management, executive function, adaptive capacity, and competence in occupational participation. Occupational therapists use a collection of tools to gather data in order to identify patterns of performance and coping that will allow children or adolescents to confidently manage their own health and

> ### Case Study 7-2
>
> Deja is entering sixth grade and was diagnosed with type 1 diabetes over the summer. Deja wears a continuous glucose monitor that tracks her glucose levels every 5 minutes throughout the day and notifies her mom through a smartphone application if Deja experiences high or low glucose levels. When Deja's blood sugar rises too high, her mom provides her with a bolus of insulin and a snack. Deja's parents are not ready to buy her a smartphone yet and are concerned about how Deja's diabetes will be managed at school. Although Deja's mom already reached out to the school principal to set up a meeting with Deja's teacher and other school personnel, Deja has her own ideas about how she can manage her condition at school. Deja prepares a list of healthy, shelf-stable snacks and beverages that could be kept in her locker or carried in her purse in case she experiences blood sugar fluctuations. She also researches an application that would allow her teachers to see data from her continuous glucose monitor.

reduce their reliance on others. Children and youth with chronic conditions develop the role of self-manager after they have acquired the knowledge and skills associated with managing their condition, experimented with behavior changes, and built a repertoire of strategies to address daily challenges (Heaton et al., 2016). Resilient self-managers believe that they have an important obligation to manage their condition and collaborate with health care providers to promote their overall health. Interventions are designed to create opportunities to learn how to self-monitor the condition, make decisions and solve daily problems, and utilize resources from the environment when needed.

Assessment

Occupational therapists often begin evaluation with a top-down approach that involves gathering information about what the child wants and needs to do in different roles and across environments. The occupational profile guides the assessment process and include information about the child's strengths, concerns, interests, and goals (AOTA, 2021). Occupational profile information can be collected from the child, the child's parents, teachers, and other health care providers (Cahill, 2020). The occupational profile is used to develop a clinical picture, determine which assessment tools are appropriate for use with the child, and begin to conceptualize goal areas.

Occupational therapists working with children and adolescents with chronic conditions evaluate those clients' readiness for assuming and performing in the self-manager role. When evaluating self-management capacity, several personal attributes are examined: self-determination, causal agency, autonomy, empowerment, and self-advocacy (Zhang et al., 2014). The occupational therapist might select a condition-specific assessment tool, such as the Diabetes Self-Management Questionnaire (Harris et al., 2000). However, several condition-neutral tools are available that address self-management knowledge and skills (Zhang et al., 2014).

Children and adolescents with a chronic condition need to demonstrate adaptive capacity and understand how to efficiently and effectively respond to contextual demands, as well as demands associated with their symptoms. Knowledge, such as understanding one's medication regimen and the severity of one's condition, is considered a predictor of successful independent condition management (Lawson et al., 2011).

The occupational therapist can assess a pediatric client's understanding of self-management–related knowledge through an informal interview or with a structured assessment tool such as the Brief Illness Perception Questionnaire (BIPQ; Broadbent et al., 2006). The BIPQ is a nine-item questionnaire that is designed to a capture a snapshot of the client's understanding about their condition and how to manage it. Some topics addressed through the BIPQ include how able the client feels to manage the condition, the client's understanding of the consequences associated with not taking care of the condition, and the client's level of concern about the severity of the condition (Broadbent et al., 2006). The BIPQ has good concurrent, predictive, and discriminant validity (Broadbent et al., 2006; Broadbent et al., 2015). Repeat administrations of the BIPQ provide the occupational therapist with information about how the client's knowledge is growing and how they are adapting during the course of intervention (Broadbent et al., 2015).

The Transition Readiness Assessment Questionnaire (TRAQ; Wood et al., 2014) is an example of a condition-neutral tool that is skill-focused. This self-report questionnaire provides an opportunity for adolescents to rate themselves on 29 self-management and self-advocacy behaviors. The TRAQ was developed based on feedback from an adolescent focus group and is thought to have good content validity, as well as excellent internal consistency (Zhang et al., 2014). The questionnaire items are organized into five domains: medication management, appointment keeping, tracking health issues, talking with providers, and managing daily activities (Wood et al., 2014).

Executive functioning highly influences one's ability to become a successful self-manager. The Weekly Calendar Planning Activity (WCPA; Toglia, 2015) is one assessment tool that occupational therapists can use to assess the executive functioning of youth with chronic conditions. One benefit of the WCPA is that the test items mirror some of the activities that the individual will need to complete on a regular basis as a self-manager (e.g., scheduling appointments). The WCPA also provides detailed information about how clients with self-management concerns approach tasks, and select and use strategies, as well as the types of challenges that are encountered and how clients adapt to overcome those challenges (Zlotnik et al., 2019).

Intervention

Children who are referred to occupational therapy specifically to address self-management of a chronic condition typically receive services in school systems, private outpatient clinics, or diagnosis-specific, hospital-run clinics (Figure 7-2). However, occupational therapy practitioners working with children and youth in any setting may encounter individuals with chronic conditions who could benefit from the development of self-management knowledge and skills. Children and youth seen for self-management are usually seen for brief intervention periods that necessitate a high level of primary caregiver involvement.

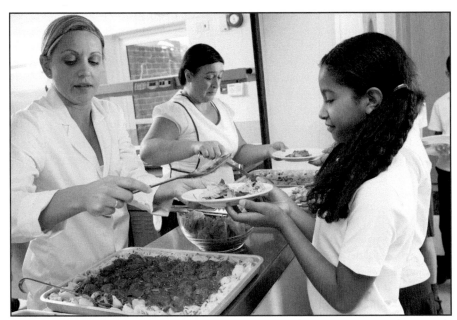

Figure 7-2. Student making healthy school lunch choices. (Monkey Business Images/shutterstock.com.)

Despite having different diagnoses, many children and youth with chronic conditions encounter similar challenges, such as experiencing fatigue and pain and needing to develop highly structured routines for medications and treatments (Lindsay et al., 2014). They also have to negotiate responsibilities related to condition management with parents, service providers, and school personnel (Lindsay et al., 2014; Polo & Cahill, 2017). Interventions for children and youth with chronic conditions address competence with medical management tasks, symptom management, and self-advocacy (Cahill et al., 2016; Lindsay et al., 2014). This competence leads to adaptation and resiliency. Occupational therapists design interventions in keeping with the child's or adolescent's developmental level and their current self-care abilities (Lindsay et al., 2014). The primary outcomes of occupational therapy intervention are increased independence and adherence to health maintenance and health promotion routines.

Functional goals are based on findings from a comprehensive evaluation and are written to measure the progress associated with the occupational therapy intervention targeting self-management. Goal attainment scaling, which is an individualized criterion-referenced process, can be used both to establish goals and to gauge progress (King et al., 2000). The goal attainment scaling process requires the occupational therapist to have a clear understanding of the steps involved in the self-management task or routine, the client's baseline level of performance, and the expected outcome of intervention. The occupational therapist first works with the client to establish a goal and then identifies a range of specific outcomes for the goal using a predetermined numerical scale. The client's progress is measured using the scale during the intervention period.

Occupational therapists use a combination of several different intervention approaches to support the coping, adaptation, and resilience of children and youth with chronic conditions. Some of the intervention approaches that can be used include psychoeducation (Saxby et al., 2019), motivational interviewing (Schaefer & Kavookjian, 2017), skills training (Piven & Duran, 2014), habit training (Gupta et al., 2018; Pérez et al., 2019), family-focused interventions (Knafl et al., 2017), and role-management training (Schmidt et al., 2020). Intervention approaches are selected based on the desired outcomes of intervention, and a combination of several different approaches is often required. Table 7-2 includes descriptions of the intervention approaches mentioned here, as well as their desired outcomes.

FAMILY COLLABORATION

Transitioning condition management from the caregivers to the child or adolescent requires intentional planning. Occupational therapists collaborate with families and other individuals in the child's social context to build adaptation, coping, and resilience. Goralski et al. (2017) recommend that the transition of responsibilities from the caregiver to the child happen early. The occupational therapy practitioner can support the transition process by working with children and their caregivers to develop a structured plan that includes the types of medical knowledge that will be shared and when, as well as helping them to match condition management skills with the child's developmental level. A personal medical history (Goralski et al., 2017) is one tool that can help children or adolescents learn more about their condition and the unique way it has affected them. The KIT: Keeping It Together tool (https://www.canchild.ca/en/research-in-practice/the-kit-keeping-it-together) developed by the CanChild Centre for Disability Research is an excellent way to organize the child's medical history, as well as other information that might be important to health providers. Using a tool like this also helps to promote self-advocacy. Working with the child to obtain this basic information is essential because many youth with chronic conditions have been protected from full knowledge of some of their health information by well-meaning health care providers and adults (Ödling et al., 2019).

Transitioning the role of condition manager is complex because the experiences of the caregivers and the child are mutually dependent (Nguyen et al., 2016). Children and youth tend to rely on their parents for support and guidance while they are becoming self-managers. Even when children and youth feel competent in their new role, parents often report having to provide reminders and additional assistance that cause them to question their child's ability to handle situations safely (Nguyen et al., 2016). Unrelated family tensions and conflicts may contribute to a caregiver's perceptions of the child's success and caregiver hesitancy to relinquish control over their child's condition management, which could ultimately limit a child's adaptation (Knafl et al., 2017). During intervention sessions, the occupational therapist should strive to engage parents as collaborators, working to help them to see their role as one of coach instead of safety net. In some cases, occupational therapists may refer families to a counselor or social worker to get assistance with addressing family dynamics or other mediating factors.

Table 7-2

Self-Management Intervention Approaches and Desired Outcomes		
Intervention Approach	**Description**	**Desired Outcomes**
Psychoeducation (Saxby et al., 2019)	Formal sequenced curriculum that includes opportunities for active participation, feedback, and collaboration with caregivers, providers, and group members. This approach emphasizes supporting the development of autonomy and independent problem solving, which is usually shaped through reinforcement and multiple opportunities to apply knowledge.	Increased knowledge about chronic condition and medical management across the lifespan.
Motivational interviewing (Schaefer & Kavookjian, 2017)	Empowers individuals to discover personal motivation and commitment to change health-related behaviors. Strategies include respectful questioning, affirmation, reflection, and sharing information. The practitioner helps to focus the client and guide the client toward goal-directed plans.	Increased adoption of positive, health-focused behaviors and development of problem-solving abilities.
Skills training (Piven & Duran, 2014)	Occupation-based and client-centered intervention activities that are specific to the management of the individual's chronic condition (e.g., teaching client with diabetes to perform daily glucose checks; Figure 7-3).	Increased psychomotor skills associated with self-management.
Habit training (Gupta et al., 2018; Pérez et al., 2019)	Supporting the individual to develop a regimented schedule and disciplined approach to manage their health condition. This can be accomplished through collaborative problem solving and low-tech (e.g., paper checklist/reminders) or high-tech (e.g., smartphone apps) strategies, or embedding the condition-related habit in another routine (e.g., pet care).	Increased use of health maintenance and health promotion habits and routines, particularly medication adherence, to manage symptoms and prevent exacerbations.
Family-focused interventions (Knafl et al., 2017)	Family members are encouraged to actively participate in the intervention to increase the child's capacity to manage the condition and enhance family functioning.	Increased collaboration and shared responsibility between caregivers and client.
Role-management training (Schmidt et al., 2020)	Empowering the client to represent their own interests to health care providers and other individuals in power. A peer-led group focused on condition-specific advocacy is one widely used strategy.	Increased competence in health consumer role and increased self-advocacy skills.

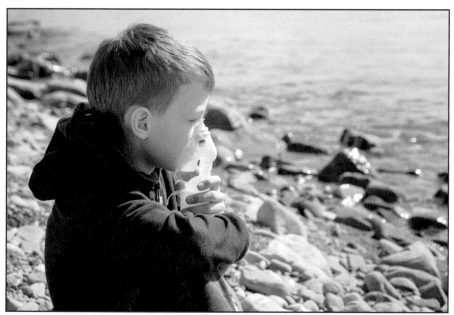

Figure 7-3. Child with cystic fibrosis nebulizing while relaxing on the beach. (Evgeniia Zakharishcheva/shutterstock.com.)

BUILDING INTERPROFESSIONAL COLLABORATIONS

In addition to working with families, occupational therapists also collaborate as part of interprofessional teams to facilitate adaptation, coping, and resilience for children and youth with chronic conditions. Members of school teams are among the most common individuals with whom occupational therapists collaborate. A study by Selekman (2017) found that teachers frequently felt that they had insufficient preparation to support children with chronic conditions at school and welcomed more communication with health care providers. Occupational therapy practitioners act as an important bridge between medical and educational systems. Occupational therapists can collaborate with teachers to increase their understanding of specific chronic conditions, the management of such conditions, and how the conditions influence a child's performance and engagement in school. Occupational therapy practitioners may also collaborate with teachers to identify appropriate times and locations for students to perform medical care routines.

School nurses often oversee school-based medical interventions (e.g., medication administration, airway clearance techniques); however, they welcome support from occupational therapists to help children and youth develop coping skills related to their condition (Polo & Cahill, 2017). Coping and problem-solving skills, as well as a child's ability to adapt to unanticipated events, are important factors associated with mental health and quality of life (Jackson et al., 2015; Matza et al., 2004). Occupational therapists can support the development of coping and adaptation at school by examining the challenges posed by the environment and the demands of the student's specific chronic condition to develop targeted interventions that build the child's capacity to manage the condition at school (Polo & Cahill, 2017).

A GLOBAL PERSPECTIVE

The United Nations Children's Fund (UNICEF) recognizes a need for education related to non-communicable diseases, some of which are acquired chronic conditions like the ones discussed in this chapter (e.g., type 2 diabetes), as well as others that are often diagnosed in middle adulthood (e.g., heart disease) but have their roots in poor childhood health practices. Non-communicable diseases account for 71% of annual deaths globally and significantly affect individuals experiencing social and economic disparities, including children (UNICEF, 2019). Preventive measures, such as diet, exercise, and the reduction of environmental risk factors, are thought to be effective in delaying or reducing the incidence of these conditions (UNICEF, 2019). Occupational therapy practitioners can help to prevent non-communicable diseases in global populations of children and youth by addressing health promotion, management, and maintenance intervention (Reitz & Scaffa, 2020).

ESSENTIAL CONSIDERATIONS FOR OCCUPATIONAL THERAPISTS

The role of self-manager is an important one for children and youth with chronic conditions. Children and youth with chronic conditions may have challenges related to coping with their disease and adapting performance patterns to accommodate necessary self-management habits and routines. Occupational therapists collaborate with children and youth with chronic conditions, their family members, and interprofessional teams to transition condition management responsibilities from caregivers to the child or adolescent. Table 7-3 includes essential considerations for occupational therapists to build adaptation, coping, and resilience in children and youth with chronic conditions. Adaptation, coping, and resilience set the foundation for self-management of chronic conditions and lead to better health outcomes and improved quality of life.

Table 7-3

Essential Considerations for Occupational Therapists to Build Adaptation, Coping, and Resilience in Children and Youth With Chronic Conditions

- Collaborate with other professionals (e.g., school nurses) to learn more about the client's medical condition and treatment.
- Assess client's readiness to assume the role of self-manager.
- Match self-management goals to the client's developmental level and self-care abilities.
- Use goal attainment scaling to establish criteria for mastery for different self-management tasks.
- Use psychoeducational strategies to provide condition-specific information to the client and the client's family.
- Use motivational interviewing strategies to support behavior change and explore the client's motivations to engage in health promotion and health maintenance.
- Use skills-training interventions to teach the client the psychomotor skills needed to safely use medical equipment.
- Use habit training interventions to encourage the adoption of self-management habits and routines.
- Support the development of self-advocacy strategies to assist the client in cultivating the resilience necessary to maintain the self-manager role.
- Explore how family dynamics support or inhibit a client's attempts at self-management.

Case Study 7-3

Maxwell is a 13-year-old boy who lives with his fathers and 8-year-old sister in a large metropolitan area. Maxwell was recently diagnosed with type 1 diabetes following a hospital stay for acute diabetic ketoacidosis and symptoms of fatigue and weight loss. After Maxwell was discharged from the hospital, he struggled to cope with the demands associated with diabetes self-management, such as being able to draw up and administer his own insulin injections and having a good understanding of how to count carbohydrates. Upon his return to school, Maxwell and one of his fathers met with the school nurse to develop a diabetes medical management plan for school, which included occupational therapy services to help facilitate Maxwell's adaptation and integrate diabetes care routines into the school day.

The occupational therapist administered the Diabetes Self-Management Questionnaire (DSMQ; Harris et al., 2000). Table 7-4 includes a summary of the items on the DSMQ and how Maxwell rated them upon self-report. The

(continued)

Case Study 7-3 (continued)

Table 7-4

Summary of Maxwell's DSMQ Ratings			
Applies to Maxwell Very Much	Applies to Maxwell to a Considerable Degree	Applies to Maxwell to Some Degree	Does Not Apply to Maxwell
Checks blood sugar with care and attention	Diet helps to maintain blood sugar levels	Takes medications as prescribed	Records blood sugar levels to analyze trends
Keeps doctors' appointments	Strictly follows diabetes diet	Occasionally eats sweets	Avoid doctors' appointments
	Skips medication	Engages in regular physical activity	Fails to check blood sugars frequently
		Avoids physical activity	Binges on restricted foods
	Skips planned physical activity	Feels diabetes care is poor	Desires to see health professionals more often

occupational therapist discusses the findings from the DSMQ with Maxwell. The boy confirms that he struggles with taking medication regularly at school, avoids physical activity throughout the day, and does not feel confident managing his diabetes.

The occupational therapist determines that more information is needed about Maxwell's executive functioning skills and administers the Weekly Calendar Planning Activity (Toglia, 2015). The occupational therapist observes Maxwell during administration of the WCPA and notes the strategies that he uses. The occupational therapist notes that Maxwell struggles to cope with stressors and does not schedule fixed appointments before flexible ones, uses self-talk to a great extent, and rereads appointments before entering them into the schedule. The occupational therapist encourages Maxwell to reflect on his WCPA performance. Maxwell indicates that the WCPA was difficult for him and that he does not frequently do tasks like this or use assignment notebooks or planners on a regular basis. He indicates that he wished he could do the task again because he might try a new approach to schedule the WCPA appointments based on the suggestions provided by the occupational therapist.

Maxwell shares that he is currently adhering to his medication regimen 2 to 3 days per week and that, although he has signed up to attend the school's daily morning open gym time, he rarely goes. The occupational therapist and Maxwell discuss how occupational therapy intervention could support his management of diabetes at school. Two goals, one related to medication adherence and one related to increasing physical activity, are collaboratively developed

(continued)

Case Study 7-3 (continued)

Table 7-5

Maxwell's Goal Attainment Scaling		
Level	Physical Activity Goal	Medication Adherence Goal
−2 Much worse than expected	Maxwell actively participates in planned physical activity (i.e., morning open gym) 0 to 1/5 days per week.	Maxwell adheres to medicine regimen at school ≤ 3/5 days per week at school.
−1 Somewhat less than expected	Maxwell actively participates in planned physical activity (i.e., morning open gym) 2/5 days per week.	Maxwell adheres to medicine regimen at school 4/5 days per week at school.
0 Expected level	Maxwell actively participates in planned physical activity (i.e., morning open gym) 3/5 days per week.	Maxwell adheres to medicine regimen at school 5/5 days per week at school.
+1 Somewhat better than expected	Maxwell actively participates in planned physical activity (i.e., morning open gym) 4/5 days per week.	Maxwell adheres to medicine regimen at school 5/5 days per week at school and 1 weekend day.
+2 Much better than expected	Maxwell actively participates in planned physical activity (i.e., morning open gym) 5/5 days per week.	Maxwell adheres to medicine regimen at school 5/5 days per week at school and 2 weekend days.

with Maxwell and documented in his diabetes self-management plan. The occupational therapist uses goal attainment scaling to establish criteria for performance. Table 7-5 includes Maxwell's goal attainment scaling.

The occupational therapist and the rest of the team determine that Maxwell will need direct occupational therapy services for at least one academic quarter, with periodic follow-ups for the rest of the school year. The occupational therapist designs an intervention to facilitate adaptive capacity using a combination of approaches, including psychoeducation, motivational interviewing, and habit training. Maxwell and the occupational therapist meet during study hall one time every week. Table 7-6 includes a description of the steps taken by the occupational therapist to implement Maxwell's intervention plan in order to support Maxwell's adaptation and independence with self-management skills at school. Maxwell eventually demonstrates resilience by independently adhering to his medication management routine and regularly including physical activity in his day.

(continued)

Case Study 7-3 (continued)

Table 7-6

Steps Taken by Occupational Therapist to Implement Maxwell's Intervention Plan

Psychoeducation

- Occupational therapist meets with school nurse to review Maxwell's diabetes medical management plan.
- Occupational therapist shares the Juvenile Diabetes Research Fund's Teen Toolkit (http://www.jdrf.org/wp-content/uploads/2013/10/JDRFTEENTOOLKIT.pdf) with Maxwell's fathers and invites dialogue about how Maxwell manages his condition at home and at school.
- Occupational therapist reviews the school medical management plan with Maxwell and answers questions.
- Occupational therapist provides Maxwell with *Type 1 Teens: A Guide to Managing Diabetes* (Hood, 2010) and opportunities to demonstrate knowledge gained through conversations and the development of a video blog for teenagers newly diagnosed with type 1 diabetes.
- Occupational therapist assesses Maxwell's knowledge about type 1 diabetes through a trivia game.

Motivational Interviewing

- Occupational therapist and Maxwell discuss his difficulties with medication adherence and attending open gym.
- Occupational therapist listens to Maxwell's perspectives without conveying judgment.
- Occupational therapist expresses empathy for Maxwell's situation, but confronts inaccurate perceptions (e.g., "I'll never be able to remember to take my medication") and points out the discrepancies between Maxwell's current health behaviors and his goal of being healthy and managing his condition independently.
- Occupational therapist and Maxwell brainstorm strategies that Maxwell can use to engage in health-supporting behaviors and review additional strategies presented in *The Diabetes Game: A Teenager's Guide to Living Well With Diabetes* (Coon, 2006), which includes a teenager's perspectives about living with diabetes and the strategies she used to overcome different challenges.
- Occupational therapist encourages Maxwell to commit to trying new strategies.
- Occupational therapist and Maxwell review strategies that were attempted and the occupational therapist reinforces Maxwell's attempts.

(continued)

Case Study 7-3 (continued)

Table 7-6 (continued)

Steps Taken by Occupational Therapist to Implement Maxwell's Intervention Plan

Habit Training

- Occupational therapist and Maxwell review his daily schedule and spaces in the school building to identify times and places where he can engage in self-management tasks, including blood glucose testing and medication administration.
- Occupational therapist and Maxwell identify already established routines (e.g., going to locker to change books) that can be used as anchors for condition-management routines.

- Occupational therapist works with Maxwell to set up the alarm and calendar features on his smartphone to schedule reminders for testing blood sugar and taking medication.
- Occupational therapist and Maxwell develop a cloud-based tracking form so he can record his daily blood sugar levels and medication regime.
- Occupational therapist introduces Maxwell to different smartphone applications, such as MyFitnessPal, to set and monitor physical activity goals throughout the week. Maxwell decides to use MyFitnessPal to track daily food intake, as well.

REFERENCES

American Occupational Therapy Association. (2020). Occupational therapy practice framework: Domain and process (4th ed.). *American Journal of Occupational Therapy, 74*(Suppl. 2), 7412410010. https://doi.org/10.5014/ajot.2020.74S2001

American Occupational Therapy Association. (2021). The Association—Improve your documentation and quality of care with AOTA's updated Occupational Profile Template. *American Journal of Occupational Therapy, 75*, 7502420010. https://doi.org/10.5014/ajot.2021.752001

Bregnballe, V., Boisen, K. A., Schiøtz, P. O., Pressler, T., & Lomborg, K. (2017). Flying the nest: A challenge for young adults with cystic fibrosis and their parents. *Patient Preference and Adherence, 11*, 229-236. https://doi.org/10.2147/PPA.S124814

Broadbent, E., Petrie, K. J., Main, J., & Weinman, J. (2006). The Brief Illness Perception Questionnaire. *Journal of Psychosomatic Research, 60*(6), 631-637. https://doi.org/10.1016/j.jpsychores.2005.10.020

Broadbent, E., Wilkes, C., Koschwanez, H., Weinman, J., Norton, S., & Petrie, K. J. (2015). A systematic review and meta-analysis of the Brief Illness Perception Questionnaire. *Psychology & Health, 30*(11), 1361-1385. https://doi.org/10.1080/08870446.2015.1070851

Cahill, S. (2020). Evaluation, interpretation, and goal writing. In J. O'Brien & H. Kuhaneck (Eds.), *Case-Smith's occupational therapy for children and adolescents* (pp.181-197). Elsevier.

Cahill, S. M., Polo, K. M., Egan, B. E., & Marasti, N. (2016). Interventions to promote diabetes self-management in children and youth: A scoping review. *American Journal of Occupational Therapy, 70*(5), 7005180020. https://doi.org/10.5014/ajot.2016.021618

Cameron, G., & Wherrett, D. (2015). Care of diabetes in children and adolescents: Controversies, changes, and consensus. *Lancet, 385*(9982), 2096-2106. https://doi.org/10.1016/S0140-6736(15)60971-0

Centers for Disease Control and Prevention. (2017). Diabetes in youth. https://www.cdc.gov/diabetestv/youth.html

Chiang, J. L., Kirkman, M. S., Laffel, L. M., Peters, A. L., on behalf of the *Type 1 Diabetes Sourcebook* authors. (2014). Type 1 diabetes through the life span: A position statement of the American Diabetes Association. *Diabetes Care, 37*(7), 2034-2054. https://doi.org/10.2337/dc14-1140

Compas, B. E., Connor-Smith, J. K., Saltzman, H., Thomsen, A. H., & Wadsworth, M. E. (2001). Coping with stress during childhood and adolescence: Problems, progress, and potential in theory and research. *Psychological Bulletin, 127*(1), 87-127. https://doi.org/10.1037/0033-2909.127.1.87

Coon, N. (2006). *The diabetes game: A teenager's guide to living well with diabetes.* Rewarding HealthSM.

Cron, R., Weiser, P., & Beukelman, T. (2019). Juvenile idiopathic arthritis. In R. Rich, T. Fleisher, W. Shearer, H. Schroeder, A. Frew, & C. Weyand (Eds.), *Clinical immunology* (5th ed., pp. 723-733). Elsevier. https://doi.org/10.1016/B978-0-7020-6896-6.00053-3

Dellon, E., Chen, E., Goggin, J., Homa, K., Marshall, B., Sabadosa, K., & Cohen, R. (2016). Advance care planning in cystic fibrosis: Current practices, challenges, and opportunities. *Journal of Cystic Fibrosis, 15*(1), 96-101. https://doi.org/10.1016/j.jcf.2015.08.004

Goralski, J. L., Nasr, S. Z., & Uluer, A. (2017). Overcoming barriers to a successful transition from pediatric to adult care. *Pediatric Pulmonology, 52*(S48), S52-S60. https://doi.org/10.1002/ppul.23778

Grajo, L. (2019). Occupational adaptation as a normative and intervention process: Schkade and Schultz's legacy. In L. C. Grajo & A. Boisselle (Eds.), *Adaptation through occupation: Multidimensional perspectives* (pp. 83-104). SLACK Incorporated.

Gupta, O. T., Wiebe, D. J., Pyatak, E. A., & Beck, A. M. (2018). Improving medication adherence in the pediatric population using integrated care of companion animals. *Patient Education and Counseling, 101*(10), 1876-1878. https://doi.org/10.1016/j.pec.2018.05.015

Harris, M., Wysocki, T., Sadler, M., Wilkinson, K., Harvey, L., Buckloh, L., Mauras, N., & White, N. (2000). Validation of a structured interview for the assessment of diabetes self-management. *Diabetes Care, 23*(9), 1301-1304. https://doi.org/10.2337/diacare.23.9.1301

Heaton, J., Räisänen, U., & Salinas, M. (2016). 'Rule your condition, don't let it rule you': Young adults' sense of mastery in their accounts of growing up with a chronic illness. *Sociology of Health & Illness, 38*(1), 3-20. https://doi.org/10.1111/1467-9566.12298

Hood, K. (2010). *Type 1 teens: A guide to managing diabetes.* American Psychology Association.

Jackson, C. C., Albanese-O'Neill, A., Butler, K. L., Chiang, J. L., Deeb, L. C., Hathaway, K., . . . Siminerio, L. M. (2015). Diabetes care in the school setting: A position statement of the American Diabetes Association. *Diabetes Care, 38*(10), 1958-1963. https://doi.org/10.2337/dc15-1418

King, G. A., McDougall, J., Palisano, R. J., Gritzan, J., & Tucker, M. A. (2000). Goal attainment scaling: Its use in evaluating pediatric therapy programs. *Physical & Occupational Therapy in Pediatrics, 19*(2), 31-52. https://doi.org/10.1080/J006v19n02_03

Knafl, K. A., Havill, N. L., Leeman, J., Fleming, L., Crandell, J. L., & Sandelowski, M. (2017). The nature of family engagement in interventions for children with chronic conditions. *Western Journal of Nursing Research, 39*(5), 690-723. https://doi.org/10.1177/0193945916664700

Knudsen, K. B., Boisen, K. A., Katzenstein, T. L., Mortensen, L. H., Pressler, T., Skov, M., & Jarden, M. (2018). Living with cystic fibrosis—A qualitative study of a life coaching intervention. *Patient Preference and Adherence, 12*, 585-594. https://doi.org/10.2147/PPA.S159306

Lawson, E. F., Hersh, A. O., Applebaum, M. A., Yelin, E. H., Okumura, M. J., & von Scheven, E. (2011). Self-management skills in adolescents with chronic rheumatic disease: A cross-sectional survey. *Pediatric Rheumatology, 9*, 35. https://doi.org/10.1186/1546-0096-9-35

Lindsay, S., Kingsnorth, S., Mcdougall, C., & Keating, H. (2014). A systematic review of self-management interventions for children and youth with physical disabilities. *Disability and Rehabilitation, 36*(4), 276-288. https://doi.org/10.3109/09638288.2013.785605

Linnemann, R., O'Malley, P., Friedman, D., Georgiopoulos, A., Buxton, D., Altstein, L., Sicilian, L., Lapey, A., Sawicki, G., & Moskowitz, S. (2016). Development and evaluation of a palliative care curriculum for cystic fibrosis healthcare providers. *Journal of Cystic Fibrosis, 15*(1), 90-95. https://doi.org/10.1016/j.jcf.2015.03.005

Lozano, P., & Houtrow, A. (2018). Supporting self-management in children and adolescents with complex chronic conditions. *Pediatrics, 141*(Suppl. 3), S233-S241. https://doi.org/10.1542/peds.2017-1284H

Matza, L. S., Swensen, A. R., Flood, E. M., Secnik, K., & Leidy, N. K. (2004). Assessment of health-related quality of life in children: A review of conceptual, methodological, and regulatory issues. *Value in Health, 7*(1), 79-92. https://doi.org/10.1111/j.1524-4733.2004.71273.x

Miller, G. F., Coffield, E., Leroy, Z., & Wallin, R. (2016). Prevalence and costs of five chronic conditions in children. *The Journal of School Nursing, 32*(5), 357-364. https://doi.org/10.1177/1059840516641190

Nguyen, T., Henderson, D., Stewart, D., Hlyva, O., Punthakee, Z., & Gorter, J. W. (2016). You never transition alone! Exploring the experiences of youth with chronic health conditions, parents and healthcare providers on self-management. *Child: Care, Health and Development, 42*(4), 464-472. https://doi.org/10.1111/cch.12334

Ödling, M., Jonsson, M., Janson, C., Melén, E., Bergström, A., & Kull, I. (2019). Lost in the transition from pediatric to adult healthcare? Experiences of young adults with severe asthma. *Journal of Asthma, 57*(10), 1119-1127. https://doi.org/10.1080/02770903.2019.1640726

Pérez, Y. I. V., Medlow, S., Ho, J., & Steinbeck, K. (2019). Mobile and web-based apps that support self-management and transition in young people with chronic illness: Systematic review. *Journal of Medical Internet Research, 21*(11), e13579. https://doi.org/10.2196/13579

Pettitt, D. J., Talton, J., Dabelea, D., Divers, J., Imperatore, G., Lawrence, J. M., . . . Hamman, R. F., for the SEARCH for Diabetes in Youth Study Group. (2014). Prevalence of diabetes in U.S. youth in 2009: The SEARCH for Diabetes in Youth Study. *Diabetes Care, 37*(2), 402-408. https://doi.org/10.2337/dc13-1838

Pinquart, M., & Pfeiffer, J. P. (2015). Solving developmental tasks in adolescents with a chronic physical illness or physical/sensory disability: A meta-analysis. *International Journal of Disability, Development and Education, 62*(3), 249-264. https://doi.org/10.1080/1034912X.2015.1020922

Piven, E., & Duran, R. (2014). Reduction of non-adherent behaviour in a Mexican-American adolescent with type 2 diabetes. *Occupational Therapy International, 21*(1), 42-51. https://doi.org/10.1002/oti.1363

Polo, K., & Cahill, S. (2017). Interprofessional collaboration to support children with diabetes. *The Open Journal of Occupational Therapy, 5*(3), Article 3. https://doi.org/10.15453/2168-6408.1338

Pyatak, E. (2011). Participation in occupation and diabetes self-management in emerging adulthood. *American Journal of Occupational Therapy, 65*(4), 462-469. https://doi.org/10.5014/ajot.2011.001453

Quittner, A. L., Goldbeck, L., Abbott, J., Duff, A., Lambrecht, P., & Solé, A. (2014). Prevalence of depression and anxiety in patients with cystic fibrosis and parent caregivers: Results of the International Depression Epidemiological Study across nine countries. *Thorax, 69*(12): 1090-1097. https://doi.org/10.1136/thoraxjnl-2014-205983

Reitz, M., & Scaffa, M. (2020). Occupational therapy in the promotion of health and well-being. *American Journal of Occupational Therapy, 74*(3): 7403420010. https://doi.org/10.5014/ajot.2020.743003

Saxby, N., Beggs, S., Battersby, M., & Lawn, S. (2019). What are the components of effective chronic condition self-management education interventions for children with asthma, cystic fibrosis, and diabetes? A systematic review. *Patient Education and Counseling, 102*(4), 607-622. https://doi.org/10.1016/j.pec.2018.11.001

Schaefer, M. R., & Kavookjian, J. (2017). The impact of motivational interviewing on adherence and symptom severity in adolescents and young adults with chronic illness: A systematic review. *Patient Education and Counseling, 100*(12), 2190-2199. https://doi.org/10.1016/j.pec.2017.05.037

Schmidt, E. K., Faieta, J., & Tanner, K. (2020). Scoping review of self-advocacy education interventions to improve care. *OTJR: Occupation, Participation and Health, 40*(1), 50-56. https://doi.org/10.1177/1539449219860583

Selekman, J. (2017). Students with chronic conditions: Experiences and challenges of regular education teachers. *The Journal of School Nursing, 33*(4), 307-315. https://doi.org/10.1177/1059840516674053

Spencer, G., Lewis, S., & Reid, M. (2019). The agentic Self and uncontrollable body: Young people's management of chronic illness at university. *Health, 25*(3), 1363459319889088. https://doi.org/10.1177/1363459319889088

Stinson, J. N., Lalloo, C., Harris, L., Isaac, L., Campbell, F., Brown, S., . . . & Buckley, N. (2014). iCan-Cope with Pain™: User-centred design of a web-and mobile-based self-management program for youth with chronic pain based on identified health care needs. *Pain Research and Management, 19*(5), 257-265. https://doi.org/10.1155/2014/935278

Stinson, J. N., Luca, N. J., & Jibb, L. A. (2012). Assessment and management of pain in juvenile idiopathic arthritis. *Pain Research and Management, 17*(6), 391-396. https://doi.org/10.1155/2012/237258

Thompson, M. (2014). Occupations, habits, and routines: Perspectives from persons with diabetes. *Scandinavian Journal of Occupational Therapy, 21*(2), 153-160. https://doi.org/10.3109/11038128.2013.85 1278

Toglia, J. (2015). *Weekly calendar planning activity?: A performance test of executive function.* AOTA Press.

United Nations Children's Fund (UNICEF). (2019). *Program guidance for early-life prevention of non-communicable diseases.* UNICEF.

Wood, D., Sawicki, G., Miller, M., Smotherman, C., Lukens-Bull, K., Livingwood, W., Ferris, M., & Kraemer, D. (2014). The Transition Readiness Assessment Questionnaire (TRAQ): Its factor structure, reliability and validity. *Academic Pediatrics, 14*(4), 415-422. https://doi.org/10.1016/j.acap.2014.03.008

Zhang, L. F., Ho, J. S., & Kennedy, S. E. (2014). A systematic review of the psychometric properties of transition readiness assessment tools in adolescents with chronic disease. *BMC Pediatrics, 14*(1), 4. https://doi.org/10.1186/1471-2431-14-4

Zimmer-Gembeck, M. J., & Skinner, E. A. (2016). The development of coping: Implications for psychopathology and resilience. *Developmental psychopathology* (vol. 4), 1-61. https://doi.org/10.1002/9781119125556.devpsy410

Zlotnik, S., Schiff, A., Ravid, S., Shahar, E., & Toglia, J. (2019). A new approach for assessing functional cognition and its unique expression in adolescents with epilepsy. *American Journal of Occupational Therapy, 73*(4, Suppl. 1), 7311500070. https://doi.org/10.5014/ajot.2019.73S1-RP401E

8

Children and Youth With Cerebral Palsy

Angela K. Boisselle, PhD, OTR

> **CHAPTER OBJECTIVES** By the end of this chapter, the reader will be able to:
> - Explain how coping and adaptive risk factors and positive strategies may affect the overall health, well-being, and participation in occupations of children and youth with cerebral palsy.
> - Describe assessment tools that can be used to evaluate coping, adaptation, and resilience in children and youth with cerebral palsy.
> - Apply intervention principles that promote coping, adaptation, and resilience in children and youth with cerebral palsy.
> - Apply elements of sense of self, connection, and adaptation to foster resilience in children and youth with cerebral palsy.

OVERVIEW OF THE POPULATION

Cerebral palsy (CP) is a non-progressive disorder that primarily affects motor abilities as a result of neurological injury before or soon after birth. Individuals with cerebral palsy may encounter a myriad of associated conditions, such as respiratory, gastrointestinal, and cognitive issues, that often result in more functional impairment than the condition of CP (Glader & Stevenson, 2019). The prevalence of cerebral palsy is approximately 1 in 500 (Novak et al., 2017). Cerebral palsy is the most common childhood motoric disability globally, with prevalence most influenced by gestational age of less than 28 weeks and/or birth weight around 2.2 pounds (Oskoui et al., 2013). Refer to Boisselle (2022) for a full overview of cerebral palsy.

Grajo, L. C., & Boisselle, A. K. (Eds.). *Adaptation, Coping, and Resilience in Children and Youth: A Comprehensive Occupational Therapy Approach* (pp. 183-208).
© 2022 Taylor & Francis Group.

Diagnosis

Diagnosis of CP can be challenging due to the complexity and broad presentation of the condition. Historically, CP is diagnosed at around 12 to 24 months of age, though in some cases later. Accurate and early diagnosis of cerebral palsy is possible with comprehensive developmental screenings and surveillance (Novak et al., 2017). If motor concerns are suspected, a combination of definitive diagnostic testing can be used, which may include brain magnetic imaging resonance (MRI), motor and developmental testing, neurological examination, cranial ultrasound, and genomic testing, as early as 6 months of age (Bosanquet et al., 2013; Novak et al., 2017). The direct causes of CP are complex and often unclear, but are a result of various risk factors present before, during, and after birth, including but not limited to: parental factors such as maternal age, multiple gestations, and genetic factors; infections; asphyxia; placental abruption; periventricular leukomalacia; hypoxic-ischemic brain injury; encephalitis; perinatal stroke; and meningitis (Bosanquet et al., 2013; Glader & Stevenson, 2019; Novak et al., 2017).

Types and Classification of Cerebral Palsy

Cerebral palsy affects muscle tone either with spasticity (also known as *velocity-dependent hypertonia*) or low muscle tone (also known as *hypotonia*). Spasticity is the most common type of CP and affects different regions of the body, most commonly: *hemiplegia* (right or left side); *diplegia* (primarily lower extremities); and *quadriplegia* (symmetrical spasticity of all four limbs). Mixed-type CP manifests with spasticity and an underlying movement disorder such as dystonia, athetosis, or ataxia (Glader & Stevenson, 2019; Novak et al., 2017).

Through an international collaborative effort, several evidence-based clinical classification systems were developed to standardize the description of motor function of children with CP on five levels, which describe minimal to moderate assistance needed for participation (I-III) to maximal assistance needed related to motor function (IV-V). Two examples are the Gross Motor Function Classification System (GMFCS; Palisano et al., 1997) and the Manual Ability Classification System (MACS; Eliasson et al., 2006). The Gross Motor Function Classification System (Palisano et al., 1997) classifies functional ambulatory abilities and assistance needed. It is the most commonly used for multidisciplinary CP practice, outcomes data, and research (Novak et al., 2013). The Manual Ability Classification System (Eliasson et al., 2006) classifies functional motor ability of the upper extremities and assistance needed in the same manner as the GMFCS and is widely used in occupational therapy practice and research.

Over the past couple of decades, the perception about disability has shifted from a biomedical focus of impairment and limitation to a focus on function and participation (Novak et al., 2013; Rosenbaum & Gorter, 2012). The World Health Organization's (WHO's) *International Classification of Functioning, Disability and Health for Children and Youth* (ICF-CY; WHO, 2007) supplements the World Health Organization's *International Classification of Functioning, Disability and Health* (ICF; WHO, 2001) and offers an international conceptual framework to identify domains of function, including body structure and function, activities, and participation as related to environmental and person factors. The ICF-CY acknowledges that child development is a dynamic process, ranging from complete dependence on family to one of some level of competence and independence, and that the child's family and the psychosocial environment are instrumental in this process. It is noteworthy for the purpose of this chapter that adaptation and resilience related to participation are closely connected to the child's health, social engagement, and overall well-being (Anaby et al., 2017; Masten, 2018; Novak et al., 2013). This chapter attempts to shift the focus from motor limitations of the child to the psychosocial perspective for occupational therapy assessment and intervention.

DEFINING ADAPTATION, COPING, AND RESILIENCE FOR CHILDREN AND YOUTH WITH CEREBRAL PALSY

Developmental resilience research appears to share focus on the individual and the family systems. Similar to the shift from biomedical to activity/participation models in rehabilitation and medicine, the concept of resilience has changed over time from one rooted in the disease process to one of dynamic and complex systems related to health and societal and global contexts (Masten, 2018; Masten & Barnes, 2018).

Coping is one's ability to manage and solve problems related to daily environmental or psychosocial stressors. Daily stressors and adversity are not necessarily negative and can promote growth when presented in a balanced manner (Majnemer et al., 2010; National Scientific Council on the Developing Child, 2015). *Adaptation* in the context of this chapter and book goes beyond that of modifying the environment or activity. It is related to the continuous internal process to respond to and overcome challenges through occupation (Grajo et al., 2019). Development of *adaptive capacity* is demonstrated by mental flexibility and the ability to solve daily problems when presented with occupational challenges (Grajo, 2019). Adaptation is also dependent upon contextual demands and dynamics of human connections (Masten & Barnes, 2018; National Scientific Council on the Developing Child, 2015). In relation to children with CP, *resilience* is the ability to cope and adapt with competence and sense of self-worth and hope in the face of adversity and occurs throughout development (Masten & Barnes, 2018; National Scientific Council on the Developing Child, 2015).

Whitney et al. (2019) conducted a comparative study of mental health of children with cerebral palsy and those without disabilities. The authors found that children with CP have an increased risk for CP-related depression, anxiety, and other mental health problems associated with cumulative issues related to reduced physical activity, poor quality of sleep, and increased pain. In a survey of parents of 61 children with CP (ages 5 to 15), Yamaguchi et al. (2014) found that 59% of those children experience some level of pain with associated pain-related anxiety, depression, or behavioral outcomes. These child-specific internal factors may not only affect the child's ability to cope with stressors, but also affect the family's ability to effectively manage stress.

Child and Family Coping and Resilience

Given that parenting is essential to child resilience, it is not surprising that much of the CP literature on adaptation and resilience is caregiver-focused. Caregivers promote positive development through co-occupations (those that are mutually engaged in by child and caregiver) that provide positive supports, protection, and facilitate regulation (American Occupational Therapy Association [AOTA], 2020a; Masten, 2018). Fairfax et al. (2019) conducted a comprehensive systematic review of quality of life (QoL) for caregivers of children with chronic illnesses. Positive coping strategies (e.g., social connection, time management) were consistent with positive QoL. The authors found that higher levels of complexity of care may result in poorer coping strategies (disengagement, substance abuse, avoidance) on behalf of the caregiver, thus resulting in disengagement of care and ultimately decreased quality of life for the child with CP. Along with complexity of care, another risk factor involves parenting that is overprotective or does not facilitate independence. Literature suggests that adaptive capacity and ultimately resilience may be related to an acknowledgement of interdependence (based on co-occupations) and an adjusted sense of "normal" rather than an acute focus on "fixing" the child (AOTA, 2020b; Rosenbaum & Gorter, 2012).

Many external stress-inducing factors can affect the family in several ways that have an impact on the child's ability to cope and exhibit resilience. Financial strain from medical management of CP can contribute to overall family stress. Overall, family burden due to out-of-pocket expenses (e.g., durable medical equipment, prescriptions, co-pays) and possible ancillary costs (e.g., travel, lodging, days off work) may affect family members' perception of stressors (Masten, 2018; Novak et al., 2013).

Children and youth with CP can present in many complex ways due to varied functional abilities, co-morbidities, and familial and psychosocial dynamics (among other factors), which can make it an arduous task to broadly and succinctly identify abilities for adaptation, coping, and resilience. For example, a child with quadriplegia may have severe motor impairments and limited ability to communicate but have typical cognitive abilities and sense of competence. Caregivers, teachers, medical providers, and/or peers may perceive that the child with CP cannot make independent decisions based on limited motor and verbal abilities. Additionally, caregivers may be hyperfocused on therapy appointments in order for the child to meet developmental milestones. The child may not be given opportunities to freely explore the environment; thus, the child may miss typical opportunities for play, peer engagement, and other leisure occupations. Lastly, the lived environment may not be physically accessible for the child, thus limiting social engagement opportunities. These aspects may leave the child with an imbalanced opportunity for successful resilience due to higher risks for learned helplessness, social isolation, and/or occupational deprivation (AOTA, 2020b; Masten, 2018).

Children with more complex medical needs have higher need for all aspects of care due to increased functional limitations, and thus, there is greater caregiver burden in terms of finances, time, psychosocial interaction, and environmental aspects (Carona et al., 2014; Yamaguchi et al., 2014). Other family factors may also influence the child's participation. Arakelyan et al. (2019) conducted a systematic review on this topic and found that lower socioeconomic status, single-parent homes, and parental stress are correlated with a significant risk for decreased participation in daily activities for the child with CP. There was also a negative relationship between families of children with physical disabilities and recreational activity participation, particularly when it was perceived as too difficult for the child to participate. Conversely, parental and community support were positively associated with the child's participation.

Despite many of these findings, it is an oversimplified error to assume that the presence of cerebral palsy or any other disability consistently negatively influences one's ability to cope and adapt to daily stressors and participate functionally. In their seminal work, Albrecht and Devlieger (1999) conducted semi-structured interviews with 153 individuals with disabilities and found that 54% presented with a phenomenon known as the *disability paradox*, in which the individual with disability views their QoL in a positive manner despite the presence of disability. The authors articulated that an effective way to address the disability paradox is through balance:

> . . . equilibrium between the body, mind and spiritual components of individuals and the relationship of persons to their physical and social environment. We conceive of health and perceptions of quality of life as a result of this balance. Illness and dissatisfaction with life are a consequence of distortions in this balance. (p. 978)

Ultimately, health, well-being, and social circumstances play a significant role in the ability to effectively manage stress, adapt to change, and overcome challenges.

Case Study 8-1

Julina is a 5-year-old Hispanic female who was diagnosed with spastic diplegia at the age of 2. She lives on the second floor of a rented, three-bedroom house with her parents, two siblings, and maternal and paternal grandparents. Julina uses a wheelchair for distances and crawls while at home. She attends public school and her wheelchair is left at school because her afterschool daycare does not have room to transport it. Julina is unable to play with her peers after school and has to be carried or ride in a wagon when out in the community. Julina states that this makes her "feel like a baby." Her mother reports that Julina has quite a bit of pain in her legs at night and she is often up with Julina when her daughter can't sleep. Her mother reports that she often feels drained and stressed about medical bills and realizes that her attitude may negatively affect Julina by being disengaged in her therapy and help with her homework.

THE ROLE OF OCCUPATIONAL THERAPY: BEST AND EVIDENCE-BASED PRACTICES FOR ASSESSMENT AND INTERVENTION

The *Occupational Therapy Practice Framework, Fourth Edition* (*OTPF-4*) highlights that the domain and process of occupational therapy is achieved through health, well-being, and participation in life through engagement in occupation (AOTA, 2020a). Much of the current research on cerebral palsy supports focus on these areas; however, there appears to be a clear divide between research aims and practice as it relates to children with cerebral palsy (Kerr et al., 2018). For instance, Anaby et al. (2017) conducted a survey of 366 occupational and physical therapists to gain their perspective on views of assessment and intervention based on the ICF domains. The authors found that occupational therapists and physical therapists alike continue to focus on interventions classified as task-related activities (e.g., self-care, mobility) at 19% to 56% of the time, as opposed to participation-related activities (leisure and community activities) at 2% to 15% of intervention time. Given that the most common reason for referral of a child with CP is to address motoric limitations, the quandary becomes how occupational therapists can sufficiently provide assessment and interventions that address the child's ability to cope and capacity to adapt. In the following sections, I propose ideas to support assessment and intervention to address the psychosocial aspects of care for children and youth with cerebral palsy.

Assessment

Assessment focused on coping, adaptive capacity, and resilience requires a bit of a shift away from traditional methods typically used for children and youth with CP. Contributing factors that may impede this shift include, and are often related to, conventional expectations by payors and other medical professionals. For example, pediatric occupational therapists are often faced with challenging demands related to current health care standards that require meeting company productivity requirements and payor documentation requirements. Additionally, the physician may refer a child with cerebral palsy to occupational therapy for specific reasons that are rooted in the biomedical model. For example, a child may be referred immediately following an upper-extremity Botulinum toxin-A (Botox) injection (medicine used to reduce spasticity) to improve range of motion. The tendency of the occupational therapist may be to select evaluation tools that are readily available and can quickly provide standardized scores and address client factors or performance skills. The drawback to these types of tools is that they may be limitation-focused and/or based on body structures and routines rather than function and participation. To address this problem, it is suggested that occupational therapists select assessment measures that are grounded in function and participation, as well as those that are intended to gather gain perceptions and desired outcomes in regard to the child and/or caregiver(s) quality of life. Only then will occupational therapists be able to truly assess factors associated with adaptation, coping, and resilience as children encounter challenges situated within the context of functional tasks or occupational performance.

Neither specific performance skills nor upper extremity assessment are addressed here. For an overview of upper extremity assessment tools appropriate for children and youth with CP, refer to a systematic review by Wagner and Davids (2012). Goal-setting, participation, and QoL tools are specifically presented because they are related to psychosocial health and well-being (Table 8-1).

Goal-Setting Measures

One method to promote adaptability for the child with CP is through thoughtful goal-setting that encourages the child to solve problems and promotes a sense of mastery and self-regulation (National Scientific Council on the Developing Child, 2015). Measures such as the Canadian Occupational Performance Measure (COPM; Law et al., 2019) and the Goal Attainment Scale (GAS; Steenbeek et al., 2007) are centered around client- and family-centered care and have long been used for research and goal setting to address participation by clinical experts in cerebral palsy. Both use an interview style and patient-reported–outcome method to generate client-centered goals that can be designed to assess adaptive capacity and resilience within the context of participation.

Function and Participation Measures

Measurements that are based in function and participation help guide occupational therapists with specific areas that may require therapeutic intervention. Information gained can also help target therapeutic activities based on identified needs, which can help facilitate effective coping and adaptive capacity. The Pediatric Evaluation of Disability Inventory Computer Adaptive Test (PEDI-CAT; Haley et al., 2005) is one example of a widely used tool that assesses cognition, social relationships, and responsibility in addition to activities of daily living and functional mobility. The School Functional Assessment (SFA; Coster et al., 1998) is centered around functional performance in the school setting while determining the child's level of participation in six school environments (e.g., classroom, playground, mealtime). The Child Occupational Self-Assessment (COSA; Kramer et al., 2014) tool is a self-assessment tool to measure perceived competence in occupational performance and participation. These measurement tools afford opportunity to explore *how* a child will perform activities while also considering the child or caregiver's *perceived quality* of participation.

Quality of Life Measures

Health-related quality of life (HRQL) measures are appropriate to assess an individual's perception about life-related activity and function. HRQL questionnaires identify

Table 8-1

Assessment Tools That Can Address Adaptation, Coping, and Resilience in Children and Youth With Cerebral Palsy

Assessment Tool	Description	Application Toward Coping, Adaptation, and Resilience
Goal-Setting Assessment Tools		
Global Attainment Scale (GAS; Steenbeek et al., 2007)	Goal-setting and scaling with a statistical analysis component. Child and/or caregiver selects the goals to guide treatment. Occupational therapists can evaluate functional progress during treatment. Applicable for all ages.	Child or caregiver works with the occupational therapist to set goals. Goals can be designed to address competence and problem-solving among other areas related to adaptive capacity and resilience.
Canadian Occupational Performance Measure, Fifth Edition (COPM; Law et al., 2019)	Interview-style assessment for occupational performance related to client satisfaction. The respondent uses 10-point scales, which can also serve as a standardized manner to measure progress.	Similar to the GAS, occupational therapists can use the COPM to develop goals for intervention. Goals can be designed around participatory activities that address aspects of participation, health, and well-being.
Functional and Participation Assessment Tools		
Pediatric Evaluation of Disability Inventory Computer Adaptive Test (PEDI-CAT; Haley et al., 2005)	Functional measurement of daily living activities, mobility, social/cognitive function, and responsibility as reported by parent or clinician for ages 0 to 20.	Insight can be gained on how the child participates and perceives involvement in daily life.
Child Occupational Self-Assessment (COSA; Kramer et al., 2014)	25-item questionnaire that assesses child's perception of competency for participation in occupations. Appropriate for ages 6 to 21.	Occupational therapists can gain insight into areas that the child perceives as the most relevant to everyday activities.
School Functional Assessment (SFA; Coster et al., 1998)	Questionnaire completed by school professionals for children in kindergarten through sixth grade that examines participation, task supports, and activity performance.	Occupational therapists can use the SFA to measure participation in the school environment and, thus, create strategies to minimize school-related stressors by providing physical and psychosocial adaptations.

(continued)

Table 8-1 (continued)

Assessment Tools That Can Address Adaptation, Coping, and Resilience in Children and Youth With Cerebral Palsy		
Assessment Tool	**Description**	**Application Toward Coping, Adaptation, and Resilience**
Children's Assessment of Participation and Enjoyment (CAPE) and Preferences for Activities of Children (PAC; King et al., 2004)	CAPE is a 55-item questionnaire that explores participation and enjoyment (recreation, physica, social, skill-based, and self-improvement domains) for ages 6 to 21. PAC is a complementary portion activity in which the child/youth indicates if they like/do not like a variety of activities (ages 6 to 12).	Child-based, self-identification method to target activities for intervention or daily life in which the child may gain satisfaction.
Quality of Life Indicators		
Cerebral Palsy Quality of Life Questionnaire (CPQOL; Waters et al., 2006)	First QoL tool specifically developed for CP. Domains include social and emotional well-being, participation, function, pain, and disability impact. Parent questionnaire for ages 4 to 12; child self-report questionnaire for ages 9 to 12.	QoL tools can be used for outcome measures and goal-setting, which provides insight into the child's/caregiver's perception of the following:
The Caregiver Priorities and Child Health Index of Life with Disabilities (CPCHILD; Narayanan et al., 2006)	Measures caregiver perception of functional limitations, health status, and well-being of children with GMFCS levels IV-V.	• Social well-being • Access to care • Impact of pain and other disability factors that may interfere with coping
The World Health Organization Quality of Life Assessment: Brief Version (WHOQOL-BREF; (WHO, 2012)	General QoL assessment that focuses on four QoL domains: physical health, psychological health, social relationships, and environment.	• Feelings of acceptance and belonging • Health management • Level of self-advocacy • Emotional well-being
Adolescent Resilience Questionnaire (ARQ; Gartland et al., 2011)	Short questionnaire for adolescents that targets personal characteristics of resilience as well as family, peer, school, and community relationships.	• Needs for community support • Parent/family connections
Child and Youth Resiliency Measure (CRYM; Resilience Research Centre, 2018)	QoL measures that are not specific to CP; however, focused on factors related to developmental resilience (child—ages 5 to 9; youth—ages 10 to 23).	

specific areas that may have to be addressed to facilitate coping and adaptive capacities for children with CP and their caregivers. For example, the Cerebral Palsy Quality of Life Inventory (CPQOL; Waters et al., 2006) was developed specifically to address well-being across life domains for children and youth with CP, and is intended to be used by clinicians and researchers. The Caregiver Priorities and Child Health Index of Life with Disabilities (CPCHILD; Narayanan et al., 2006) was developed to specifically target QoL for children with GMFCS IV-V (that is, children with more functional limitations). The WHOQOL-BREF (WHO, 2012) and the Child and Youth Resiliency Measure (CRYM; Resilience Research Centre, 2018) are not specific to cerebral palsy, but do encompass individual, social, and contextual aspects of QoL. Overall, the assessment tools mentioned in this chapter are not a comprehensive list; however, they do offer a variety of tools that can be utilized to establish goals, measure outcomes, and supplement research on adaptation, coping skills, and resilience in children and youth with CP. These measures are listed and described in Table 8-1.

Intervention

As discussed in the preceding section, resilience is a dynamic and interconnected process of adaptive capacity in the face of adversity that continues to occur throughout development (Gartland et al., 2011; Masten & Barnes, 2018; National Scientific Council on the Developing Child, 2015). Adversity for children with CP begins with motoric limitations, and may also be exacerbated by numerous other issues: co-morbid conditions and complications; family/peer dynamics; socioeconomic issues; global-health concerns such as pandemics; access to environments; and governmental policies, among other things (Novak et al., 2013; Masten & Barnes, 2018). Resilience is highly dependent on internal and external factors that have little to do with the mere presence of physical limitations. Further, it is important to understand that resilience depends on adaptive capacity for a specific situation at hand across various contexts. Resilience in one situation does not automatically translate to resilience in all situations.

The Resilience Triad is proposed to focus occupational therapy intervention on coping and adaptive strategies for children and youth with cerebral palsy (Figure 8-1). It is developmentally based, dynamic, and highly dependent on the child's sense of self, social connection, and engagement in occupation. The Resilience Triad is foundationally connected to the definition of occupational adaptation by Grajo, Boisselle, and DaLomba (2019):

1. A product of engagement in occupation.
2. A transaction with the environment.
3. A manner of responding to change and life transitions.
4. And a process of forming a desired sense of self (p. 3).

Overall, the Resilience Triad is a visual and descriptive framework that supplements the principles of occupational adaptation by proposing intervention methods designed to guide the child with CP toward resilience. It does not offer a prescriptive list of existing interventions, but rather encompasses psychosocial aspects of CP intervention that draw upon a summation of studies from the international fields of occupational therapy, psychology, and cerebral palsy research.

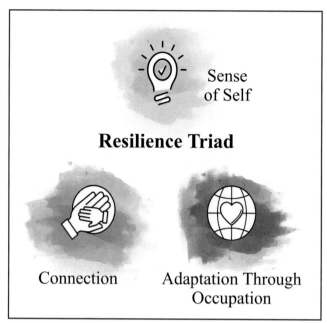

Figure 8-1. Resilience Triad: A framework for occupational therapy intervention to support adaptation, coping, and resilience in children and youth with cerebral palsy. Three elements of resilience: (1) Sense of self: motivation, problem solving, and competence; (2) connection: family, peers, and community; and (3) adaptation through occupation: physical and attitudinal environments, advocacy, and health management

Element 1—Sense of Self: Motivation, Problem Solving, and Competence

Personal factors influence the dynamic process of resilience. Characteristics such as motivation and gaining competence through self-regulation and problem solving are indicative of strong resilient traits (Gartland et al., 2011; Masten, 2018). A qualitative study by Kramer and Hammel (2011) found that competence develops when the child is permitted to work through problems in order to solve them and frequently practices new skills. Renowned psychologist Alfred Adler (1992), known as the father of modern psychology, advocated that allowing children to explore their environment through play allows them to push themselves forward in development, provides an opportunity to express themselves, and also helps them to navigate social expectations. To facilitate coping strategies and adaptive capacity, occupational therapists should work with children to identify occupations that have close and meaningful connections to their everyday lives. Research also supports the contention that "fun" and meaningful activities are fundamental in eliciting functional and participatory engagement (AOTA, 2020b; Kramer & Hammel, 2011; Rosenbaum & Gorter, 2012). Empowering the child to collaborate in the design of activities used for treatment not only addresses meaning, but also gives the child a sense of control, which may contribute improved quality of life and resilience (Öhrvall et al., 2019). Additionally, occupational therapists should not shy away from creative activities, as they provide an effective way to expose the child to a balanced opportunity for trial and error, reinforcement of self-regulation, and sense of mastery (Masten, 2018).

Novak et al. (2013) conducted a systematic review specifically related to intervention methods for children with CP in which outcomes-based, context-focused therapy with child-centered goal-based functional activities and home programming were graded with a "green light" for CP-based interventions. Their findings further support that the child should be actively engaged in identifying specific goals and activities to be used during treatment sessions and for the home program. Through this client-centered process, occupational therapists can offer the enjoyable yet challenging activities within a safe environment that allows the child to problem-solve and gain competency (Majnemer et al., 2010). Cognitive-based interventions such as the Cognitive Orientation to daily Occupational Performance (CO-OP) may also be used to create and implement an intentional plan for participation using the global strategy of Goal-Plan-Do-Check (Dawson et al., 2017). In a small qualitative study, Öhrvall et al. (2019) confirmed that CO-OP may be an effective intervention for adolescents with MACS level I-II to promote motivating challenges and self-efficacy, as participants were given the opportunity make decisions about the goals and activities and were allowed time to practice.

It is advocated here that children with CP be provided with opportunities for choice during occupational interventions regardless of GMFCS levels or cognitive ability. Occupational therapists can foster opportunities to allow children to have a voice in their treatment, thereby creating opportunities for successful adaptation. Some ideas for promoting voice and mutual respect include:

- Communicating at eye level with the child.
- Allowing time for responses.
- Working collaboratively with speech-language pathologists to give the child a means to access alternative communication methods.
- Utilizing real-world contexts to create opportunities for competence building and appropriate adaptive responses (Foley et al., 2012; Piggot et al., 2002).

An example of utilizing natural contexts is shown in Figure 8-2: a home-health occupational therapist accompanies an adolescent to the grocery store to obtain lunch items for school in order to provide strategies for navigating the physical environment while offering opportunities for self-regulation and problem-solving. While an internal sense of self is important, supportive relationships are also key in the development of resilience.

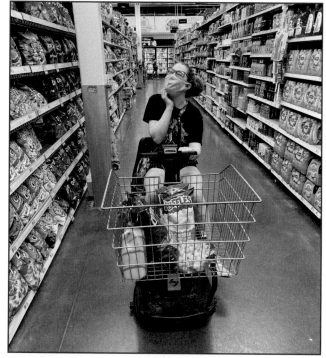

Figure 8-2. Elizabeth shopping in preparation for the online school year.

Element 2—Connection: Family, Peers, and Community

In *Understanding Human Nature,* Adler (1992) explored the deep connection between human adaptation and social connection:

> The human mind could render immediate first aid and compensate for physical deficiencies. Constant feelings of inadequacy stimulate humanity's foresight and ability to avoid danger, and caused the mind to develop to its present condition of thinking, feeling, and acting. Society has played an essential role in the process of adaptation, and the mind must interact from the very beginning with the conditions of communal life. All its faculties are developed upon one fundamental principle: the logic of communal life. (p. 37)

There is strong evidence that social support and connection with family, peers, and the community are instrumental for the coping and quality of life of a child with CP (Bedell et al., 2013; Carona et al., 2014; Masten, 2018; Saleh et al., 2008). Occupational therapists are in a unique position to provide a balanced view and genuine portrayal of expectations with positive social support that can foster adaptive capacity for children with CP and their caregivers. Social skills are also highly correlated with successful resilience; therefore, social skills training is a beneficial technique for developing deeper relationships with family and peers (Gartland et al., 2011). Realistic goal setting,

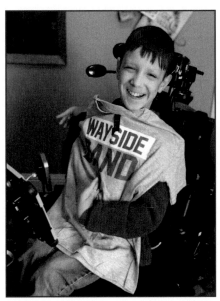

Figure 8-3. Daniel proudly showing his school band t-shirt.

evidence-based practice, and provision of community resources are some ways to ensure balanced family support (Carona et al., 2013; Novak et al., 2013). Further examples include establishment of sleep routine schedules; time management and organization strategies; development of pain-reducing strategies such as meditation and yoga; and facilitation of creative arts, recreation, and sporting activities (Figure 8-3). Occupational therapists can also help balance adaptive capacities of both the child and caregiver by providing strategies and community resources to help prioritize family demands, establish healthy routines and habits, and guard against negative perceptions of others (Foley et al., 2012; Rosenbaum & Gorter, 2012).

Element 3—Adaptation Through Occupation

Adaptation, for the purpose of the Resilience Triad, involves the dynamic process of the child's successful use of their adaptive capacity for self-mastery and connection to others while navigating the broader societal, attitudinal, and built environments in order to participate in occupations despite adversity. Masten (2018) identifies external yet interconnected factors, such as family structure, economic circumstances, and normative development, that contribute to resilience. Thus, motivation and competency building are directly related to expectations of others and the demands of the environment that match their abilities (Kramer & Hammel, 2011).

It is well documented that negative attitudinal perspectives from caregivers, friends, and society may influence the child's ability to efficiently and effectively cope and

Case Study 8-2

Barrett is a 16-year-old adolescent with spastic diplegia (GMFCS and MACS Level II) who attends occupational therapy in an outpatient clinic. While goal-setting using the GAS, he revealed that he had recently been hired for his first job as a cashier at a home improvement store. He mentioned he was concerned that the other employees and customers might view him differently and that he was anxious about possibly getting fatigued from standing throughout the shift. He was also worried about asking for modification, as he did not want to be viewed differently. The occupational therapist collaboratively analyzed the activities Barrett would be expected to do and created simulated scenarios so that he had the opportunity to practice and problem-solve, which allowed him to safely and independently perform his job. They also worked to develop solutions to address potential negative attitudes. As part of the home program, Barrett was tasked with researching the American with Disabilities Act (ADA) so that he was knowledgeable about his rights and could self-advocate while on the job. Lastly, Barrett developed a plan as to what to discuss with his manager about his needs for his job shifts (e.g., availability of a stool, rest breaks).

participate in occupations (AOTA, 2020a; Carona et al., 2014; Colver et al., 2011; Grajo, 2019; Rosenbaum & Gorter, 2012). In a culmination of personal negative coping factors, attitudinal barriers, and physical barriers, children with CP may be deprived of everyday occupations. Occupational therapists can model positive attitudes when addressing the child directly and/or caregivers. Empowerment opportunities can be created for the child to self-advocate in school, community, and work environments. Further details of occupational therapists' role in helping a child or youth engage in occupation through collaboration and, on a global scale, are described in the following sections.

INTERPROFESSIONAL AND FAMILY COLLABORATION: OCCUPATIONAL THERAPISTS AS TRANSFORMATIVE LEADERS

Care for the child or youth with cerebral palsy often requires an expansive collaborative effort among the client, caregivers, rehabilitation therapists, educators, medical providers, and community organizations. In the educational setting, the occupational therapist provides support to clients directly or through consultations with teachers, paraprofessionals, school psychologists, school nurses, and other members of the rehabilitation team. The occupational therapist can take an active role, not only in adapting the physical environment and educational materials, but also by facilitating the generation of coping strategies and methods to promote psychological growth, well-being, and independence (Carona et al., 2014). The occupational therapist may offer a variety of strategies to help the child cope with school-related stressors that may arise due to barriers of accessing the physical environment or the educational curriculum that impede participation. For example, a kindergartener with spastic quadriplegia who is in a wheelchair may not be able to get on the floor with peers for circle time. This may, in turn, cause the child to disengage or misbehave during that time. The occupational therapist can offer suggestions to modify the activity (suggest that the class stand to be more at eye level) or environment (such as having a beanbag seat available for the child to sit in) to promote social engagement with peers.

Many children and youth with cerebral palsy experience frequent hospitalizations for various reasons, such as orthopedic surgeries; gastrointestinal, respiratory, or tone management; and hip surveillance, among other things. Some of these interventions require extended lengths of stay in the hospital. Occupational therapists can play a crucial role during the hospital visit, as well as when preparing the child to return home. Collaborative efforts to minimize stressors during the stay can be made through close coordination of care with the family and among occupational therapists, physicians, nurses, dieticians, child life specialists, and psychologists. Examples include working with therapeutic recreation, music, and/or physical therapists to identify activities that may promote participation, relaxation, and enjoyment in daily living, school, and leisure activities while in the hospital; collaborating with child-life specialists to help the child understand what to expect from surgery; working with nurses, speech-language pathologists, and/or caregivers so that the child has a method to communicate needs (e.g., for pain medication, food and water) to ease anxiety; and collaborating with physical therapists and the family to discuss expectations following surgery and modifications that may be needed within the home (Figure 8-4).

A less conventional, yet crucial role is for occupational therapists to strategically position themselves to become transformative leaders when advocating for children and youth with CP and other conditions with their employer, local, state, or international entities and policy. In his 2007 Slagle Lecture, Hinojosa showed tremendous predictive insight in his assertions that we are living in a time of rapid and unpredictable change with advances in knowledge and technology that have made our lives more interconnected and complex. Recently, the global pandemic introduced innumerable stressors for most individuals, including children with CP, caregivers, and rehabilitation therapists. It further highlighted Hinojosa's view of the significance of human adaptability and technology to continue the delivery of occupational therapy services. For example, many children were suddenly attending school from home, putting an extra burden on caregivers to be both teachers and rehabilitation therapists. Many families (and healthcare workers) were affected by stressors such as loss of employment, limitations of community activities and social opportunities with family members and peers, and closed day-care facilities. The most obvious repercussion was a significant reduction of occupational engagement in typical activities due to the necessity of quarantine (WHO, 2020). Therapy agencies were required to discover innovative ways to manage caseloads while being cognizant of social distancing and the medical fragility of their clients. Occupational therapists had to navigate how each payor would handle payment for telehealth, understand webinar platforms and privacy issues, have an understanding of accessibility

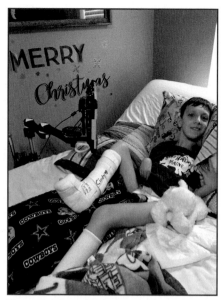

Figure 8-4. Daniel in the hospital for hip surgery.

to technology for each client, and develop methods to virtually administer assessments and deliver services. Collaborative problem solving and flexibility became paramount with the child, caregivers, and rehabilitation therapists in the effort to provide services efficiently and safely.

It is the position of the World Federation for Occupational Therapists (WFOT, 2019a; WFOT, 2019b) that a holistic and psychosocial approach of occupational therapists can facilitate occupational engagement and participation with clients and that there are "increasing opportunities that enable occupational therapists to practice with communities aims to strengthen the design and facilitation of initiatives that promote health, prevent injury and illness, improve well-being and inclusion, and reduce burden of disease" (WFOTa, 2019, p. 2). For example, in Texas, occupational therapists are employed as subject-matter experts with some Medicaid-based, managed-care organizations (MCOs) to determine medical necessity for occupational therapy that is based on health, safety, and independence (Texas Medicaid and Health Partnership [TMHP], 2021). Occupational therapists can concurrently ensure that practitioners use evidence-based interventions specific to cerebral palsy (and other conditions) to promote activity and participation, while also advocating for policy that supports positive occupation-based interventions through participation, health promotion, and well-being. Additionally, value-based payment programs, which are rooted in quality services rather than fee-for-service methods, offer new opportunities for occupational therapists in the medical setting to collaborate with MCO occupational therapists and case managers to support quality services and public health initiatives that address quality of life and well-being. For example, home-health occupational therapists are frequently in the home and work in close proximity to the family. They may be able to establish a level of trust and transparency needed to identify family stressors and coping risk factors, such as abuse and neglect (Foley et al., 2012; Piggot et al., 2016). In turn, the home-health occupational therapists can communicate concerns to the MCO in order to coordinate programs focused on stress reduction, family resources, respite care, skilled nursing, and behavioral health. Beyond local coordination of care, occupational therapists also have a significant role on an international level to address developmental resilience.

A GLOBAL PERSPECTIVE

Availability of the health care, support, and accessibility required for the care of children and youth with cerebral palsy can vary globally. In developed countries, CP appears to be well studied. Some literature exists on pediatric CP well-being and quality of life, with a majority from the caregiver perspective. Literature searches reveal a majority of studies from North America, Europe, and Australia. Goldsmith et al. (2016) conducted an online survey with 37 CP surveillance programs and found similar concentration of CP experts. Participants were from 11 countries in the aforementioned continents and tend to be highly focused on the medical perspective related to body structures and functions. The authors found that barriers to international consistency with CP surveillance were related to funding, conflicting data collection methods, and differing research initiatives. The survey did not seek feedback from clients and caregivers, although many programs include both as part of the program (e.g., the Cerebral Palsy Research Network [CPRN] in the United States). All programs from the study reported use of the GMFCS. The MACS was used less often and tended to be centralized geographically. Some programs are beginning to explore functional outcomes. The addition of QoL aspects is acknowledged to be needed for the future as a surveillance initiative.

Studies specific to Canada, Europe, and Africa contribute some insight into broad issues that may affect resilience in children with CP. Saleh et al. (2008) conducted a Canada-wide survey of physical and occupational therapists treating children with CP. It revealed that although physical therapists focus more on body and structures, both physical and occupational therapists show a deficit in addressing participation in leisure activities and play. In a study by Colver et al. (2011), the European Child Environment Questionnaire was given to 818 families of children with CP across eight regions in Europe to explore environmental, social, and attitudinal constructs. Children with higher GMFCS levels had fewer social opportunities and negative attitudes from family and friends, but the attitudes of therapists were consistent regardless of the severity of disability (Colver et al., 2011). Levels of participation and social engagement were found to depend greatly on access to the physical environment, government policy, and social programs. For example, Denmark and Sweden have greater access to inclusive after-school programs and social events. Little research is conducted in developing countries on the resilience and well-being of children with CP. For example, Donald et al. (2015) documented conversations with 22 physicians from five countries in Africa that revealed African barriers and needs:

- Access to services—lack wheelchair accessibility, sparse resources and limited access due to poor infrastructure and medication availability; financial barriers to health care.
- Quality of care—limited treatments for spasticity management; inconsistency in treatment approaches and local guidelines, in general.
- Education—Need education for clients, caregivers, and clinicians; need for innovative approaches to treatment; limited availability of teaching hospitals and training for clinicians at the university level; and lack of access to evidence-based practice resources.

These studies indicate global disparities that may impede development of resilience in children with CP, such as lack of focus on rehabilitation interventions centered around participation, connection, and opportunities for engagement in occupations. For future studies, more focus on aspects of developmental resilience in children and youth with CP may be warranted.

ESSENTIAL CONSIDERATIONS FOR OCCUPATIONAL THERAPISTS USING THE RESILIENCE TRIAD

Table 8-2 provides occupational therapists with essential considerations for assessment and intervention. The provided considerations draw upon the Resilience Triad in the areas of the child's sense of self, connection, and engagement in occupation.

Table 8-2

Essential Considerations for Occupational Therapy Assessment and Intervention Using the Resilience Triad	
Facilitate growth in the child's sense of self	• Select goal-setting tools in order to establish goals that promote opportunities for problem solving and competency building • Present age-appropriate mindfulness, creative arts, and/or fitness activities to promote stress reduction • Offer pain management strategies to improve coping and reduce symptoms of anxiety • Promote self-regulation and coping strategies to adapt efficiently through participation in daily activities • Provide strategies to establish health and sleep routines and schedules

(continued)

Table 8-2 (continued)

Essential Considerations for Occupational Therapy Assessment and Intervention Using the Resilience Triad

Encourage the establishment of connection	• Utilize participation-based assessment tools to gain insight on how the child interacts with family, peers, and community • Encourage caregivers to share the caregiving burden with relatives or friends • Provide therapeutic and community resources, including coping-related educational opportunities and ideas for family respite • Offer child-centered social skills groups that promote positive peer/sibling relationships • Create coaching strategies that teach coping with bullying and conflict resolution • Promote positive aspects of interdependence and co-occupation to foster family coping and resilience
Address aspects related to engagement in occupation	• Provide QoL measures to gain perspective from the child/caregiver • Present culturally relevant occupations in the context of real-world situations whenever possible • Address health disparities through promotion of inclusive activities within the home, community, and school settings • Foster activities centered around health management and self-advocacy in order to promote the voice of the child/youth with CP • Demonstrate empathetic listening strategies and speak at eye level while giving the child time to respond • Coordinate or provide resources for community recreation and leisure activities that the child identifies as engaging and motivating • Advocate for CP-related resilience initiatives through evidence-based practice (EBP), quality care, and legislation • Provide coping strategies and support related to care provision during COVID-19 (see https://www.who.int/publications-detail/critical-preparedness-readiness-and-response-actions-for-covid-19)

Adapted from AOTA, 2020b; Masten, 2018; National Scientific Council on the Developing Child, 2015; Rosenbaum & Gorter, 2012; Whitney et al., 2019; and WHO, 2020.

Case Study 8-3

Destiny: Occupational Services Using the Resilience Triad

Client History

Destiny is a 17-year-old Black female with mixed-type spastic quadriplegia with dystonia. She was referred to home-health occupational therapy following a deep brain stimulation procedure in which the occupational therapist was asked to monitor functional changes in both posture and bilateral manual abilities. Destiny has significant dysarthria, so she needs extra time to provide verbal responses. Review of her medical record reveals that she has typical cognitive abilities. Her mother or stepsister are often present during her occupational therapy appointments. Destiny currently has a caregiver-dependent manual wheelchair. She relies on family members for all activities of daily living. She expressed disrupted sleep routines due to pain-associated spasticity. Destiny's mother also has disrupted sleep because she helps Destiny with tube feedings. Destiny is very social and active at school and church. She said she would like to do activities with people her age, but often does not get invited to participate in extracurricular activities. She has a boyfriend and hopes he will ask her to prom.

Evaluation

The occupational therapist gathered information as requested by the neurologist, which included assessment of body functions and client factors, such as range of motion, tone assessment, and upper-extremity functional analysis needed for outcomes data for deep brain stimulation (DBS). In collaboration with Destiny's neurologist and physical therapist, GMFCS and MACS level V was assigned, signifying the need for assistance with and modification of all daily life activities. The PEDI-CAT was given to the mother, who indicated that Destiny was either unable to do or required a lot of help for performance in daily activity and mobility, needed some help for social cognitive activities, and assumed some shared responsibility for organizing and planning daily activities, but that the mother takes care of much of it. Destiny and her mother were interviewed through the semi-structured format of the COPM, which revealed several areas that could be addressed in occupational therapy, including those specific to self-care. Destiny perceived her overall performance as 2.0 and satisfaction as 3. Destiny and her mother were also given the Child and Youth Resiliency Measure (CRYM); both of them rated Destiny on the lower end in resilience, but interestingly Destiny rated herself higher than her mother did.

Identified areas related to sense of self, connection, and occupational engagement were as follows:

1. Destiny stated that she previously had a power wheelchair and would like to explore using one again because she is tired of needing her family or peers to propel the chair for her. She also indicated that it embarrassed her to need someone to push her in order to participate in dances. The mother

(continued)

Case Study 8-3 (continued)

stated that one barrier is that Destiny's wheelchair vendor feels she is not appropriate for power mobility due to behavior issues. They described that at the last visit, Destiny knocked off the vendor's glasses. Destiny reported that the vendor dropped a tool on the ground and that she was unable to control her reaction (her mother described it as extensor-tone startle reflex).

2. Destiny explained that she loves to watch nature documentaries and sit-coms on television, but she cannot use the remote control; therefore, her younger brother always gets to decide on the shows, "which is usually cartoons." The mother stated that there are often arguments over what is on the television and Destiny often gets mad and retreats to her room.

Destiny and her mother reported that the mom typically takes care of all of Destiny's health management decisions and that she has not involved Destiny in aspects related to adulthood transition needs regarding health care and education.

Intervention

Table 8-3 is a summary of some intervention strategies designed to foster coping strategies and capacity to adapt to a variety of situations.

Table 8-3

Intervention Strategies for Destiny	
Facilitate growth in Destiny's sense of self	• Destiny and the occupational therapist discussed pain management strategies to improve coping and reduce symptoms of anxiety. Destiny verbalized that she would try a meditation app prior to bedtime or when her pain was exacerbated. Destiny and the occupational therapist were able to locate an app for her tablet that Destiny seemed motivated to use. • Promote self-regulation and coping strategies to adapt efficiently through participation in daily activities. • Provide strategies to establish healthy sleep routines and schedules.
Encourage the establishment of connection	• Destiny had a seating and mobility appointment with a new vendor. Destiny explained up front that she has a startle reflex, so the vendor was aware during transfers and positioning. She showed good success with independent mobility using controls in her head rest. • The occupational therapist also discussed with the vendor Destiny's desire to use a TV remote so that she can choose programs at home. The occupational therapist and the vendor were able to program her wheelchair head rest to control her tablet. Not only was she able to use the remote independently, she could turn her bedroom lights and ceiling fan on and off, and she was able to post to social media without asking her siblings or mother.

(continued)

Case Study 8-3 (continued)

Table 8-3 (continued)

Intervention Strategies for Destiny	
	• The occupational therapist and Destiny's mom discussed options for her to share caregiving duties, particularly at night. Destiny's mom contacted her MCO case manager and was able to obtain skilled nursing for g-tube feedings and positioning; the case manager also referred her for respite care. • The occupational therapist provided coaching strategies to Destiny for conflict resolution. The occupational therapist invited Destiny's siblings to participate in group activities to allow opportunities for Destiny to navigate solutions for when she became frustrated.
Address aspects related to engagement in occupation	• Destiny and the occupational therapist created a list of health management needs to prepare for transition to adulthood. Destiny and her mom selected and made visits to potential adult family practitioners. • As part of Destiny's home program, she agreed to call her neurologist to specifically discuss pain-management options to supplement DBS. • The occupational therapist and Destiny co-taught the nurse range-of-motion and stretching routines, positioning, and ADL strategies, so that the mom would not need to do these daily. Destiny learned to advocate for herself when she was uncomfortable or needed something done a different way. • The occupational therapist and Destiny located a city community program for teens with special needs to participate in dances and community outings. Destiny attended every weekend and reported that she was very happy she could dance independently using her power wheelchair.

Destiny demonstrated measurable gains throughout treatment. Both she and her mom reported higher satisfaction (5) and performance (6) on the COPM, as well as improved and significantly higher QoL scores on the CYRM. She also showed improved PEDI-CAT scores in all areas. The mom reported that they are having less conflict at home and both of them feel more rested. Destiny stated she is happy that she is able to do more for herself and that she no longer has to rely on her mother to push her wheelchair or to chat with her friends on social media. She also reported with excitement that she is thinking for the first time that she can get a job after high school.

REFERENCES

Adler, A. (1992). *Understanding human nature.* OneWorld.

Albrecht, G. L., & Devlieger, P. J. (1999). The disability paradox: High quality of life against all odds. *Social Science & Medicine, 48*(8), 977-988. https://doi.org/10.1016/S0277-9536(98)00411-0

American Occupational Therapy Association. (2020a). Occupational therapy practice framework: Domain and process (4th ed.). *American Journal of Occupational Therapy, 74*(Suppl. 2), 7412410010. https://doi.org/10.5014/ajot.2020.74S2001

American Occupational Therapy Association. (2020b). Occupational therapy in the promotion of health and well-being. *American Journal of Occupational Therapy, 74*(3), 7403420010. https://doi.org/10.5014/ajot.2020.743003

Anaby, D., Korner-Bitensky, N., Steven, E., Tremblay, S., Snider, L., Avery, L., & Law, M. (2017). Current rehabilitation practices for children with cerebral palsy: Focus and gaps. *Physical & Occupational Therapy in Pediatrics, 37*(1), 1-15. https://doi.org/10.3109/01942638.2015.1126880

Arakelyan, S., Maciver, D., Rush, R., O'hare, A., & Forsyth, K. (2019). Family factors associated with participation of children with disabilities: A systematic review. *Developmental Medicine & Child Neurology, 61*(5), 514-522. https://doi.org/10.1111/dmcn.14133

Bedell, G., Coster, W., Law, M., Liljenquist, K., Kao, Y. C., Teplicky, R., Anaby, D., & Khetani, M. A. (2013). Community participation, supports, and barriers of school-age children with and without disabilities. *Archives of Physical Medicine and Rehabilitation, 94*(2), 315-323. https://doi.org/10.1016/j.apmr.2022.09.024

Boisselle, A. (2022). Cerebral palsy. In B. Atchison & D. Dirette (Eds.), *Conditions in occupational therapy.*

Bosanquet, M., Copeland, L., Ware, R., & Boyd, R. (2013). A systematic review of tests to predict cerebral palsy in young children. *Developmental Medicine & Child Neurology, 55*(5), 418-426. https://doi.org/10.1111/dmcn.12140

Carona, C., Moreira, H., Silva, N., Crespo, C., & Canavarro, M. C. (2014). Social support and adaptation outcomes in children and adolescents with cerebral palsy. *Disability and Rehabilitation, 36*(7), 584-592. https://doi.org/10.3109/09638288.2013.804596

Carona, C., Pereira, M., Moreira, H., Silva, N., & Canavarro, M. C. (2013). The disability paradox revisited: Quality of life and family caregiving in pediatric cerebral palsy. *Journal of Child & Family Studies, 22*, 971-986. http://doi.org/10.1007/s10826-012-9659-0

Colver, A. F., Dickinson, H. O., Parkinson, P., Arnaud, C., Beckung, E., Fauconnier, J., Marcelli, M., Mcmanus, V., Michelsen, S. I., Parkes, J., & Thyen, U. (2011). Access of children with cerebral palsy to the physical, social and attitudinal environment they need: A cross-sectional European study. *Disability and Rehabilitation, 33*(1), 28-35. https://doi.org/10.3109/09638288.2010.485669

Coster, W., Deeney, T. A., Haltiwanger, J. T., & Haley, S. M. (1998). *School Functional Assessment user's manual.* Therapy Skill Builders.

Dawson, D., McEwen, S. E., & Polatajko, H. J. (2017). *Cognitive orientation to daily occupational performance in occupational therapy: Using the CO-OP approach™ to enable participation across the lifespan.* AOTA Press.

Donald, K. A., Kakooza, A. M., Wammanda, R. D., Mallewa, M., Samia, P., Babakir, H., Bearden, D., Majnemer, A., Fehlings, D., Shevell, M., Chugani, H., & Wilmshurst, J. M. (2015). Pediatric cerebral palsy in Africa: Where are we? *Journal of Child Neurology, 30*(8), 963-971. https://doi.org/10.1177/0883073814549245

Eliasson, A. C., Krumlinde-Sundholm, L., Rösblad, B., Beckung, E., Arner, M., Öhrvall, A. M., & Rosenbaum, P. (2006). The Manual Ability Classification System (MACS) for children with cerebral palsy: Scale development and evidence of validity and reliability. *Developmental Medicine & Child Neurology, 48*(7). 549-554. https://doi.org/10.1111/j.1469-8749.2006.tb01313.x

Fairfax, A., Brehaut, J., Colman, I., Sikora, L., Kazakova, A., Chakraborty, P., Potter, B. K., in collaboration with the Canadian Inherited Metabolic Diseases Research Network. (2019). A systematic review of the association between coping strategies and quality of life among caregivers of children with chronic illness and/or disability. *BMC Pediatrics, 19*, 215. https://doi.org/10.1186/s12887-019-1587-3

Foley, K.-R., Blackmore, A. M., Girdler, S., O'Donnell, M., Glauert, R., Llewellyn, G., & Leonard, H. (2012). *To feel belonged*: The voices of children and youth with disabilities on the meaning of wellbeing. *Child Indicators Research, 5*, 375-391. https://doi.org/10.1007/s12187-011-9134-2

Gartland, D., Bond, L., Olsson, C. A., Buzwell, S., & Sawyer, S. M. (2011). Development of a multi-dimensional measure of resilience in adolescents: the Adolescent Resilience Questionnaire. *BMC Medical Research Methodology, 11*, 134. https://doi.org/10.1186/1471-2288-11-134

Glader, L. J., & Stevenson, R. D. (2019). Overview of cerebral palsy: Definition, classification and impact. In L. Glader & R. Stevenson (Eds.), *Children and youth with complex cerebral palsy* (pp. 1-14).

Goldsmith, S., McIntyre, S., Smithers-Sheedy, H., Blair, E., Cans, C., Watson, L., & Yeargin-Allsopp, M. (2016). An international survey of cerebral palsy registers and surveillance systems. *Developmental Medicine & Child Neurology, 58*(S2), 11-17. https://doi.org/10.1111/dmcn.12999

Grajo, L. (2019). Occupational adaptation as a normative and intervention process: Schkade and Schultz's legacy. In L. C. Grajo & A. Boisselle (Eds.), *Adaptation through occupation: Multidimensional perspectives*. SLACK Incorporated.

Grajo, L., Boisselle, A., & DaLomba, E. (2019). Defining the construct of occupational adaptation. In L. C. Grajo & A. Boisselle (Eds.), *Adaptation through occupation: Multidimensional perspectives*. SLACK Incorporated.

Haley, S. M., Raczek, A. E., Coster, W. J., Dumas, H. M., & Fragala-Pinkham, M. A. (2005). Assessing mobility in children using a computer adaptive testing version of the Pediatric Evaluation of Disability Inventory. *Archives of Physical Medicine & Rehabilitation, 86*(5), 932-939. https://doi.org/10.1016/j.apmr.2004.10.032

Hinojosa, J. (2007). Becoming innovators in an era of hyperchange [Eleanor Clarke Slagle Lecture]. *American Journal of Occupational Therapy, 61*(6), 629-637. https://doi.org/10.5014/ajot.61.6.629

Kerr, C., Bowe, S. J., Miyazaki, K., & Imms, C. (2018). Psychometric evaluation of the 'Evidence Based Practice Competencies Questionnaire—Cerebral palsy'. *Physical & Occupational Therapy in Pediatrics, 38*(3), 305-315. https://doi.org/10.1080/01942638.2017.1420002

King, G. A., King, S., Rosenbaum, P., Kertoy, P., Law, M., & Hurley, P. (2004). *CAPE/PAC manual: Children's assessment of participation and enjoyment & preferences for activities of children*. PsychCorp.

Kramer, J. M., & Hammel, J. (2011). "I do lots of things": Children with cerebral palsy's competence for everyday activities, *International Journal of Disability, Development and Education, 58*(2), 121-113. https://doi.org/10.1080/1034912X.2011.570496

Kramer, J. M., Velden, M., Kafkes, A., Basu, S., Federico, J., & Kielhofner, G., (2014). *Child Occupational Self-Assessment (COSA) version 2.2*. The Model of Human Occupation Clearinghouse.

Law, M., Baptiste, S., Carswell, A., McColl, M. A., Polatajko, H., & Pollock, N. (2019). *Canadian Occupational Performance Measure* (5th ed. rev.). COPM, Inc.

Majnemer, A., Shevell, M., Law, M., Poulin, C., & Rosenbaum, P. (2010). Level of motivation in mastering challenging tasks in children with cerebral palsy. *Developmental Medicine & Child Neurology, 52*(12), 1120-1126. http://doi.org/10.1111/j.1469-8749.2010.03732.x

Masten, A. S. (2018). Resilience theory and research on children and families: Past, present, and promise. *Journal of Family Theory & Review, 10*(1), 12-31. https://doi.org/10.1111/jftr.12255

Masten, A. S., & Barnes, A. J. (2018). Resilience in children: Developmental perspectives. *Children, 5*(7), 98. https://doi.org/10.3390/children5070098

Narayanan, U. G., Fehlings, D., Weir, S., Knights, S., Kiran, S., & Campbell, K. (2006). Initial development and validation of the Caregiver Priorities and Child Health Index of Life with Disabilities (CPCHILD). *Developmental Medicine & Child Neurology, 48*(10), 804-812. https://doi.org/10.1111/j.1469-8749.2006.tb01227.x

National Scientific Council on the Developing Child. (2015). Supportive relationships and active skill-building strengthen the foundations of resilience: Working paper 13. https://developingchild.harvard.edu/resources/supportive-relationships-and-active-skill-building-strengthen-the-foundations-of-resilience/

Novak, I., Morgan, C., Adde, L., Blackman, J., Boyd, R. N., Brunstrom-Hernandez, J., Cioni, G., Damiano, D., Darrah, J., Eliasson, A., DeVries, L. S., Einspieler, C., Fahey, M., Fehlings, D., Ferriero, D. M., Fetters, L., Fiori, S., Forssber, H., Gordon, A. M., . . . Badawi, N. (2017). Early, accurate diagnosis and early intervention in cerebral palsy: Advances in diagnosis and treatment. *JAMA Pediatrics, 171*(9), 897-907. https://doi.org/10.1001/jamapediatrics.2017.1689

Novak, I., Mcintyre, S., Morgan, C., Campbell, L., Dark, L., Morton, N., Stumbles, E., Wilson, S. A., & Goldsmith, S. (2013). A systematic review of interventions for children with cerebral palsy: State of the evidence. *Developmental Medicine & Child Neurology, 55*(10), 885-910. https://doi.org/10.1111/dmcn.12246

Öhrvall, A., Bergqvist, L., Hofgren, C., & Peny-Dahlstrand, M. (2019). "With CO-OP I'm the boss"— experiences of the cognitive orientation to daily occupational performance approach as reported by young adults with cerebral palsy or spina bifida. *Disability and Rehabilitation, 42*(25), 1-8. https://doi.org/10.1080/09638288.2019.1607911

Oskoui, M., Coutinho, F., Dykeman, J., Jetté, N., & Pringsheim, T. (2013). An update on the prevalence of cerebral palsy: A systematic review and meta-analysis. *Developmental Medicine & Child Neurology, 55*(6), 509-519. https://doi.org/10.1111/dmcn.12080

Palisano, R., Rosenbaum, P., Walter, S., Russell, D., Wood, E., & Galuppi, B. (1997). Development and reliability of a system to classify gross motor function in children with cerebral palsy. *Developmental Medicine & Child Neurology, 39*(4), 214-223. https://doi.org/10.1111/j.1469-8749.1997.tb07414.x

Piggot, J., Paterson, J., & Hocking, C. (2002). Participation in home therapy programs for children with cerebral palsy: Compelling challenge. *Qualitative Health Research, 12*(8), 1112-1129. https://doi.org/10.1177/104973202129120476

Resilience Research Centre. (2018). *CYRM and ARM user manual.* Resilience Research Centre, Dalhousie University. http://www.resilienceresearch.org

Rosenbaum, P., & Gorter, J. W. (2012). The 'F-words' in childhood disability: I swear this is how we should think! *Child: Care, Health and Development, 38*(4), 457-463. https://doi.org/10.1111/j.1365-2214.2011.01338.x

Saleh, M. N., Korner-Bitensky, N., Snider, L., Malouin, F., Kennedy, E., & Roy, M. A. (2008). Actual vs. best practices for young children with cerebral palsy: A survey of paediatric occupational therapists and physical therapists in Quebec, Canada. *Developmental Neurorehabilitation, 11*(1), 60-80. https://doi.org/10.1080/17518420701544230

Steenbeek, D., Ketelaar, M., Galama, K., & Gorter, J. W. (2007). Goal attainment scaling in paediatric rehabilitation: A critical review of the literature. *Developmental Medicine & Child Neurology, 49*(7), 550-556. https://doi.org/10.1111/j.1469-8749.2007.00550.x

Texas Medicaid and Health Partnership. (2021). *Provider Handbooks: Physical Therapy, Occupational Therapy, and Speech Therapy Services Handbook (Texas Medicaid Provider Procedures Manual, vol. 2).* https://www.tmhp.com/resources/provider-manuals/tmppm

Wagner, L. V., & Davids, J. R. (2012). Assessment tools and classification systems used for the upper extremity in children with cerebral palsy. *Clinical Orthopaedics & Related Research, 470*(5), 1257-1271. https://doi.org/10.1007/s11999-011-2065-x

Waters, E., Davis, E., Boyd, R., Reddihough, D., Mackinnon, A., Graham, H. K., Lo, S. K., Wolfe, R., Stevenson, R., Bjornson, K., Blair, E., & Ravens-Sieberer, U. (2006). *Cerebral Palsy Quality of Life Questionnaire for Children (CP QOL-Child) manual.* Deakin University.

Whitney, D. G., Warschausky, S. A., & Peterson, M. D. (2019). Mental health disorders and physical risk factors in children with cerebral palsy: A cross-sectional study. *Developmental Medicine & Child Neurology, 61*(5), 579-585. https://doi.org/10.1111/dmcn.14083

World Federation of Occupational Therapists. (2019a). *Position statement: Occupational therapy and community-centered practice.* https://www.wfot.org/resources/occupational-therapy-and-community-centred-practice

World Federation of Occupational Therapists. (2019b). *Position Statement: Occupational therapy and mental health.* https://wfot.org/resources/occupational-therapy-and-mental-health

World Health Organization. (2012). *WHOQOL: User Manual.* World Health Organization. https://www.who.int/publications/i/item/WHO-HIS-HSI-Rev.2012.03

World Health Organization. (2001). *International classification of functioning, disability and health (ICF).* World Health Organization.

World Health Organization. (2007). *International classification of functioning, disability and health: children and youth version: ICF-CY.* https://apps.who.int/iris/handle/10665/43737

World Health Organization. (2020). Disability considerations during the COVID-19 outbreak. https://www.who.int/publications/i/item/WHO-2019-nCoV-Disability-2020-1

Yamaguchi, R., Perry, K. N., & Hines, M. (2014). Pain, pain anxiety and emotional and behavioural problems in children with cerebral palsy. *Disability and Rehabilitation, 36*(2), 125-130. https://doi.org/10.3109/09638288.2013.782356

Children and Youth With Cancer or Terminal Illness

Laura Stimler, OTD, OTR/L, BCP, C/NDT and
Jessica Sparrow, OTD, OTR/L, BCP

CHAPTER OBJECTIVES By the end of this chapter, the reader will be able to:

- Describe the pediatric oncology population and occupational barriers that may result after cancer and its treatment.
- Illustrate the psychological impact of cancer and its treatment and the influence of adaptation, coping, and resilience in pediatric oncology clients and their families.
- Explain the occupational therapy process along the pediatric cancer care continuum, and describe strategies to implement a collaborative approach with families, social environments, educators, health care teams, and other professionals.

OVERVIEW OF THE POPULATION

The National Cancer Institute (NCI; 2015) describes *cancer* as a collection of related diseases that involve cell division and invasion of other tissues. According to the American Childhood Cancer Organization (2019), approximately 15,780 children aged 0 to 19 years are diagnosed with cancer in the United States annually. In 2015, the United States had approximately 429,000 childhood cancer survivors (CCSs) aged 0 to 19 years (NCI, 2019). In most cases, causes of childhood cancers are unknown, although approximately 5% are hereditary (NCI, 2019). Children diagnosed with cancer differ from adults diagnosed with this disease, as children frequently respond differently to

Grajo L. C., & Boisselle, A. K. (Eds.). *Adaptation, Coping,
and Resilience in Children and Youth: A Comprehensive
Occupational Therapy Approach* (pp. 209-236).
© 2022 Taylor & Francis Group.

standard treatments due to their growing bodies. Younger children are usually more susceptible to late effects of cancer and its treatment (American Cancer Society [ACS], 2016). Also, cells of origin are different for childhood and adult cancers (Ambati & Boulad, 2019). The most common childhood cancers include leukemia and central nervous system tumors (brain and spinal cord). Other types of childhood cancers include neuroblastoma, Wilm's tumor, Hodgkin's and Non-Hodgkin's lymphoma, rhabdomyosarcoma, and retinoblastoma (ACS, 2019).

Diagnosis and treatment for childhood cancer require a specialized, multidisciplinary approach. Most children receive care at the NCI-supported Children's Oncology Group (COG) affiliated facilities (NCI, 2019). Initial diagnosis can be difficult, as many early symptoms mirror those similar to benign pediatric conditions (e.g., fever, lymphadenopathy, loss of appetite). Diagnostic procedures include biopsy, imaging modalities, blood work, and extent-of-disease evaluation. Common treatments include radiation, steroids, stem cell transplantation (SCT), surgery, and targeted immune therapy (Ambati & Boulad, 2019).

Toxic cancer treatments targeting body systems and structures are inextricably intertwined with the complex developmental domains of young children, which pose unique risks and challenges (Donnan et al., 2015). Vincristine, cisplatin, methotrexate, and cyclophosphamide are chemotherapy agents commonly used to treat pediatric cancers. Side effects may include, but are not limited to, hair loss, loss of deep tendon reflexes, weakness, numbness, tingling, myelosuppression, nausea, vomiting, neurotoxicity, and cardiotoxicity (Gilchrist & Tanner, 2013; Green & Makker, 2019). Occupational therapy services are established or emerging in many NCI-supported institutions. Pediatric occupational therapy services focus on the developmental, educational, emotional-behavioral, and injury-related needs of children and youth; they also address self-determination and self-advocacy along with role transition (AOTA, 2014). Hence, occupational therapists are well positioned to monitor the developmental needs of CCSs.

ADAPTATION, COPING, AND RESILIENCE IN CHILDREN AND YOUTH WITH CANCER

The physical and psychosocial burden of childhood cancer and its treatment weighs heavily on the entire family. CCSs are at risk for medical complications, some activities are potentially life-threatening, and precautions may be required. Diagnosis and treatment for childhood cancer require specialized medical care provided in NCI-supported institutions. Consequently, families must adapt to their child's cancer diagnosis, as the disease process and side effects of treatment may impede typical roles and routines. For example, caregivers and families often relocate to enable a child to receive necessary treatments, resulting in parental job loss. When active treatment begins, caregivers are expected to assume an active role in treating and monitoring complex medical needs of the child. In the absence of a parent or caregiver, siblings frequently take on the burden of fulfilling these new roles and responsibilities in their family system (Peikert et al., 2018).

Psychosocial issues related to childhood cancer throughout the continuum of care are well documented. Post-traumatic stress disorder (PTSD), distress, depression, and anxiety may occur as part of the cancer continuum of care and disrupt familiar roles and routines (Coughtrey et al., 2017; Long et al., 2018; Lyons, 2020; Peikert et al., 2018). Unique trends may occur during specific phases of care. Immediately after diagnosis, children and families need to adapt quickly after the initial shock of a cancer diagnosis. Parents must become accustomed to the overwhelmingly complex medical environment while feeling helpless and immobilized in their parental role. Active treatment phases may cause distress due to the high need for and frequency of intense medical care. In everyday life, challenges during the initial phases of treatment may significantly alter daily roles and routines, such as school, work, and social interaction. Although studies on CCSs have reported improved psychosocial outcomes after diagnosis, psychological distress and PTSD symptoms may still remain (Peikert et al., 2018). Siblings of children with cancer often experience uncertainty and fear, as well as interrupted daily life and academic participation. For example, when parents are emotionally unavailable or at the hospital for their child's treatment, siblings often take on caretaker roles (Long et al., 2018).

Nearly 32 million children have a chronic condition that prevents full participation on a daily basis (Mullins et al., 2015). This includes CCSs who may experience occupational challenges that impose barriers on adaptation, coping, and resilience. Various models, including the Wallander and Varni Disability-Stress-Coping Model, the Thompson and Gustafson Transactional Stress and Coping Model, and Kazak et al.'s Social Ecological Model, show possible relationships and trends between each of these constructs among this population (Mullins et al., 2015). For example, a common theme among these models is the correlation between family functioning (e.g., family relations, perceived burden of care, depressive symptoms, and doctor-parent relationship) and child adjustment (e.g., coping strategies, psychosocial issues). Similarities among models include interpersonal and intrapersonal parent variables, illness parameters and severity, and child demographics. Parent adjustment can directly affect the adjustment of children with juvenile rheumatoid disease, cancer, diabetes, or sickle cell disease (Mullins et al., 2015). Illness uncertainty is linked to adjustment outcomes in children with cancer, those receiving solid organ transplants, and adolescents with type 1 diabetes (Mullins et al., 2015). A study by Monti et al. (2017) on associations between maternal and paternal coping and depressive symptoms and children's coping during and after a cancer diagnosis showed that CCSs need to respond to changing demands and stressful treatments and procedures repeatedly throughout the cancer care continuum. The following case stories illustrate examples of parental concerns of CCSs.

Case Study 9-1

Omar

Omar is a 2-year-old male (Figure 9-1) who resides in Washington, DC, with his two mothers and two older siblings. He was recently diagnosed with neuro-blastoma after a mass was identified in his abdominal region during a routine check-up with the pediatrician. Upon diagnosis, he was noted to have bony metastatic disease in his lower extremities. His treatment included surgical resec-tion of primary tumor, chemotherapy (vincristine, cisplatin, cyclophosphamide, and doxorubicin), radiation, and autologous stem cell transplantation. Prior to his diagnosis, Omar attended daycare full time and participated in a soccer program. Omar's family used public transportation daily for community mobility. Due to his compromised immune system, Omar may no longer attend daycare or take public transportation. His mother quit her job due to his complex medical needs and frequent appointments. When asked about important roles she would like the occupational therapy practitioner to address, Omar's mother replied, "I want my son to play and engage in activities that he previously loved to do. He does not seem interested in toys or challenging himself. Some of his chemo-therapy causes cardiac issues, and I am nervous to push him over his limit. I feel like I have too many roles now. In addition to being a mother and wife, I feel like Omar's home nurse and therapist."

Figure 9-1. Omar.

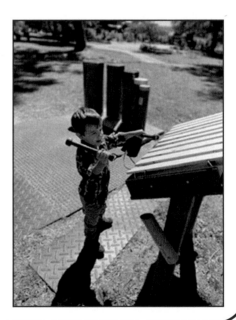

Case Story 9-2
Yaakov

Yaakov is an 8-year-old male who lives in Brooklyn, New York, with his mother, father, and siblings in an Orthodox Jewish community. His mother took him to the pediatrician after he complained of headaches, vision changes, and decreased coordination. The pediatrician recommended going to the emergency room immediately for testing. Magnetic resonance imaging (MRI) and cerebrospinal fluid analysis confirmed a diagnosis of medulloblastoma. Yaakov's treatment included resection of the primary tumor, chemotherapy, and radiation therapy. His course of treatment was complicated by posterior fossa syndrome resulting in loss of speech, irritability, and ataxia. Prior to his diagnosis, Yaakov enjoyed attending Hebrew school, weekly synagogue services on the Sabbath, and riding his bike with his siblings. While collecting information for Yaakov's occupational profile, his mother expressed feeling "exhausted trying to meet Yaakov's needs, as well as his siblings'. He does not communicate well and has low frustration tolerance. He gives up quickly when trying new things, and pushes games away that are difficult for him. He wants to play with his brothers and sisters, but he cannot keep up. I am tired all the time."

THE ROLE OF OCCUPATIONAL THERAPY: BEST AND EVIDENCE-BASED PRACTICES FOR ASSESSMENT AND INTERVENTION THROUGHOUT THE PEDIATRIC CANCER CARE CONTINUUM

The Occupational Therapy Process Throughout the Cancer Care Continuum

Occupational therapy services for the CCS should be holistic and client centered and focus on reducing stressors associated with cancer and building capacity for successful occupational performance. As the role of the occupational therapist in pediatric oncology is relatively new, evidence describing occupational therapy intervention programs consists mostly of descriptive studies and expert opinions. Interventions should be provided based on clinical judgment and client preferences.

As occupational therapists initiate the occupational therapy process and seek to identify barriers to, and interventions that will promote, adaptation, coping, and resilience in CCSs, there are important diagnosis- and treatment-related considerations that they must be aware of. Information about the child's past medical history, current medical status, and treatment plan are necessary to develop a safe plan of care that meets the child's rehabilitation needs. Fluctuations in the child's medical status may be frequent and, thus, should be monitored throughout the cancer care continuum. Members of the child's medical care team, comprising physicians, nurse practitioners, and/or nurses, are all valuable sources for obtaining this important information.

Occupational Profile

Obtaining a thorough occupational profile that identifies the child's preferences, roles, routines, perceived functional strengths and limitations, and participation in various environments will immensely influence the effectiveness of occupational therapy services provided to CCSs. The child's and family's values, beliefs, spirituality, priorities, and goals for occupational performance, quality of life (QoL), and participation will substantially influence and guide the occupational therapy process. For example, the family of a child recently diagnosed with a brain tumor may not be ready to begin occupational therapy services, preferring to spend their time receiving support from close family and friends. However, another family may be eager to receive support services that assist with and enhance the child's ability to adapt and cope. Each family and child is unique, and the occupational therapist should specifically identify their readiness to take in new information, their current perceived level of and satisfaction with occupational performance, reported stressors that influence occupational performance, and their level of motivation and readiness to participate actively in the occupational therapy process. See Table 9-1 for assessment tools that will guide development of the child's occupational profile.

EVIDENCE-BASED APPROACHES FOR ASSESSMENT AND INTERVENTION

Assessment

The number of stressors a CCS and their family may experience throughout the cancer care continuum is substantial. Stress and anxiety surrounding the initial diagnosis, illness, invasive procedures, fear of relapse, separation from family, intense treatment schedules, economic problems such as with insurance and finances, managing home and family demands including the care of other children, and worries about the child's health and prognosis affect the entire family (Kupst & Patenaude, 2016; Pai, 2007). The child may also experience occupational deprivation due to hospitalizations, illness, and immunosuppression (Miralles et al., 2016). Both the CCS and family members must find ways to cope with the diagnosis- and treatment-related sequelae (Kupst & Patenaude, 2016). Health care professionals need to be aware of possible psychosocial stressors that long-term CCSs may experience, as well as related treatment options (Bitsko et al., 2016). As part of the multidisciplinary care team, occupational therapists can help identify psychosocial stressors that restrict occupational performance and are barriers to successful

Table 9-1

Client Factor Assessment Tools to Identify Barriers for Adaptation, Coping, and Resilience in CCS

Domain	Assessment Tool
Psychosocial functions	• Distress Thermometer (adapted pediatric version; Wiener et al., 2017) • Psychosocial Assessment Tool (Alderfer et al., 2009) • Child Behavior Checklist (Achenbach & Rescorla, 2001) • Behavior Assessment System for Children (Reynolds & Kamphaus, 2004) • PROMIS (Hinds et al., 2013) • NIH Toolbox for Neurological and Behavioral Functioning Measure: Emotion Battery (Gershon et al., 2013)
Fatigue and activity tolerance	• PROMIS Fatigue (Hinds et al., 2013) • PedsQL Multidimensional Fatigue Scale (Varni et al., 2002)
Pain	• Pediatric Quality of Life Inventory Emotional Functioning and Pain Scales (Varni et al., 2004)
Cognitive capacity	• Behavior Rating Inventory of Executive Functioning, Second Edition (Gioia et al., 2000) • Children's Kitchen Task Assessment (Rocke et al., 2008) • Weekly Calendar Planning Activity (Toglia, 2015)
Development	• Ages and Stages Questionnaire (Squires et al., 2009) • Battelle Developmental Inventory (Newborg, 2005)
Social	• Social Emotional Assets and Resilience Scales (SEARS; Merrell, 2008)
Participation	• Children's Assessment of Participation and Enjoyment & Preferences for Activities of Children (King et al., 2004) • School Function Assessment (Coster et al., 1998) • Preschool Activity Card Sort (Berg & LaVesser, 2006) • Child Occupational Self-Assessment (Kramer et al., 2014) • Pediatric Evaluation of Disability Inventory (Haley, 1992). • Canadian Occupational Performance Measure (Law et al., 2019)

(continued)

Table 9-1 (continued)

Client Factor Assessment Tools to Identify Barriers for Adaptation, Coping, and Resilience in CCS	
Domain	Assessment Tool
Quality of Life	• The PedsQL Generic Core Scales (Varni et al., 2001) • The PedsQL Condition-Specific Modules: 　　▪ Cancer Module (Varni et al., 2002) 　　▪ Brain Tumor Module (Palmer et al., 2007) 　　▪ Stem Cell Transplant Module (Lawitschka et al., 2014) • PROMIS Quality of Life Measure (Hinds et al., 2013)

Abbreviations: PROMIS, Patient-Reported Outcomes Measurement Information System

coping, adaptation, and resilience. The *Children's Oncology Group Long-Term Follow-Up Guidelines for Survivors of Childhood, Adolescent and Young Adult Cancers* (version 5.0; 2018) recommends a yearly psychosocial assessment of a CCS that assesses depression, anxiety, post-traumatic stress, suicidal ideation, social withdrawal, and risky behaviors that could lead to serious illness or injury. Occupational therapists can use tools such as the National Comprehensive Cancer Network (NCCN) Distress Thermometer to screen for psychosocial issues and guide referral to appropriate psychosocial support services. The adapted version of the NCCN Distress Thermometer (2020) has been validated and used in the identification of psychosocial difficulties experienced by children with cancer (Wiener et al., 2017). The brief screen completed by the caregiver provides a distress rating between 0 (No Distress) to 10 (High Distress), and includes a symptom checklist where raters can indicate the reason for their distress. Additionally, assessment of health-related quality of life with tools such as the Pediatric Quality of Life Inventory (PedsQL) can identify CCSs experiencing, or at risk for experiencing, restrictions in QoL as a result of their diagnosis and treatment (Varni et al., 2001). See Table 9-1 for additional assessment tools to assist in identifying barriers to adaptation, coping, and resilience in CCSs.

Health Promotion and Maintenance Interventions

Health maintenance—including occupational engagement and the development of health routines, responsibilities, and roles—has been associated with increased resilience, coping, and adaptation in children (Usaite & Cameron, 2015). Sposito and colleagues described the self-reported coping strategies of children with cancer hospitalized for chemotherapy (2015). Children reported that health maintenance behaviors, such as gaining knowledge about their disease and treatment, easing the burden of side effects, finding joy in eating, engaging in play and leisure, and maintaining hope and religious practices, were all sources of coping (Sposito et al., 2015). While most CCS tend to cope well, the importance of standard-of-care comprehensive supportive care practices, including the services of multidisciplinary psychosocial support teams, in supporting this at-risk population has been emphasized (Phipps et al., 2012). Occupational therapists can collaborate with the child's multidisciplinary team (including medical providers, psychology services, chaplain services, and child life services) to develop interventions that support the child's development of these and other coping strategies that promote psychosocial wellness.

Health-related knowledge about disease and its treatment may be an important component of a child's ability to cope with and adjust to a cancer diagnosis. When children and families confirm that they are ready to receive this information, provision of developmentally appropriate information about diagnosis, treatment, functional impairments, prognosis for functional improvements, risk factors for late effects of cancer, and availability of support resources will empower the child and family to become well-informed and active participants in their rehabilitation and cancer care journey.

CCSs may have difficulty following structured routines and developing new roles and responsibilities after diagnosis, due to hospitalizations, illness, intense treatment schedules, and spending significant amounts of time away from home and school. Occupational therapists can facilitate development of new roles, routines, and responsibilities by developing and facilitating adherence to a new daily schedule and routine that include participation in activities of daily living (ADLs) and other meaningful activities while in the hospital. Measures such as the COPM (Law et al., 2019) or Pediatric Evaluation of Disability Inventory (Haley, 1992) can be very useful tools to help identify meaningful activities and current level of performance and satisfaction with those activities. Discussion of the child's schedule, activities, and goals should be included in multidisciplinary discussions about the child's care, as collaborative support will be required to facilitate goal achievement.

A holistic approach guides occupational therapists to interventions that ease the burden of diagnosis and treatment-related side effects through a multifaceted approach that includes facilitation of engagement in meaningful occupations, development of health management strategies, and addressing impairments in body function. Cancer-associated pain is a distressing side effect of cancer and treatment that may limit the ability of CCSs to participate in meaningful activities (including difficulty walking, eating, moving, and playing) and negatively affect their quality of life (Alberts et al., 2018). Cancer-related pain is reported by up to 52% to 60% of CCSs and their parents (Hedén et al., 2013; Jibb et al., 2015). Pain can originate from several sources, including diagnostic and treatment procedures, underlying malignancy, or other factors not associated with the disease process (Tutelman et al., 2018). Non-pharmacological pain management strategies have been recommended as an important part of a comprehensive pain management plan, and integrative, supportive, and rehabilitative therapies, including occupational therapy, are an expected part of the treatment protocol (Friedrichsdorf & Nugent, 2013). For example, relaxation, massage, and guided imagery have been reported as effective pain-management interventions that lead to improved self-reported coping abilities in CCSs (Sposito et al., 2015).

CCSs are at risk for developing secondary cancers, cardiovascular disease, osteoporosis, sleep deficiencies, and diabetes, among other adverse effects of their disease and treatment (Children's Oncology Group, 2018). Furthermore, CCSs with these conditions have been reported to experience a significantly higher prevalence of symptoms of emotional distress (Vuotto et al., 2017). When approved by a physician, exercise and a healthy diet are recommended as safe and noted to play a valuable role in reducing obesity, reducing fatigue and sleep disturbance, and increasing physical function in CCSs (Children's Oncology Group, 2018; Huang & Ness, 2011; Morales et al., 2020). Unfortunately, CCSs report barriers to exercise and following a healthy diet, including being too tired, being too busy, lack of experience with exercise, worry about injury, and lack of knowledge about how to make healthy (especially low-fat) food choices (Arroyave et al., 2008). Occupational therapists can guide the CCS in developing safe and effective wellness practices through interventions that include education, collaborative goal development, and development of routines that promote healthy habits and minimize distress associated with side effects of cancer and treatment.

Enhancing Functional Cognitive Capacity

The risk of cognitive impairment and the need to monitor neurocognitive functioning in children with cancer are well established (Conklin et al., 2017; Hanzlik et al., 2015; Moore, 2005). Cancer-related cognitive impairment (CRCI), including problems with attention, processing speed, working memory, and visual motor integration, varies in severity and deficits may occur over the cancer care continuum; therefore, repeated serial monitoring of cognitive skills is recommended (Castellino et al., 2014; Krull et al., 2008). Multiple members of the child's care team can monitor the child's cognitive abilities. When available, a comprehensive neurocognitive evaluation with a neuropsychologist and follow-up are recommended for CCSs at risk of cognitive impairments. Occupational therapists can evaluate the child's functional cognitive skills and related occupational performance across various contexts and environments (e.g., home, school, and community). For example, the occupational therapist may identify that a CCS experiences difficulty organizing her school assignments within the classroom or difficulty sequencing the tasks within her morning routine at home. Performance-based functional cognitive assessments such as the Children's Kitchen Task Assessment (Rocke et al., 2008) can measure the capacity of the child with, or at risk of, CRCI to participate in everyday life activities and provide valuable insights on the child's cognitive functioning. Metacognitive strategy training (Patel et al., 2009), social skills training (Barrera et al., 2018), and compensatory training (Tanner et al., 2020) have been found to improve functional cognitive skills, metacognition, and executive functioning. In turn, the child's participation in meaningful occupations, social confidence, satisfaction with activities, and quality of life may improve.

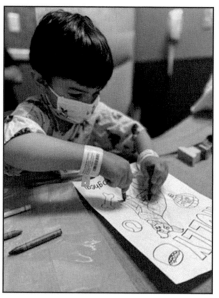

Figure 9-2. Child engaging in developmentally appropriate activity.

Support Engagement in Age-Appropriate Occupations

Childhood Development

Young children with cancer are at high risk of delays in cognitive development, fine and gross motor skills, social–emotional development, and behavioral functioning due to their diagnosis and treatment (Harman et al., 2018). Prolonged periods of hospitalization, illness, and cancer-related precautions restrict these children's access to age-appropriate environments, activities, and social experiences, in turn limiting opportunities for play and learning and thus their capacity for coping, adaptation, and resilience. Developmental skills should be closely monitored throughout the cancer care continuum.

Successful occupational development and adaptation in infants and toddlers requires opportunities for play, social interaction, and exploring and interacting with the environment (Case-Smith, 2010; National Research Council, Institute of Medicine, 2000). Children less than 3 years old with cancer should be referred to intervention services early in the cancer care continuum (Harman et al., 2018). Occupational therapists can support the child's ability to participate in age-appropriate activities and roles through environmental adaptation, activity modification, and family education about developmentally appropriate activities (Figure 9-2).

Education

The CCS may also require support to facilitate adjustment and coping with changes in their educational roles and routines. Participation in both the academic and social aspects of school are often immediately disrupted when a child is diagnosed with cancer. School attendance may be precluded by lengthy and intense treatments, illness, or relocation to another city or state for treatment. Reintegration into school after treatment may also be complicated by anxiety and stressors for the CCS, such as cognitive and physical challenges, worry about peer acceptance, and ongoing disruptions to school attendance by medical appointments (Stimler & Skuller, 2020). Occupational therapy practitioners can help to reduce the stressors associated with changes in the child's academic participation by identifying barriers to successful school reintegration. The School Function Assessment (Coster et al., 1998) can help identify classroom performance strengths and challenges for children returning to school after completing cancer treatment. Interventions to support adaptation, coping, and resilience should focus on minimizing stressors associated with disruptions in school and fostering engagement in educational activities. School connectedness—the "belief by students that adults and peers in the school care about their learning, as well as about them as individuals"— has been correlated with students' psychosocial adjustment and academic success (Dovi et al., 2019). Promoting school connectedness in the CCS may enhance resilience and should be collaboratively addressed by the multidisciplinary psychosocial care team, including teachers, psychologists, child life specialists, and occupational therapists. Occupational therapists can foster educational engagement and engagement in school activities through education, advocacy, development of accommodations, modifications, and education that will reduce stressors and barriers as the child transitions back to school. School reintegration efforts have been found to lead to enhanced academic achievement, lower levels of depression, increases in peers' willingness to interact with children, and decreased worry and anxiety (Helms et al., 2016). Provision of education to the parent, peers, and educator to assist them in understanding the child's illness and needs, anticipated challenges, and need for support is recommended (Castellino et al., 2014). Accommodations and modifications such as participation in virtual academic or social school activities (Figure 9-3; e.g., Skype, phone calls, or emails from teachers/ peers) and recommending changes to the child's daily school schedule to allow for shorter days or for breaks due to fatigue or illness may help promote participation and minimize stressors and barriers as the child transitions back to school (Kupst & Patenaude, 2016).

Leisure Activities

For some children and adolescents with cancer, participation in preferred leisure activities such as sports, low-demand physical activities (e.g., walking), crafting, or drawing was likely a primary way to cope with stress prior to diagnosis (Kupst & Patenaude, 2016). For CCSs, environmental restrictions (e.g., hospitalization) and side effects of cancer treatment (e.g., medical precautions, nausea, musculoskeletal or neurological impairments) are common and may preclude them from participation in these meaningful pursuits that are important to their coping and resilience. If engagement in these meaningful activities is limited by medical restrictions or performance limitations, the occupational therapist should work with the child and care team to eliminate environmental barriers to performance and identify accommodations or alternative means of participation. Assessments such as the Child Occupational Self-Assessment (Kramer et al., 2014) will be helpful in identifying activity preferences, challenges, and strengths, so that interventions can be designed to support participation and engagement. Occupational therapists can also use engagement in leisure activities as a tool to promote coping, adaptation,

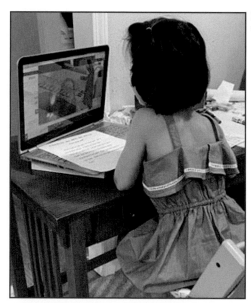

Figure 9-3. School reintegration through virtual participation.

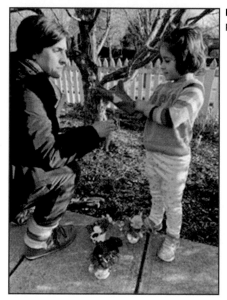

Figure 9.4. Leisure activities can be a tool to promote coping, adaptation, and resilience in CCSs.

and resilience in CCSs (Figure 9-4). For example, it has been suggested that art and music interventions promote the well-being of children undergoing cancer treatment by reducing anxiety, fear, and pain and promoting collaborative behaviors; enhancing communication with the treatment team; and counteracting the disruption of selfhood that cancer treatment evokes (Derman & Deatrick, 2016; Uggla et al., 2018).

Social Engagement

Environmental and contextual barriers such as being physically separated from friends and family, limited school participation, limited ability to attend community or religious events, as well as medical and physical symptoms such as changes in appearance, neurological sequelae pain and fatigue, reduce the opportunities of the CCS for social engagement (Barrera et al., 2020; Donnan et al., 2015; Sodergren et al., 2017). Family and social supports are also affected if cancer care is not near the child's home, as many individuals feel removed from understanding partners, family, and community (Walling et al., 2019). Social interaction can be beneficial in increasing knowledge, decreasing isolation, and improving adjustment for CCSs, and therefore, provision of opportunities for social interaction during cancer treatment and into long-term survivorship are strongly recommended (Christiansen et al., 2015). The occupational therapist has a role in the assessment of social needs, strengths, and preferences, as well as in the provision of social-skills interventions that collaboratively (along with families, peers, and the cancer care team) build capacity for adaptation, coping, and resilience.

Social-skills interventions for CCSs are designed to promote social-developmental skills, prevent or reduce social-competence deficits, and improve CCSs' QoL (Barrera et al., 2020). Social-skills training programs may include capacity building for making friends, conflict resolution, social cognitive problem solving, and assertiveness training, among other skills (Barrera et al., 2020; Christiansen et al., 2015). CCSs participating in social skills training programs have reported improved self-control and self-acceptance, reduced feelings of sadness, improved problem solving, increased social confidence with peers, and reduced acting-out (Barrera et al., 2020). Hospitalized children receiving chemotherapy reported that connecting with people outside the hospital was beneficial in coping with hospitalization (Sposito et al., 2015).

See Table 9-2 for interventions to promote social-skills development, provide opportunities for social engagement, and support the development of new social roles for the CCS during and after cancer treatment.

SPECIAL CONSIDERATIONS FOR ADAPTATION, COPING, AND RESILIENCE IN CHILDREN AND YOUTH WITH CANCER

Palliative Care and End of Life

Although survival rates for many childhood cancers have risen significantly, some children with cancer cannot be cured. The holistic and family-centered approach of the occupational therapy practitioner, in collaboration with other members of the care team, provides valuable insights into the needs of children and their families at the end of life. Occupational therapists believe that maintaining function and involvement in desired life activities contributes to improved quality of life, including through enhancing spiritual well-being and an individual's ability to cope (American Occupational Therapy

Table 9-2

Interventions to Build Capacity for Adaptation, Coping, and Resilience in Childhood Cancer Survivors

Health Promotion and Maintenance

Provide Education

- Disease- and treatment-specific education (Sposito et al., 2015)
- Anticipatory guidance focused on risk factors for secondary conditions and functional impairments
- Value of occupational engagement (Sposito et al., 2015)
- Patient education resources include the book *Childhood Cancer Survivors: A Practical Guide to Your Future* (Keene et al., 2012) and Children's Oncology Group Health links (Children's Oncology Group, n.d.)

Mitigate Distressing Symptoms

- Reduce cancer-associated pain:
  - Physical interventions: Massage, comfort positioning, educating family in benefits of and techniques for close contact/touch (Friedrichsdorf & Nugent, 2013; Jibb et al., 2015; Sposito et al., 2015; Tutelman et al., 2018)
  - Cognitive behavioral interventions: Distraction (e.g., video games or listening to music), deep breathing exercises, relaxation and sleep, guided imagery, art therapy, aromatherapy (Friedrichsdorf & Nugent, 2013; Jibb et al., 2015; Sposito et al., 2015; Tutelman et al., 2018)
- Improve sleep:
  - Massage (Jacobs et al., 2016)
  - Sleep hygiene, including limiting naps to 1 hour so as not to interfere with nighttime sleep (NCCN, 2015)
- Manage fatigue and improve physical activity:
  - Yoga (Danhauer et al., 2019; Weaver & Darragh, 2015; Wurz et al., 2014)
  - Provide safe and effective exercise, energy conservation, and nutrition programs and related education (Arroyave et al., 2008; Baumann et al., 2012; Huang & Ness, 2011; NCCN, 2015)

Facilitate Development of Routines, Roles, and Responsibilities

- Collaborative development of daily schedule and occupational goals during hospitalizations
- Engagement in activities of daily living (Baumann et al., 2010)
- Promote independence and self-management skills
- Enlist the child's entire care team to support the child's goals and engagement

(continued)

Table 9-2 (continued)

Interventions to Build Capacity for Adaptation, Coping, and Resilience in Childhood Cancer Survivors

Enhancing Functional Cognitive Capacity

- Metacognitive strategy training program (Patel et al., 2009)
- Internal or external memory aids, such as visualizations, alarms, lists, or calendars (Tanner et al., 2020)

Engagement in Age-Appropriate Occupations

Promote Attainment of Developmental Milestones

- Early intervention services (Harman et al., 2018)
- Promote normalization of the environment and opportunities for play, social interaction, and explore options when the child is without access to these opportunities naturally (e.g., provide opportunities for fantasy/imaginative play; create play space in hospital room with supplies including floor mat, age-appropriate toys; use what is in the environment in new and creative ways, such as making a balloon out of a medical glove; Kupst & Patenaude, 2016; Mohammadi et al., 2017; Sposito et al., 2015)
- Provide parent education to foster development

Promote Engagement in Educational Activities

- Facilitate school connectedness (Dovi et al., 2019)
- Use school reintegration programs, including information about cancer for teachers and peers (Helms et al., 2016)
- Provide parent and educator education about anticipated deficits and need for support services (Castellino et al., 2014)
- Minimize barriers to school participation through technology (e.g., tele-education; Kupst & Patenaude, 2016)
- Minimize barriers to school participation through accommodations and modifications (e.g., reduced workload, extended time for tests and assignments, using elevator instead of stairs, advocating for permission for the child to wear a hat/scarf in the classroom due to hair loss)
- Advocate for necessary educational supports (Castellino et al., 2014)
- Contribute to development of 504 plan or Individualized Education Plan (IEP)
- Address functional deficits affecting educational performance and participation

(continued)

Table 9-2 (continued)

Interventions to Build Capacity for Adaptation, Coping, and Resilience in Childhood Cancer Survivors
Promote Engagement in Leisure Activities
• Facilitate engagement in meaningful leisure activity through development of new roles and responsibilities (e.g., change from goalie to manager on soccer team; Anaby et al., 2016; Sposito et al., 2015)
• Art therapy (Derman & Deatrick, 2016)
• Music therapy (Uggla et al., 2018)
• Camps for children with cancer (Neville et al., 2019; Wu et al., 2016)
Social Engagement
• Social-skills training (Barrera et al., 2018; Barrera et al., 2020)
• Facilitate maintenance of the CCS's relationships with family and friends outside the hospital (Sposito et al., 2015; Willard et al., 2019)
• Use technology such as texting, Skype, sharing photos, email, or social media to facilitate virtual engagement in school, events, and social relationships and reduce the sense of isolation (Kupst & Patenaude, 2016)
• Collaborate with multidisciplinary care team to plan celebrations of milestones and events in ways that allow the CCS to engage (e.g., graduation ceremony, birthday celebrations, end of chemotherapy)
• Facilitate networking among CCSs and their families who have had similar cancer experiences
• Hospital-based social groups (e.g., teen groups, play groups, tween groups, craft groups, cooking/nutrition groups)
• CCS peer mentoring programs or family mentoring programs in which newly diagnosed patients and families who are interested in meeting other families are paired up with established patients or long-term cancer survivors
• Camps for children with cancer (Neville et al., 2019; Wu et al., 2016)

Association [AOTA], 2011). For children at the end of life, the occupational therapist can facilitate the child's engagement in activities that are meaningful, including those related to school activities, community activities, play, and mobility. Engagement in these typical occupations of childhood can provide children with a sense of control, identity, and competence. Because children may experience pain, fatigue, reduced mobility, anxiety, depression, and fear during this phase of the cancer care continuum, modification to previous occupations, modification to the environment, and training of the child or family in coping strategies to allow for continued participation and meaningful family interactions may be necessary (AOTA, 2011; Jalmsell et al., 2006). Additionally, symptom-based interventions such as pain-management services; support of neurologic, cognitive, musculoskeletal, and psychosocial needs; or education in energy-conservation strategies may be valuable (Tester, 2006).

Childhood Cancer and Long-Term Survivorship

As the number of long-term cancer survivors increases, so does the need for interventions addressing long-term late effects of cancer and its treatment. As CCSs transition out of active treatment and return to their homes, their schools, and their communities, they will once again require support to adapt and cope with their new situations. Years after completing cancer treatment, patients may require physical, cognitive, and/or psychosocial support for success in academics, vocational plans, and independent living (Kupst & Patenaude, 2016). CCSs are less likely to be employed, attain education beyond high school, or live independently, and report difficulties with driving and attending community events (Berg et al., 2009; Ness et al., 2006). Survivors may benefit from services like occupational therapy, which facilitate the acquisition of adult skills and independence and promote QoL. This includes mastering normative social functioning, coping strategies, emotional development, and working toward educational or vocational goals (Bitsko et al., 2016).

Per Bitsko et al. (2016), survivor self-report is the most accurate method of assessing functioning within these domains. Examples include survivor self-report of poor physical functioning, extent of late effects, cancer-related pain, and health beliefs. Tools assessing participation and promoting goal setting, such as the Canadian Occupational Performance Measure, Fifth Edition (Law et al., 2019) and the Pediatric Quality of Life Inventory (Varni et al., 2002), can guide long-term cancer survivors to self-identify performance and satisfaction with independent living, higher education, employment, and QoL, and develop related goals.

For CCSs, occupational therapists facilitate improved occupational performance through remediation or compensation for functional limitations; they also act as transition navigators assisting the long-term cancer survivor and family (Sparrow, 2020). Vocational rehabilitation can provide survivors and employers with tools and strategies to promote educational and vocational attainment (Tanner et al., 2020). Refer to Tables 9-2 and 9-3 for evidence-based approaches to occupational therapy assessment and intervention for CCSs.

BUILDING INTERPROFESSIONAL COLLABORATIONS

A multidisciplinary approach to occupational therapy services for CCSs is recommended, as members of the child's care team can provide valuable information about their medical status, treatment plan, psychosocial circumstances, and needs of the child and family. The care team may include an oncologist and/or radiologist, nurse practitioner, physician assistant, nurse, social worker, child life specialist, music therapist, audiologist, physical therapist, speech therapist, chaplain, psychologist, neuropsychologist, and school teacher.

Many CCSs reside in rural communities and travel long distances for specialized, multidisciplinary care. A qualitative survey by Walling et al. (2019) reported families' frustration with the lack of regard for the specialized needs of their children at local hospitals. Establishing communication between the cancer specialty institution and local community hospital at diagnosis can help identify and provide complex resources for appropriate care. Collaboration among health care providers (HCPs) may improve the family's trust that their child is receiving appropriate specialized care at local facilities (Walling et al., 2019). Cross-disciplinary communication may also improve client outcomes by maximizing carryover of tailored strategies.

A Global Perspective

Childhood cancer presents unique challenges globally for clients, caregivers, and HCPs. The International Agency for Research on Cancer (IARC, 2016) reported that worldwide, approximately 300,000 children under 19 years of age are annually diagnosed with cancer. In developed countries, childhood cancer is less than 1% of all cancer diagnoses; however, in developing countries where children compose almost half the population, these rates can be five times higher. Survival rates for children with cancer are improving, but major disparities exist (survival rate 80% in developed vs. 10% to 15% in developing countries; IARC, 2016). Also, there are significant variations in the distribution of diagnoses internationally, due to missed diagnoses, exposure to different treatments, and poor access to appropriate/expensive diagnostic tools or to major government-funded hospitals (IARC, 2016; Walubita et al., 2018). There are multifaceted cultural influences along the childhood cancer continuum of care that affect adaptation, coping, and resilience. Occupational therapy practitioners are called to practice culturally sensitive care and understand the perspective of international HCPs (Taleghani et al., 2012). Refer to Table 9-3 on essentials for occupational therapy practitioners to consider in building adaptation, coping, and resilience with CCSs.

Essential Considerations for Occupational Therapists to Build Adaptation, Coping, and Resilience

Table 9-3

Essentials to Build Adaptation, Coping, and Resilience for Childhood Cancer Survivors		
Essential Considerations	Barriers to Adaptation, Coping, and Resilience	Strategies
1) Create a culture and environment that promotes occupation participation	• Children's complex medical needs may result in caregivers and parents becoming overprotective, limiting the child's development of self-determination and independence due to learned helplessness.	• Set up automatic referrals for high-risk clients. • Provide preventive care and education. • Initiate the occupational therapy process early in continuum of care. • Use a formal screening process for new clients.
2) Recognize unique precautions and side effects related to cancer and its treatment	• When children receive cancer treatment or have a weakened immune system, they may not be allowed to leave the hospital room due to risk for infection. Strict protective isolation precautions may result in physical and social isolation, limiting a child's opportunity to participate in childhood occupations in natural environments and contexts with family and peers. • Abnormal lab values, cancer treatment-related side effects, and dependency on medical equipment (central lines, oxygen support) can create barriers to engagement in age-appropriate play, social	• Obtain parameters and information related to critical lab values from the primary team and medical chart. • Clients with thrombocytopenia and anemia should be monitored for nausea, pain, headache, pallor, bruising, petechiae, abnormal resting vital signs, and fatigue. These symptoms may require a modification of assessment or interventions (Gilchrist & Tanner, 2017). • Monitor cancer metastases or disease progression. • Clients with central lines should avoid contact sports and heavy lifting, to avoid damage or dislodgement. Therapists should keep the surrounding area dry and clean and ensure that the line is secured properly to avoid dislodging during activity.

(continued)

Table 9-3 (continued)

Essentials to Build Adaptation, Coping, and Resilience for Childhood Cancer Survivors		
Essential Considerations	**Barriers to Adaptation, Coping, and Resilience**	**Strategies**
	interaction, and attainment of physical and psychosocial milestones.	Maximize comfort by using pillows, blankets, or other props for positioning, and maintain comfortable upper-extremity range-of-motion activities. • Adhere closely to infection-control guidelines.
3) Recognize the cancer continuum of care	• A CCS's and the family's ability to adapt and cope often fluctuate, and may be dependent on the cancer care continuum. For example, during pretreatment, children and families may experience anxiety related to adjustments to moving near an NCI-supported institution for care, as well as role transitions; during the survivorship phase these individuals may experience anxiety due to fear of recurrence.	• Occupational therapists should recognize differences in unique life roles, habits, and routines for CCSs and their family system along the cancer care continuum. • Modify the occupational therapy process as needed with respect to where the client is in their journey.
4) Bridge the gap in service delivery	• Evidence highlighting a CCS's increased risk for distress, anxiety, post-traumatic stress, and depression is well established. These psychosocial issues may result in avoidance behavior and limited occupational engagement (Lyons, 2020). Recognition of how occupational therapy services can support adaptation, coping, and resilience is limited in many clinical and community-based settings.	• Maximize communication between rural community settings and NCI-supported COG-affiliated cancer institutions. • Stay current on NCCN guidelines, NCI guidelines, etc. • Determine an appropriate and qualified individual to act as a client liaison between the cancer-specialty institution, community hospital, school, and family.

Case Study 9-3
Francesca

Occupational Profile

Francesca, a 14-year-old Latina female, lives with her mother in Memphis, Tennessee. They relocated to allow Francesca to receive specialized care at an NCI-supported, COG-affiliated hospital. Her father stayed in Puerto Rico for his current job and to allow her 10-year-old sister to finish the school year. Francesca was diagnosed after experiencing night sweats, fever, weight loss, and bruising. Francesca loves to read and swim. She was excited to plan her quinceañera, but sad that she may not be able to celebrate in Puerto Rico.

Medical Treatment

Francesca has undergone multiple phases of central nervous system (CNS)-directed (intrathecal) and systemic chemotherapy (remission induction, consolidation/intensification, and maintenance), CNS radiation, corticosteroids, and allogeneic stem cell transplantation (SCT) from an 8/10 HLA unmatched unrelated donor. Chemotherapy agents included vincristine, doxorubicin, cyclophosphamide, cytarabine, mercaptopurine, and methotrexate. Francesca's course of treatment was complicated by graft-vs.-host disease (GVHD) with severe skin involvement 30 days after the SCT, as well as steroid myopathy and osteonecrosis.

Analysis of Occupational Performance

The SCT medical team initiated a referral for occupational therapy to address decreased participation in activities of daily living (ADLs), fatigue, and depression during Francesca's hospitalization. The occupational profile was developed using the COPM (Law et al., 2019). Francesca reported decreased scores in performance and satisfaction socializing with friends and participation in self-care activities, specifically dressing and bathing. ADL performance was assessed through skilled observation and the Functional Independence Measure Instrument (Uniform Data System for Medical Rehabilitation, 2012). Francesca required moderate assistance dressing and bathing due to cancer-related fatigue and limited overhead-reaching precautions due to a newly placed mediport. The PedsQL Stem Cell Transplant Module Teen-Self and Parent Reports were used to screen and monitor physical, psychosocial, and overall health-related quality of life (Lawitschka et al., 2014). Francesca and her mother indicated concerns about her coping, feelings of sadness, and anxiety related to missing age-appropriate opportunities related to school, socialization, and her quinceañera.

Occupational Therapy Intervention Plan

The occupational therapist created a plan to treat Francesca 2 days per week, for 30 minutes per session. Together, they develop a daily schedule including

(continued)

Case Study 9-3 (continued)

her ADL routine (e.g., dressing, bathing, tooth-brushing). Education was provided regarding compensatory strategies and energy conservation during her ADL routine to minimize the impact of fatigue. The benefits of walking to the bathroom for all self-care needs instead of performing them at the bedside were highlighted. Supports were put into place, including the use of a loaner laptop to promote increased social interaction with family and friends using Skype, to participate in school virtually online, and to create digital stories about her personal journey. Guided imagery was used as a preparatory strategy to decrease the impact of Francesca's anxiety during her daily routine (Wilson et al., 2016). Finally, behavioral approaches were also incorporated by allotting time for Francesca to plan for her quinceañera after completion of non-preferred activities.

Occupational Therapy Outcomes

Upon discharge from the hospital following her SCT, Francesca required close supervision during dressing and bathing. Outpatient occupational therapy was recommended to monitor her splinting needs, functional status in relation to range-of-motion restrictions, and cancer-related fatigue (CRF) management. The outpatient occupational therapist collaborated with Francesca to reclaim her occupational identity after experiencing occupational disruption due to her cancer diagnosis. This process involved identifying potential challenges as a CCS when re-engaging in previously meaningful social and school-based occupations (Stanley, 2019). In addition, an adolescent CCS community support group was recommended.

REFERENCES

Achenbach, T. M., & Rescorla, L. A. (2001). *Manual for the ASEBA School-Age Forms & Profiles.* University of Vermont, Research Center for Children, Youth, & Families.

Alberts, N. M., Gagnon, M. M., & Stinson, J. N. (2018). Chronic pain in survivors of childhood cancer: A developmental model of pain across the cancer trajectory. *Pain, 159*(10), 1916-1927. https://doi.org/10.1097/j.pain.0000000000001261

Alderfer, M. A., Mougianis, I., Barakat, L. P., Beele, D., DiTaranto, S., Hwang, W.-T., Rielly, A. T., & Kazak, A. E. (2009). Family psychosocial risk, distress, and service utilization in pediatric cancer: Predictive validity of the Psychosocial Assessment Tool (PAT). *Cancer, 115*(S8), S4339-S4349. https://doi.org/10.1002/cncr.24587

Ambati, S. R., & Boulad, F. (2019). Evaluation and management of pediatric cancers. In M. D. Stubblefield (Ed.), *Cancer rehabilitation: Principles and practice* (2nd ed., pp. 359-373). Demos Medical.

American Cancer Society. (2019). *Types of cancer that develop in children.* https://www.cancer.org/cancer/cancer-in-children/types-of-childhood-cancers.html

American Childhood Cancer Organization. (2019). *US childhood cancer statistics.* https://www.acco.org/us-childhood-cancer-statistics

American Occupational Therapy Association. (2011). The role of occupational therapy in end-of-life care. *American Journal of Occupational Therapy, 65*(Suppl.), s66-s75. https://doi.org/10.5014/ajot.2011.65s66

American Occupational Therapy Association. (2014). *AOTA fact sheet: Occupational therapy's role with children and youth.* https://www.aota.org/-/media/Corporate/Files/AboutOT/Professionals/WhatIsOT/CY/Fact-sheets/Children%20and%20Youth%20fact%20sheet.pdf

Anaby, D. R., Law, M. C., Majnemer, A., & Feldman, D. (2016). Opening doors to participation of youth with physical disabilities: An intervention study/Favoriser la participation des adolescents ayant des handicaps physiques: Étude d'intervention. *Canadian Journal of Occupational Therapy, 83*(2), 83-90. https://doi.org/10.1177/0008417415608653

Arroyave, W. D., Clipp, E. C., Miller, P. E., Jones, L. W., Ward, D. S., Bonner, M. J., Rosoff, P. M., Snyder, D. C., & Demark-Wahnefried, W. (2008). Childhood cancer survivors' perceived barriers to improving exercise and dietary behaviors. In *Oncology Nursing Forum, 35*(1), 121-130. https://doi.org/10.1188/08.onf.121-130

Barrera, M., Atenafu, E. G., Sung, L., Bartels, U., Schulte, F., Chung, J., Cataudella, D., Hancock, K., Janzen, L., Saleh, A., Strother, D., Downie, A, Zelcer, S., Hukin, J., & McConnell, D. (2018). A randomized control intervention trial to improve social skills and quality of life in pediatric brain tumor survivors. *Psycho-Oncology, 27*(1), 91-98. https://doi.org/10.1002/pon.4385

Barrera, M., Hancock, K., Bartels, U., Solomon, A. & Desjardins, L. (2020). "I'm with my people!" *Cancer Nursing, 44*(3), 197-204. https://doi.org/10.1097/NCC.0000000000000779

Baumann, F. T., Bloch, W., & Beulertz, J. (2012). Clinical exercise interventions in pediatric oncology: A systematic review. *Pediatric Research, 74,* 366-374. https://doi.org/10.1038/pr.2013.123

Baumann, F. T., Kraut, L., Schüle, K., Bloch, W., & Fauser, A. A. (2010). A controlled randomized study examining the effects of exercise therapy on patients undergoing haematopoietic stem cell transplantation. *Bone Marrow Transplantation, 45*(2), 355-362. https://doi.org/10.1038/bmt.2009.163

Berg, C., & LaVesser, P. (2006). The preschool activity card sort. *OTJR: Occupation, Participation and Health, 26*(4), 143-151. https://doi.org/10.1177/153944920602600404

Berg, C., Neufeld, P., Harvey, J., Downes, A., & Hayashi, R. J. (2009). Late effects of childhood cancer, participation, and quality of life of adolescents. *OTJR: Occupation, Participation and Health, 29*(3), 116-124. https://doi.org/10.3928/15394492-20090611-04

Bitsko, M. J., Cohen, D., Dillon, R., Harvey, J., Krull, K., & Klosky, J. L. (2016). Psychosocial late effects in pediatric cancer survivors: A report from the Children's Oncology Group. *Pediatric Blood & Cancer, 63*(2), 337-343. https://doi.org/10.1002/pbc.25773

Case-Smith, J. (2010). Development of childhood occupations. In J. Case-Smith & J. O'Brien (Eds.), *Occupational therapy for children* (6th ed., pp. 56-83). Mosby.

Castellino, S. M., Ullrich, N. J., Whelen, M. J., & Lange, B. J. (2014). Developing interventions for cancer-related cognitive dysfunction in childhood cancer survivors. *Journal of the National Cancer Institute, 106*(8), dju186. https://doi.org/10.1093/jnci/dju186

Children's Oncology Group. (n.d.). Children's Oncology Group health links. http://www.survivorship-guidelines.org

Children's Oncology Group. (2018). Long-term follow up guidelines for survivors of childhood, adolescent, and young adult cancers, version 5.0. http://www.survivorshipguidelines.org

Christiansen, H. L., Bingen, K., Hoag, J. A., Karst, J. S., Velázquez-Martin, B., & Barakat, L. P. (2015). Providing children and adolescents opportunities for social interaction as a standard of care in pediatric oncology. *Pediatric Blood & Cancer, 62*(S5), S724-S749. https://doi.org/10.1002/pbc.25774

Conklin, H. M., Ashford, J. M., Clark, K. N., Martin-Elbahesh, K., Hardy, K. K., Merchant, T. E., Ogg, R. J., Jeha, S., Huang, L., & Zhang, H. (2017). Long-term efficacy of computerized cognitive training among survivors of childhood cancer: A single-blind randomized controlled trial. *Journal of Pediatric Psychology, 42*(2), 220-231. https://doi.org/10.1093/jpepsy/jsw057

Coster, W., Deeney, T., Haltiwanger, J., & Haley, S. M. (1998). *School function assessment.* Pearson Education.

Coughtrey, A. E., Millington, A., Bennett, S., Christie, D., Hough, R., Su, M., Constantinou, M., & Shafran, R. (2017). The effectiveness of psychosocial interventions for psychological outcomes in pediatric oncology: A systematic review. *Journal of Pain and Symptom Management, 55*(3), 1004-1017. https://doi.org/10.1016/j.jpainsymman.2017.09.022

Danhauer, S. C., Addington, E. L., Cohen, L., Sohl, S. J., Van Puymbroeck, M., Albinati, N. K., & Culos-Reed, S. N. (2019). Yoga for symptom management in oncology: A review of the evidence base and future directions for research. *Cancer, 125*(12), 1979-1989. https://doi.org/10.1002/cncr.31979

Derman, Y. E., & Deatrick, J. A. (2016). Promotion of well-being during treatment for childhood cancer. *Cancer Nursing, 39*(6), E1-E16. https://doi.org/10.1097/NCC.0000000000000318

Donnan, B. M., Webster, T., Wakefield, C. E., Dalla-Pozza, L., Alvaro, F., Lavoipierre, J., & Marshall, G. M. (2015). What about school? Educational challenges for children and adolescents with cancer. *The Australian Educational and Developmental Psychologist, 32*(1), 23-40. https://doi.org/10.1017/edp.2015.9

Dovi, A., Lindwall, J., Sato, T., Brigden, J., & Phipps, S. (2019). Perceived school connectedness as it relates to parent-reported behavior and adaptive skills in youth with recently diagnosed cancer. *Children's Health Care, 49*(3), 233-246. https://doi.org/10.1080/02739615.2019.1686982

Friedrichsdorf, S. J., & Nugent, A. P. (2013). Management of neuropathic pain in children with cancer. *Current Opinion in Supportive and Palliative Care, 7*(2), 131-138. https://doi.org/10.1097/spc.0b013e3283615ebe

Gershon, R. C., Wagster, M. V., Hendrie, H. C., Fox, N. A., Cook, K. F., & Nowinski, C. J. (2013). NIH toolbox for assessment of neurological and behavioral function. *Neurology, 80*(11, Suppl. 3), S2-S6. https://doi.org/10.1212/WNL.0b013e3182872e5f

Gilchrist, L. S., & Tanner, L. (2013). The pediatric-modified total neuropathy score: a reliable and valid measure of chemotherapy-induced peripheral neuropathy in children with non-CNS cancers. *Supportive Care in Cancer, 21*(3), 847-856. https://doi.org/10.1007/s00520-012-1591-8

Gilchrist, L. S., & Tanner, L. R. (2017). Safety of symptom-based modification of physical therapy interventions in pediatric oncology patients with and without low blood counts. *Rehabilitation Oncology, 35*(1), 3-8. https://doi.org/10.1097/01.reo.0000000000000042

Gioia, G., Isquith, P., Guy, S., & Kenworthy, L. (2000). Behaviour rating inventory of executive function. *Child Neuropsychology, 6*(3), 235-238. https://doi.org/10.1076/chin.6.3.235.3152

Green, A. K., & Makker, V. (2019). Principles of antineoplastic therapeutics. In M. D. Stubblefield (Ed.), *Cancer rehabilitation: Principles and practice* (2nd ed., pp. 38-58). Springer.

Haley, S. M. (1992). *Pediatric Evaluation of Disability Inventory (PEDI): Development, standardization and administration manual.* PEDI Research Group.

Hanzlik, E., Woodrome, S. E., Abdel-Baki, M., Geller, T. J., & Elbabaa, S. K. (2015). A systematic review of neuropsychological outcomes following posterior fossa tumor surgery in children. *Child's Nervous System, 31*(10), 1869-1875. https://doi.org/10.1007/s00381-015-2867-3

Harman, J. L., Wise, J., & Willard, V. W. (2018). Early intervention for infants and toddlers: Applications for pediatric oncology. *Pediatric Blood & Cancer, 65*(5), e26921. https://doi.org/10.1002/pbc.26921

Hedén, L., Pöder, U., von Essen, L., & Ljungman, G. (2013). Parents' perceptions of their child's symptom burden during and after cancer treatment. *Journal of Pain and Symptom Management, 46*(3), 366-375. https://doi.org/10.1016/j.jpainsymman.2012.09.012

Helms, A. S., Schmiegelow, K., Brok, J., Johansen, C., Thorsteinsson, T., Simovska, V., & Larsen, H. B. (2016). Facilitation of school re-entry and peer acceptance of children with cancer: A review and meta-analysis of intervention studies. *European Journal of Cancer Care, 25*(1), 170-179. https://doi.org/10.1111/ecc.12230

Hinds, P. S., Nuss, S. L., Ruccione, K. S., Withycombe, J. S., Jacobs, S., DeLuca, H., Faulkner, C., Liu, Y., Cheng, Y. I., Gross, H. E., Wang, J., & DeWalt, D. A. (2013). PROMIS pediatric measures in pediatric oncology: Valid and clinically feasible indicators of patient-reported outcomes. *Pediatric Blood & Cancer, 60*(3), 402-408. https://doi.org/10.1002/pbc.24233

Huang, T. T., & Ness, K. K. (2011). Exercise interventions in children with cancer: A review. *International Journal of Pediatrics, 2011.* https://doi.org/10.1155/2011/461512

International Agency for Research on Cancer. (2016). *World Health Organization Press Release No. 241: International childhood cancer day: Much remains to be done to fight childhood cancer.* https://www.acco.org/wp-content/uploads/2016/02/pr241_E.pdf

Jacobs, S., Mowbray, C., Cates, L. M., Baylor, A., Gable, C., Skora, E., Estrada, M., Cheng, Y., Wang, J., Lewin, D., & Hinds, P. (2016). Pilot study of massage to improve sleep and fatigue in hospitalized adolescents with cancer. *Pediatric Blood & Cancer, 63*(5), 880-886. https://doi.org/10.1002/pbc.25902

Jalmsell, L., Kreicbergs, U., Onelov, E., Steineck, G., & Henter, J. I. (2006). Symptoms affecting children with malignancies during the last month of life: A nationwide follow-up. *Pediatrics, 117*(4), 1314-1320. https://doi.org/10.1542/peds.2005-1479

Jibb, L. A., Nathan, P. C., Stevens, B. J., Seto, E., Cafazzo, J. A., Stephens, N., Yohannes, L., & Stinson, J. N. (2015). Psychological and physical interventions for the management of cancer-related pain in pediatric and young adult patients: An integrative review. *Oncology Nursing Forum, 42*(6), E339-357. https://doi.org/10.1188/15.ONF.E339-E357

Keene, N., Hobbie, W., & Ruccione K. (2012). *Childhood cancer survivors: A practical guide to your future.* Childhood Cancer Guides.

King, G. A., King, S., Rosenbaum, P., Kertoy, M., Lay, M., & Hurley, P. (2004). *CAPE/PAC manual: Children's Assessment of Participation and Enjoyment & Preferences for Activities of Children.* PsychCorp.

Kramer, J., Velden, M. T., Kafkes, A., Basu, S., Federico, J., & Kielhofner, G. (2014). *Child occupational self assessment.* Model of Human Occupation Clearinghouse.

Krull, K. R., Okcu, M. F., Potter, B., Jain, N., Dreyer, Z., Kamdar, K., & Brouwers, P. (2008). Screening for neurocognitive impairment in pediatric cancer long-term survivors. *Journal of Clinical Oncology, 26*(25), 4138-4143. https://doi.org/10.1200/jco.2008.16.8864

Kupst, M. J., & Patenaude, A. F. (2016). Coping and adaptation in pediatric cancer: current perspectives. In A. N. Abrams, A. C. Muriel, & L. Wiener (Eds.), *Pediatric psychosocial oncology: Textbook for multidisciplinary care* (pp. 67-79). Springer International Publishing.

Law, M., Baptiste, S., Carswell, A., McColl, M. A., Polatajko, H., & Pollock, N. (2019). *Canadian occupational performance measure* (5th ed. rev.). COPM, Inc.

Lawitschka, A., Güçlü, E. D., Varni, J. W., Putz, M., Wolff, D., Pavletic, S., Greinix, H., Peters, C., & Felder-Puig, R. (2014). Health-related quality of life in pediatric patients after allogeneic SCT: Development of the PedsQL Stem Cell Transplant module and results of a pilot study. *Bone Marrow Transplantation, 49,* 1093-1097. https://doi.org/10.1038/bmt.2014.96

Long, K. A., Lehmann, V., Gerhardt, C. A., Carpenter, A. L., Marsland, A. L., & Alderfer, M. A. (2018). Psychosocial functioning and risk factors among siblings of children with cancer: An updated systematic review. *Psycho-Oncology, 27*(6), 1467-1479. https://doi.org/10.1002/pon.4669

Lyons, K. (2020). Psychosocial issues. In B. Braveman & R. Newman (Eds.), *Cancer and occupational therapy: Enabling performance and participation across the lifespan* (pp. 253-264). AOTA Press.

Merrell, K. W. (2008). Social emotional assets and resilience scales (SEARS). PAR.

Miralles, P. M., Ramón, N. C., & Valero, S. A. (2016). Adolescents with cancer and occupational deprivation in hospital settings: A qualitative study. *Hong Kong Journal of Occupational Therapy, 27*(1), 26-34. https://doi.org/10.1016/j.hkjot.2016.05.001

Mohammadi, A., Mehraban, A. H., & Damavandi, S. A. (2017). Effect of play-based occupational therapy on symptoms of hospitalized children with cancer: A single subject study. *Asia-Pacific Journal of Oncology Nursing, 4*(2), 168-172. https://doi.org/10.4103/apjon.apjon_13_17

Monti, J. D., Winning, A., Watson, K. H., Williams, E. K., Gerhardt, C. A., Compas, B. E., & Vannatta, K. (2017). Maternal and paternal influences on children's coping with cancer-related stress. *Journal of Family Studies, 26,* 2016-2025. https://doi.org/10.1007/s10826-017-0711-y

Moore III, Bartlett D. (2005). Neurocognitive outcomes in survivors of childhood cancer. *Journal of Pediatric Psychology, 30*(1): 51-63. https://doi.org/10.1093/jpepsy/jsi016

Morales, J. S., Santana-Sosa, E., Santos-Lozano, A., Baño-Rodrigo, A., Valenzuela, P. L., Rincón-Castanedo, C., Fernández-Moreno, D., González Vicent, M., Pérez-Somarriba, M., Madero, L., Alvaro Lassaletta, A., Fiuza-Luces, C., & Alejandro Lucia. (2020). Inhospital exercise benefits in childhood cancer: A prospective cohort study. *Scandinavian Journal of Medicine & Science in Sports, 30*(1), 126-134. https://doi.org/10.1111/sms.13545

Mullins, L., L., Molzon, E. S., Suorsa, K. I., Tackett, A. P., Ahna, L. H. P., & Cheney, J. M. (2015). Models of resilience: Developing psychosocial interventions for parents of children with chronic health conditions. *Family Relations: Interdisciplinary Journal of Applied Family Studies, 64*(1), 176-189. https://doi.org/10.1111/fare.12104

National Cancer Institute. (2015). *What is cancer?* https://www.cancer.gov/about-cancer/understanding/what-is-cancer

National Cancer Institute. (2019). *Childhood cancers.* https://www.cancer.gov/types/childhood-cancers

National Comprehensive Cancer Network. (2015). Guidelines version 2.2015 panel members cancer-related fatigue. NCCN clinical practice guidelines in oncology: Cancer-related fatigue.

National Comprehensive Cancer Network. (2020). NCCN clinical practice guidelines in oncology: Distress management version 2.2020. http://www.nccn.org/professionals/physician_gls/pdf/distress.pdf

National Research Council, Institute of Medicine. (2000). *From neurons to neighborhoods: The science of early childhood development.* National Academy Press.

Ness, K., Wall, M., Oakes, J., Robinson, L., & Gurney, J. (2006). Physical performance limitations and participation restrictions among cancer survivors: A population-based study. *Annals of Epidemiology, 16*(3), 197-205. https://doi.org/10.1016/j.annepidem.2005.01.009

Neville, A. R., Moothathamby, N., Naganathan, M., Huynh, E., & Moola, F. J. (2019). A place to call our own: The impact of camp experiences on the psychosocial wellbeing of children and youth affected by cancer—A narrative review. *Complementary Therapies in Clinical Practice, 36,* 18-28. https://doi.org/10.1016/j.ctcp.2019.04.007

Newborg, J. (2005). *Battelle developmental inventory* (2nd ed.). Riverside Publishing.

Pai, A. L., Greenley, R. N., Lewandowski, A., Drotar, D., Youngstrom, E., & Peterson, C. C. (2007). A meta-analytic review of the influence of pediatric cancer on parent and family functioning. *Journal of Family Psychology, 21*(3), 407-415. https://doi.org/10.1037/0893-3200.21.3.407

Palmer, S. N., Meeske, K. A., Katz, E. R., Burwinkle, T. M., & Varni, J. W. (2007). The PedsQL™ brain tumor module: Initial reliability and validity. *Pediatric Blood & Cancer, 49*(3), 287-293. https://doi.org/10.1002/pbc.21026

Patel, S. K., Katz, E. R., Richardson, R., Rimmer, M., & Kilian, S. (2009). Cognitive and problem solving training in children with cancer: A pilot project. *Journal of Pediatric Hematology/Oncology, 31*(9), 670-677. https://doi.org/10.1097/mph.0b013e3181b25a1d

Peikert, M. P., Inhestern, L., & Bergelt, C. (2018). Psychosocial interventions for rehabilitation and reintegration into daily life of pediatric cancer survivors and their families: A systematic review. *Public Library of Science ONE, 13*(4), e0196151. https://doi.org/10.1371/journal.pone.0196151

Phipps, S., Peasant, C., Barrera, M., Alderfer, M. A., Huang, Q., & Vannatta, K. (2012). Resilience in children undergoing stem cell transplantation: results of a complementary intervention trial. *Pediatrics, 129*(3), e762-e770. https://doi.org/10.1542/peds.2011-1816

Reynolds, C. R., & Kamphaus, R. W. (2004). *Behavior assessment system for children.* American Guidance Service.

Rocke, K., Hays, P., Edwards, D., & Berg, C. (2008). Development of a performance assessment of executive function: The Children's Kitchen Task Assessment. *American Journal of Occupational Therapy, 62*(5), 528-537. https://doi.org/10.5014/ajot.62.5.528

Sodergren, S. C., Husson, O., Robinson, J., Rohde, G. E., Tomaszewska, I. M., Vivat, B., Dyar, R., & Darlington, A.-S. (2017). Systematic review of the health-related quality of life issues facing adolescents and young adults with cancer. *Quality of Life Research, 26*(7), 1659-1672. https://doi.org/10.1007/s11136-017-1520-x

Sparrow, J. (2020). Special considerations for children with cancer. In B. Braveman & R. Newman (Eds.), *Enabling performance and participation for cancer survivors across the life course* (ch. 4). AOTA Press.

Sposito, A. M. P., Silva-Rodrigues, F. M., Sparapani, V. D. C., Pfeifer, L. I., de Lima, R. A. G., & Nascimento, L. C. (2015). Coping strategies used by hospitalized children with cancer undergoing chemotherapy. *Journal of Nursing Scholarship, 47*(2), 143-151. https://doi.org/10.1111/jnu.12126

Squires, J., Bricker, D., Twombly, E., Nickel, R., Clifford, J., Murphy, K., Hoselton, R., Potter, L., Mounts, L., & Farrell, J. (2009). *Ages & stages questionnaires* (3rd ed.). Paul H. Brookes.

Stanley, M. (2019). The lived experience of occupational adaptation: Adaptation in the wake of adversity, life transitions, and change. In L. C. Grajo & A. K. Boisselle (Eds.), *Adaptation through occupation: Multidimensional perspectives* (pp. 175-192). SLACK Incorporated.

Stimler, L., & Skuller, J. (2020). Education. In B. Braveman & R. Newman (Eds.), *Enabling performance and participation for cancer survivors across the life course.* AOTA Press.

Taleghani, F., Fathizadeh, N., & Naeri, N. (2012). The lived experiences of parents of children diagnosed with cancer in Iran. *European Journal of Cancer Care, 21*(3), 340-348. https://doi.org/10.1111/j.1365-2354.2011.01307.x

Tanner, L., Keppner, K., Lesmeister, D., Lyons, K., Rock, K., & Sparrow, J. (2020). Cancer rehabilitation in the pediatric and adolescent/young adult population. *Seminars in Oncology Nursing, 36*(1), 150984. https://doi.org/10.1016/j.soncn.2019.150984

Tester, C. (2006). Occupational therapy in paedatric oncology and palliative care. In J. Cooper (Ed.), *Occupational therapy in oncology and palliative care* (pp. 107-124). Whurr Publishers.

Toglia, J. (2015). *Weekly calendar planning activity: A performance test of executive function* (p. 176). AOTA Press.

Tutelman, P. R., Chambers, C. T., Stinson, J. N., Parker, J. A., Fernandez, C. V., Witteman, H. O., Nathan, P. C., Barwick, M., Campbell, F., Jibb, L. A., & Irwin, K. (2018, March). Pain in children with cancer: Prevalence, characteristics, and parent management. *The Clinical Journal of Pain, 34*(3), 198-206. https://doi.org/10.1097/AJP.0000000000000531

Uggla, L., Bonde, L. O., Hammar, U., Wrangsjö, B., & Gustafsson, B. (2018). Music therapy supported the health-related quality of life for children undergoing haematopoietic stem cell transplants. *Acta Paediatrica, 107*(11), 1986-1994. https://doi.org/10.1111/apa.14515

Uniform Data System for Medical Rehabilitation (UDSMR). (2012). *The FIM® instrument: Its background, structure, and usefulness.* UDSMR.

Usaite, K., & Cameron, J. (2015). Participation in enjoyable structured activities can promote resilience in young people. *British Journal of Occupational Therapy, 78*, 2-3.

Varni, J. W., Burwinkle, T. M., & Katz, E. R. (2004). The PedsQL™ in pediatric cancer pain: A prospective longitudinal analysis of pain and emotional distress. *Journal of Developmental & Behavioral Pediatrics, 25*(4), 239-246. https://doi.org/10.1097/00004703-200408000-00003

Varni, J. W., Burwinkle, T. M., Katz, E. R., Meeske, K., & Dickinson, P. (2002). The PedsQL™ in pediatric cancer: Reliability and validity of the Pediatric Quality of Life Inventory™ generic core scales, multidimensional fatigue scale, and cancer module. *Cancer, 94*(7), 2090-2106. https://doi.org/10.1002/cncr.10428

Varni, J. W., Seid, M., & Kurtin, P. S. (2001). PedsQL™ 4.0: Reliability and validity of the Pediatric Quality of Life Inventory™ Version 4.0 generic core scales in healthy and patient populations. *Medical Care, 39*(8), 800-812. https://doi.org/10.1097/00005650-200108000-00006

Vuotto, S. C., Krull, K. R., Li, C., Oeffinger, K. C., Green, D. M., Patel, S. K., Srivastava, D., Stovall, M., Ness, K. K., Armstrong, G. T., Robison, L. L., & Brinkman, T. M. (2017). Impact of chronic disease on emotional distress in adult survivors of childhood cancer: A report from the Childhood Cancer Survivor Study. *Cancer, 123*(3), 521-528. https://doi.org/10.1002/cncr.30348

Walling, E. B., Fiala, M., Connolly, A., Drevenak, A., & Gehlert, S. (2019). Challenges associated with living remotely from a pediatric cancer center: A qualitative study. *Journal of Oncology Practice, 15*(3), e219-e229. https://doi.org/10.1200/JOP.18.00115

Walubita, M., Sikateyo, B., & Zulu, J. M. (2018). Challenges for health care providers, parents and patients who face a childhood cancer diagnosis in Zambia. *BMC Health Services Research, 18,* 314. https://doi.org/10.1186/s12913-018-3127-5

Weaver, L. L., & Darragh, A. R. (2015). Systematic review of yoga interventions for anxiety reduction among children and adolescents. *American Journal of Occupational Therapy, 69*(6), 6906180070p1-6906180070p9. https://doi.org/10.5014/ajot.2015.020115

Wiener, L., Battles, H., Zadeh, S., Widemann, B. C., & Pao, M. (2017). Validity, specificity, feasibility and acceptability of a brief pediatric distress thermometer in outpatient clinics. *Psycho-Oncology, 26*(4), 461-468. https://doi.org/10.1002/pon.4038

Willard, V. W., Russell, K. M., Long, A., & Phipps, S. (2019). The impact of connectedness on social functioning in youth with brain tumors. *Pediatric Blood & Cancer, 66*(5), e27607. https://doi.org/10.1002/pbc.27607

Wilson, D. K., Hutson, S. P., Hall, J. M., & Anderson, K. M. (2016). Examining the digital story created by an adolescent with cancer: Insights and ideas from a case story. *Open Journal of Nursing, 6*(5), 426-434. https://doi.org/10.4236/ojn.2016.65044

Wu, Y. P., McPhail, J., Mooney, R., Martiniuk, A., & Amylon, M. D. (2016). A multisite evaluation of summer camps for children with cancer and their siblings. *Journal of Psychosocial Oncology, 34*(6), 449-459. https://doi.org/10.1080/07347332.2016.1217963

Wurz, A., Chamorro-Vina, C., Guilcher, G. M., Schulte, F., & Culos-Reed, S. N. (2014). The feasibility and benefits of a 12-week yoga intervention for pediatric cancer out-patients. *Pediatric Blood & Cancer, 61*(10), 1828-1834. https://doi.org/10.1002/pbc.25096

10

Children and Youth With Visual Impairments

Tammy Bruegger, OTD, MSE, OTR/L, ATP

CHAPTER OBJECTIVES By the end of this chapter the reader will:

- Recognize symptoms of low vision and blindness and their impact on adaptation, coping, and resilience.
- Distinguish between strategies of adaptation, coping, and resilience in children with visual impairment
- Determine strategies to assist children and youth with visual impairment with adaptation, coping, and resilience.

OVERVIEW OF THE POPULATION

According to Varma et al. (2017, p. 2), "[v]isual impairment (VI) in early childhood can significantly impair development of visual, motor, and cognitive function and lead to adverse psychosocial consequences." This chapter discusses children and youth who have visual impairment (VI) due to low vision and blindness, with emphasis on the occupational therapy practitioner's roles in facilitating the client's ability to adapt, cope, and demonstrate resilience in various contexts of occupational participation.

Coping is an important aspect of self-regulation, emotion, cognition, behavior, physiology, and interaction with the environment (Compas et al., 2001). *Coping* may be defined as an ongoing dynamic process that changes in response to the demands of a stressful situation. In addition, coping is a purposeful response directed toward resolving the stressful relationship between the person and the environment by decreasing negative emotions that arise as a result of stress. Compas et al. (2001) suggest that both problem-focused coping and emotion-focused coping occur in stressful situations. As

Grajo L. C., & Boisselle, A. K. (Eds.). *Adaptation, Coping, and Resilience in Children and Youth: A Comprehensive Occupational Therapy Approach* (pp. 237-259).
© 2022 Taylor & Francis Group.

a result, the person's way of dealing with stress, which may be based on temperament, family or parent support, and positive or negative outlook, affects their coping (Prior, 2015). For example, in problem-based coping, the person, family, or child may come up with possible solutions to the issue at hand. If the child is diagnosed with a chronic condition, such as visual impairment, the parents may look for information or ways to address or treat the visual impairment by seeking answers or learning from health care professionals. The child may address it by seeking information or being taught strategies by the parent, occupational therapist, other health care professional, or educator. With emotion-based coping, the person may react with an emotional response. The response may be negative, such as in anger or stress, but could also involve positive strategies for coping, such as taking a walk to calm oneself, listening to music, or other strategies (Compas et al., 2001). With appropriate support, this leads to adaptation by the client. According to Grajo (2019) and Grajo et al. (2018), adaptation through occupation has four essential themes:

1. It is an internal human process that is a product of engagement in human occupation and a process by which humans overcome challenges in the environment while participating in occupations.

2. It is manifested when the person transacts with the environment.

3. Adaptation becomes more apparent when the person responds to change and experiences life transitions.

4. As the person continuously adapts, they form a desired sense of self.

A part of this is the concept of resilience, which may be an internal component of coping and adaptation. *Resilience* is the ability to recover and "bounce back" after an incident that disrupts typical life functions (Compas et al., 2001). These concepts are intrinsically intertwined when a child is facing a difficult situation, and learns to cope by utilizing coping strategies and developing their ability to adapt: the outcome is resilience. However, a question remains: How do occupational therapists facilitate coping, adaptability, and resilience with clients who have low vision and blindness? To answer this question, we must find out more about children who have low vision and blindness, their occupational performance needs as determined by appropriate assessment, and the interventions used to increase occupational performance and participation in occupations.

Low vision and blindness are the leading cause of disability in the United States and most developing countries (Chan et al., 2017). The World Health Organization (2019) reports that there are at least 2.2 billion people with low vision or blindness worldwide, with 1 billion of these cases preventable or treatable. In the United States alone there are more than 3.4 million people over age 40 with blindness, 21 million who have "vision problems," and 80 million who have potentially blinding diseases, according to the Centers for Disease Control and Prevention (CDC, 2017). A report by Varma et al. (2017) states that more than 174,000 children who are 3 to 5 years of age were visually impaired in the United States in 2015. More than 121,000 of these cases (69%) involved simple uncorrected refractive error, and 43,000 (25%) had bilateral amblyopia. The number of children aged 3 to 5 years with VI is projected to increase by 26% by 2060 due to inequity in health care services for children with visual impairment and multiple health care needs of those who are of multiracial backgrounds. Children with

Hispanic and white backgrounds are the largest groups, followed by children of African American and Asian American heritage (Varma et al., 2017). In addition, children with VI often have other disabling conditions and multiple disabilities that require special education and more extensive vision and therapy services. Due to this inequity, children with African American, Hispanic/Latino, and multiracial backgrounds who have special health care needs were two to three times as likely to have unmet vision care needs as white children with special health care needs. This inequity remains even after controlling for differences in household structure, socioeconomic status, health status, use of health services, and perceptions of service professionals (Varma et al., 2017).

These numbers do not account for the numbers of older children and adults who currently have visual impairments or those who will become visually impaired from accidents and illness. In the United States in 2015, among people 40 years of age or older, there were 3.22 million people who had low vision and 1.02 million who were legally blind. This number is expected to increase by 25% per decade, predicting 6.95 million people with VI and 2.01 million people with blindness in 2050 due to an increase in the aging Baby Boomer generation (Varma et al., 2016). In a more recent study, Chan et al. (2017) estimated that low vision and blindness would increase by 30% by 2050. In addition, occurrences in women, especially those of Hispanic descent, will increase the most due to the longevity of women as compared to men and an increase in this group's population. Women are also reported to not receive treatment for blinding conditions such as glaucoma. Furthermore, the criteria for blindness are based on visual field loss, and visual field loss is not included in the report by Varma et al. (2017) or other prevalence reports; therefore, this may be an underestimation of blindness caused by progressive or degenerative diseases such as glaucoma or retinal degeneration.

Early intervention is critical for better visual outcomes. A large percentage of preschool VI can be prevented or treated by low-cost refractive correction. In addition, vision screening in preschool-age children and follow-up care will have a significant, prolonged effect on both visual function and academic and social achievements, and, therefore, should be recommended for all children (Varma et al., 2017).

The high prevalence of VI among Hispanic white, African American, and multiracial children is of particular concern, because children of these groups were shown to receive less vision care (Varma et al., 2017). According to U.S. Census projections, during the next 45 years, the multiracial, Asian, and Hispanic populations will be the fastest-growing groups, and by 2060, 64% of children younger than 18 years of age will be racial and ethnic minorities. This shift in the groups most affected by preschool VI resulting from the projected trend indicates an increasingly racially and ethnically diverse child population in the United States.

In summary, given a projected doubling of the prevalence of VI and blindness over the next 35 years, vision screening and intervention for refractive error and early eye disease may prevent and/or reduce a high proportion of individuals from suffering from these conditions, enhance their quality of life, and potentially decrease direct and indirect costs to the U.S. economy (Chan et al., 2017; Varma et al., 2016; Varma et al., 2017).

Types of Visual Conditions

Low vision is defined as a reduction in visual acuity no better than 20/70 but better than 20/200 in the better eye with correction (American Foundation for the Blind, 2020). *Legal blindness* is defined as visual acuity no better than 20/200 in the better eye with the best correction and a central visual field that is no greater than 20 degrees (American Foundation for the Blind, 2020). In addition, the International Statistical Classification of Diseases further defines visual impairment into mild, moderate, and severe VI (Dandona & Dandona, 2006). Cortical/cerebral visual impairment (C/CVI, also called neurological visual impairment) is the leading cause of visual impairment in children around the world (Lueck & Dutton, 2015). C/CVI is associated with other neurological conditions such as anoxia, traumatic brain injury, and cerebral palsy, and affects the visual processing that occurs throughout the dorsal and ventral vision pathways and other areas of the brain. Because children who have uncorrected refraction errors or neurological visual impairment will be affected developmentally over a lifetime, this is significant and will increase the number of persons of all ages with visual impairment.

Children with visual impairment may have an ocular-based visual condition, a neurological visual impairment, or a combination of ocular and neurological visual impairment in addition to other neurological conditions. Cortical/cerebral visual impairment is a neurological visual impairment that occurs due to damage to the brain and visual pathways (Lueck & Dutton, 2015, Roman-Lantzy, 2018), as opposed to an ocular visual impairment, which occurs in the structures of the eye to the optic chiasm. C/CVI involves not only the eye, but also the optic nerve, dorsal and ventral optic pathways, lateral geniculate body, and the brain, including the occipital, temporal, parietal, and frontal lobes (Lueck & Dutton, 2015). More than 22% of the children reported to have low vision or blindness are diagnosed with C/CVI . Diagnosis of cortical/cerebral visual impairment typically occurs through observation of the child, interview of the parent, review of medical records, and completion of a checklist by an ophthalmologist. Christine Roman-Lantzy (2018), a teacher of the visually impaired (TVI), has developed an assessment called the Cortical Visual Impairment Range, which has a list of symptoms and traits seen in CVI and is used to determine if a particular child has C/CVI. This assessment is usually conducted by a TVI, therapist, or other professional who has been trained to use the instrument. Typical symptoms that indicate a need for assessment include the need for a preferred color, usually red or yellow; need for movement; visual latency; visual field preference; difficulty with visual complexity; absent or atypical visual reflexes (blink and nasopalpebral); difficulty with visual novelty; absence of visually guided reach; light gazing or need for light/reflective materials; and difficulty with distance viewing. Sometimes magnetic resonance imaging (MRI) reveals changes (Roman-Lantzy, 2018). Cortical/cerebral visual impairment is the leading cause of low vision and blindness in children worldwide, yet it is often not identified or is misidentified (Chokron & Dutton, 2016; Kong et al., 2012; Roman-Lantzy, 2018). It may be seen in conjunction with or caused by other neurological or brain-based conditions such as cerebral palsy, periventricular leukomalacia, traumatic brain injury, hydrocephalus, and anoxia (Kong et al., 2012). Ocular conditions may also occur with neurological visual impairment, such as hemianopsia (visual field deficit), strabismus (misalignment of the eyes), or amblyopia (loss of vision in one eye). Cerebral visual impairment, retinopathy of prematurity, and optic nerve hypoplasia are the most common diagnoses seen in children besides general acuity issues.

Occupational Profile

Vision significantly affects development and learning of all children, and these effects are amplified in children who have low vision and blindness (Brémond-Gignac et al., 2011). Most resources state that more than 80% of learning occurs through vision (Project IDEAL, 2013); therefore, anything that affects vision either prenatally or postnatally may affect development in all other areas. Occupations—what a child does throughout their day—are strongly affected by lack of vision. Learning to navigate the typical activities of childhood without effective visual skills requires coping and adaptive responses in order to optimize outcomes and function (Auigestad, 2017). Several studies discuss the impact of visual impairment on psychosocial function and relate successful and unsuccessful coping, adaptability, and resilience to the development of self-esteem (Auigestad, 2017; Yuan et al., 2017). In a systematic review by Auigestad (2017), the majority of the studies suggested that children and young adults with visual impairments had more emotional problems than did their sighted peers and that boys experience more serious depression than girls. In Australia, Cochrane et al. (2011) conducted a study of adults with low vision and blindness to determine what influenced their successful outcomes. They found that avoidant coping has a detrimental impact on visual-related quality of life (VRQoL) over time. The researchers indicated that low-vision specialists should be aware of their clients' coping strategies and encourage clients to engage in active rather than avoidant coping to deal with the effects of their vision impairment. This is important information for occupational therapy practitioners in adopting strategies for clients with visual impairment, low vision, and blindness based on occupational supports and barriers (Table 10-1).

Occupational Supports

Early identification, accurate assessment, and appropriate intervention are critical to provide a developmental foundation for occupational performance throughout childhood and adult life with children who have visual impairment. Many factors serve as occupational supports for children with visual impairment, including early intervention, parent education and parental attachment, development of exploration, communication, joint attention, and self-concept (van den Broek et al., 2017), development of tactile and auditory skills, and development of persistence (Yuan et al., 2017). A focus on occupational strengths, particularly persistence, is consistent with the concept of using active coping, because persistence is an active strategy for coping, adaptability, and resilience efforts.

Table 10-1

Occupational Profile of Children With Visual Impairment	
Supports	Barriers
• Development of tactile skills • Development of auditory skills • Development of persistence • Development of hardiness • Early intervention to improve development of motor and speech-language skills • Secure parent-child attachment, social engagement, parental coaching and education	• Lack of vision to initiate motor responses • Lack of vision to initiate and modify social interactions • Lack of vision for visually guided reach • Lack of vision to take advantage of modeling and imitation • Lack of ability to pick up incidental information from environment to adapt or modify responses • Difficulty with self-regulation of sensory processing areas
Synthesized from Augestad (2017), Bakke et al. (2019), Lueck and Dutton (2015), and Yuan et al. (2017).	

Occupational Barriers

Occupational therapy practitioners address occupation as reported in the *Occupational Therapy Practice Framework: Domain and Process, Fourth Edition* (American Occupational Therapy Association [AOTA], 2020), which defines *occupation* as the daily life activities in which people engage. Occupations of children occur in context and are influenced by the child's performance skills and performance patterns. *Occupational performance skills* are those skills that are observable (e.g., motor, process, and social interactions) and are key aspects of successful occupational participation. Children's early occupations include self-help, rest and sleep, social participation, play and leisure, communication, learning, and literacy. Without intact vision, all of these areas will be affected (Lueck & Dutton, 2015; Roman-Lantzy, 2018). Children with visual impairment have context-based variability in performance that affects their occupational profile.

The timing of the appearance of the condition that affects vision is important, because if it occurs during a critical time in development, it affects not only vision, but other areas of development as well. Studies of neuroplasticity and vision show that many other areas of the brain are involved in visual development (Lueck & Dutton, 2015; Merebet et al., 2017). Visual impairment, thus, affects typical development, including motor skills, activities of daily living (ADLs), play, cognition, and communication (Lueck & Dutton, 2015; Merebet et al., 2017; Oluonye & Sargent, 2018). In addition, because 80% of what is learned comes from visual input, future development is hindered by the child's inability to learn incidentally, and thus, the child is disadvantaged due to loss of visual learning. Challenges include lack of vision to stimulate initiation of a motor response, or to initiate and modify a social interaction; lack of visually guided reach;

lack of ability to take advantage of modeling and imitation; and lack of ability to pick up incidental information from the environment for self-regulation (Auigestad, 2017; Lueck & Dutton, 2015; Yuan et al., 2017).

Social Skills

Children with visual impairment have difficulty with eye contact, and therefore, emotional bonding with the parent may be difficult. In addition, the parent or caregiver does not get the reciprocal input and reinforcement from the child necessary to establish a bond. Vision also allows for anticipation of movement. If the child sees the caregiver walking toward her when she is crying or needs help, she may pause in anticipation of being picked up or touched. If the child with a visual impairment does not see the person approaching, he may startle when picked up or touched. To help the child anticipate being touched or moved, the adult needs to speak prior to touching the child and provide touch cues to the child prior to providing care or picking the child up. Behaviors that are adaptive to enable the child to cope, or are reactive owing to the stress caused by certain environments or conditions that exceed the child's mental processing capacity, can resemble a range of disorders such as autism spectrum disorder (ASD) and attention deficit hyperactivity disorder (ADHD). Engagement in activities, parental attachment, and coaching of the child may reduce repetitive behaviors such as eye poking or head shaking. Persistence of these behaviors can negatively affect development of self-concept and social connectivity (van den Broek et al., 2017). Secure parent-child relationships are as important for the quality of life of children with visual impairments as they are for other children, and may be an important resilience factor for mitigating the psychosocial risks to development faced by children with visual impairment (van den Broek et al., 2017).

Learning

Cognitive development depends on a child's early sensory experiences from vision, hearing, movement, and tactile exploration. In typical development, the ability to localize and explore visually develops before the abilities to localize sound, to move, and to explore tactilely. Without vision to help connect the various types of sensory input, it is more difficult for the child with visual impairment to perceive objects or situations that are apparent to sighted children. Children who have visual impairment may have different patterns of development related to attention and exploration (they may not understand or be aware of an object if they have no tactile experience with the object), object permanence (knowing that objects exist when they are not seen), object constancy (recognizing similarities in objects), categorization (identifying similarities and differences in objects and events), spatial relationships (understanding where objects are in relation to one another), and orientation (understanding where they are in relation to other people and objects in the environment; Lueck & Dutton, 2015).

Motor Skills

A child's vision significantly affects the development of fine and gross motor skills. Vision affects the child's stimulus and ability to move around in the environment, because children are motivated to move, sit up, get on all fours, crawl, pull to stand, and walk mainly by visual input (Lueck & Dutton, 2015). Vision is critical in development of the mental constructs of cause/effect, object permanence, and function object use (Lueck & Dutton, 2015). Visually guided reach in all positions is reduced when a child's vision is impaired. In addition, due to lack of movement and play in a variety of positions, children with visual impairment may have decreased strength in their hands, arms, shoulders, and trunk, as well as decreased trunk rotation during ambulation or other movements (Bakke et al., 2019). This further hinders their development of reach, grasp, and fine motor/manipulation skills.

Play Skills

Children develop imitation and play skills through incidental learning and observation. Without vision, it is difficult for a child to learn through incidental means. Thus, it is important to provide other ways of learning through tactile, auditory, and kinesthetic sensory modes by touching, manipulating, and helping the child experience play and functional skills.

DEFINING ADAPTATION, COPING, AND RESILIENCE FOR CHILDREN WITH VISUAL IMPAIRMENTS

In a systematic review by Auigestad (2017), studies showed that children with visual impairment have more emotional and psychological issues than children and young adults without visual impairment. These studies established that social support, friendship, and independence in mobility are important for enhancing the mental health of all children. The studies showed, however, that children with earlier onset and more severe visual impairments may be less likely to experience a reduction in their mental health over time. A study by Yuan et al. (2017) found that children with visual impairment who were well adjusted (37% of 400 people) demonstrated more independence, were more mobile, maintained appropriate home and community activities, and had successful employment. Others who were maladjusted (29%) demonstrated more dependence, were mobility dependent, engaged in limited home and community activities, and had no recorded work history. The well-adjusted group also showed higher scores on intelligence, manual dexterity, emotional stability, and realistic acceptance of their visual impairment. They also attained higher educational levels than the maladjusted group. In an exploratory study by Bruegger et al. (2021), there were positive correlations among

Case Study 10-1
Eddie

Eddie has an ocular condition called *optic atrophy* (Figure 10-1). His vision is measured at 20/200 in both eyes. He has some vision for color and shape but is unable to see detail or even letters in words. He is learning to use Braille with a refreshable Braille display and iPad (Apple). He also is using a Perkins Brailler. He is learning to use a white cane to improve his functional mobility and has shown very good progress in this area. Eddie is very bright and has good communication skills. He gets very frustrated and is embarrassed that he has to use Braille. He wants to do what other students in his kindergarten class do. As a result, he is happy to use the iPad by itself to access digital books with text-to-speech output to read stories and books through Bookshare, Tar Heel Reader, and Audible. At times, Eddie will throw tantrums if he doesn't want to work on Braille or if something doesn't work perfectly for him. Often this emotional reaction will affect his cooperation and performance all day. Recently, he has seen that he can teach others about Braille and how to operate the refreshable Braille display with a digital tablet, so he works on Braille more readily. He is learning to be more adaptable and his coping skills have improved due to his increased confidence and self-esteem with his classroom activities.

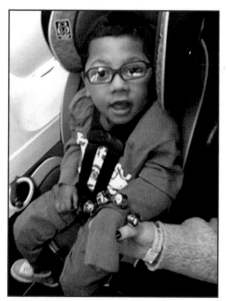

Figure 10-1. Eddie has optic atrophy.

Case Study 10-2

Lily

Lily is 4 years old and has cortical/cerebral visual impairment, cerebral palsy, seizure disorder, and several other medical impairments and needs. Early in her time in preschool or at home, she would fall asleep, refuse to participate, or cry due to lack of engagement or participation in daily activities. Today, she is socially connected and motivated to participate in the classroom and at home. Her family is very supportive. She receives attention and positive feedback from her parents, therapists/teachers, and extended family. All of these things support her development of her self-image, coping, and resilience. Lily has little movement in her trunk and extremities; her best achievement in movement is turning her head side to side and elbow movement in one arm. She uses a tilt-in-space wheelchair with head support and a tray. Lily is dependent for all ADLs. She is able to activate a single button switch to turn on switch-adapted musical toys to play with her friends. Because she does not have verbal speech, she communicates using a speech-generating device (SGD) connected to adaptive switches. She has good receptive language and cognitive abilities when she is exposed to new concepts and has the opportunity for adapted learning activities (Figure 10-2). She appears to be happy and have good self-esteem, especially after learning to use her communication device and access digital books and learning activities on her dynamic-display SGD. The visual display on her SGD has been adjusted to be less complex, with larger, simpler pictures that use only two or three colors, less detail, and a plain black or white background. She uses two-switch scanning, advancing the scan across the pictures with a proximity switch at her head and a button switch by her hand. When the device scans, it

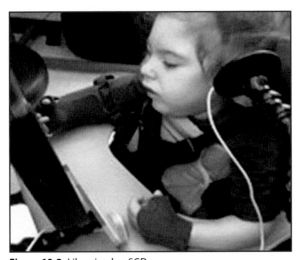

Figure 10-2. Lily using her SGD.

(continued)

Case Study 10-2 (continued)

highlights each picture with a red border and says the name of the picture with voice output in a different voice. When she pushes the button switch with her hand, a female-child voice "talks" her selection for her. Prior to getting her SGD, she responded by facial expressions, such as smiling, looking toward things that she wanted if they were placed within 6 inches from her eyes, crying, and vocalization. She was unable to communicate verbally or make her wants and needs known without the SGD and did not interact with other children or adults prior to receiving the device. Now, she is better able to participate in school and literacy activities and talk with others around her at school and home. She is able to answer questions to demonstrate that she understands. Her early intervention and independence with some skills and the family's inclusion of her in many activities at home has aided in development of her self-image. Lily is now more able to cope with difficulties in her day, and does not throw tantrums, refuse to participate, or fall asleep due to lack of engagement in activities, thus demonstrating growth in her coping, resilience, and adaptability throughout her day.

sensory processing, coping, participation, and quality of life with children who had visual impairment. Similar relationships have been found by other researchers (Chien et al., 2016; Hamed-Daher & Engel-Yeger, 2019).

THE ROLE OF THE OCCUPATIONAL THERAPIST: ASSESSMENTS FOR COPING, ADAPTABILITY, AND RESILIENCE

With children who have low vision and blindness, occupational therapy practitioners typically address sensory processing, fine motor skill development, self-care (including feeding and other ADLs and IADLs), use of residual vision, and access to literacy using assistive technology. Because occupational therapists are holistic and concerned with occupations and occupational performance, abilities related to mental health and psychosocial adjustment are appropriate areas of intervention for occupational therapists to address (AOTA, 2020).

Assessment

Only a limited number of assessments have been developed for use with children who have visual impairment. However, several assessments have been used effectively to establish an occupational profile or assessment of occupational performance for such clients. These include the Functional Independence Measure for Children (WeeFIM), the Activities Scale for Kids (ASK), and the Pediatric Evaluation of Disability Inventory

(PEDI). These assessments are used to measure functional performance in self-care, functional mobility, cognition, and social abilities through observation of the child or an interview format (Cordier et al., 2016). The Canadian Occupational Performance Measure (COPM) and the AOTA Occupational Performance Template are used for establishing an occupational profile. The COPM has good reliability and validity and is client focused and individualized for the child's needs (Cordier et al., 2016). The Oregon Project for Preschoolers with Visual Impairment is one type of assessment that measures motor skills, language/communication, cognition, ADLs, and compensatory skills in the preschool population (The Oregon Project for Children, 2020). It was specifically developed for use with children who have visual impairment. The Callier-Azusa Scale (The Callier Center for Communication Disorders, 2020) was created to assess children with visual impairment and other multiple needs, including deaf-blindness. The Brigance Developmental Scales and the Boehm Test of Basic Concepts both have tactile and large-picture versions for children with visual impairment (available through the American Printing House for the Blind). Children with visual impairment often have difficulty processing sensory information, but there are no sensory-processing assessments made for children with visual impairment. Dean et al. (2018) reported that children with sensory avoiding behaviors showed more externalizing behaviors, depression, resilience, and adaptability. In their study, which compared the Child Sensory Profile 2 with the Behavior Assessment System for Children and Parent Rating Scales, they found that sensory seeking is related to depression and resilience, whereas sensory sensitivity is related to externalizing behaviors in typical children. Evidence of sensory processing in children with visual impairment is limited and warrants further study.

The Brief COPE (Coping Orientation to Problems Experienced) instrument stands out because it is intended to assess the core aspects of coping in children with visual impairment. A study by Yuan et al. (2017) discussed the development of the assessment for adolescents in China from the Brief Coping Scale, which was adapted to reflect the cultural differences in children in China and titled the Brief COPE Revised, and then changed to the COPE-Revised. The COPE-Revised initially measured 14 coping strategies: active coping, positive reframing, planning, use of emotional support, use of instrumental support, venting, self-distraction, acceptance, self-blame, behavioral disengagement, humor, denial, religion, and substance use. These strategies were then narrowed down to three: self-directed coping, other-directed coping, and relinquished-control coping. The researchers compared the COPE-Revised with the Brief Coping Scale and the differences among populations of children with visual impairment. In the study, Yuan et al. found that self-esteem was not always associated with positive coping and that there were other factors occurring with children with visual impairment that warranted further study. The first study preliminarily explored the applicability of the Brief COPE to Chinese adolescent students with visual impairments. Based on the results, the Brief COPE was modified and renamed COPE-Revised. The second study tested the internal psychometric properties and the criterion-related validity of the COPE-Revised. Criterion-related validity was obtained through investigating the correlation between coping and self-esteem (Yuan et al., 2017). There are many assessments of coping, resilience, stress, depression, and adaptability, but there are very few that were developed specifically for clients or children with visual impairment. As noted earlier, children with visual impairment develop in unique ways in motor, sensory, perceptual, cognitive, and social-emotional areas. Results from standard assessments will not be appropriate or valid for a child who has a visual impairment, due to the lack of experimental research with this population in these areas. Nevertheless, assessments of adults and children without visual impairment in these areas are useful to gain insight into the unique ways that children who have visual impairment may think and react regarding coping. The measurement of coping and emotion regulation has been developed primarily by four approaches: questionnaires completed by children and adolescents or parents, interviews, observations of behavior, and measures of physiological processes (Compas et al., 2001). Interview measures are found to be more appropriate for young children with limited reading ability. They provide opportunity to ensure comprehension and to probe for details about the coping strategies. Self-reporting measures may be used as the child gets older and is able to understand nuances of language (Compas et al., 2001).

Intervention

In infancy and toddler stages, children's emotional reactions are controlled by the parent. During early childhood, children's increased understanding of emotions enables the parents to move from directly controlling children's emotional reactions to coaching the children in emotional regulation strategies (Compas et al., 2001). In middle to late childhood, children begin to use cognitive-based strategies such as cognitive reappraisal or distraction. For stress reduction, they may use relaxation strategies and deep breathing or mindfulness to reduce physiological arousal. From middle childhood into adolescence, peer relationships become important and serve as a source of support. In addition, further learning about emotional experiences and emotional regulation strategies occurs. During middle and late adolescence, increased ability to think and consider one's emotions allows for more awareness and independent management of one's own and others' emotions and the beginning development of executive function skills (Compas et al., 2001).

COLLABORATIVE APPROACH WITH FAMILIES AND THE SOCIAL ENVIRONMENT

Occupational therapy practitioners can facilitate and foster a collaborative approach with children, peers, and children's families by supporting social interactions and interaction with their lived environments and communities. This approach involves modeling and guiding social interactions with peers throughout daily occupations such as play, school, and community activities. In addition, interprofessional collaboration with parents, teachers, paraprofessionals, and other professionals (such as speech pathologists, social workers, and psychologists) is critical to ensure that adaptation, coping, and resilience are supported in all environments and occupations. Early intervention services are provided in the natural environment such as the home. Therefore, communication and collaboration with parents is important and helps ensure that any intervention is carried out in all settings in which the child participates. Research suggests that early intervention services should follow a service delivery model that is family centered rather than teacher or therapist directed (Hatton et al., 2013; Pletcher & Younggren, 2013). In addition, services may be provided in preschools and in community settings, such as parks, restaurants, and playgrounds. This allows the child with a visual impairment to experience learning in real settings (experiential learning) through interaction with real materials and objects.

BUILDING INTERPROFESSIONAL COLLABORATIONS

It is important that occupational therapy practitioners collaborate and work as a team with other professionals, especially if they are new to work with this population, in order to increase their comfort level and effectiveness. Children with low vision and blindness in early childhood may receive services from occupational therapy, physical therapy, speech pathology, early-childhood education, special education, ophthalmology/optometry, and other medical or educational services. Other professionals who may be part of the team for children who have visual impairment include a teacher of the visually impaired (a teacher who specializes in instruction and strategies for low vision and blindness) and an orientation and mobility instructor (a teacher trained in white cane use and other vision-related mobility skills). Occupational therapists can foster a collaborative approach with interdisciplinary teams to facilitate adaptation, coping, and resilience through team assessments, team goals, and team interventions. Interventions may occur in multiple environments, such as home, school, hospital/clinic, and community settings. The collaborative approach may be used with a team involving educational, health care, and other community-based professionals. Occupational therapy practitioners work with other disciplines to structure environments, teach cognitive strategies, and develop social and emotional skills that promote self-regulation, competence development, trust building and confidence, and resilience through participation.

A GLOBAL PERSPECTIVE

In countries other than the United States, professionals have addressed coping and resilience in a variety of ways. For instance, Yuan and associates (2017) completed a study using the COPE and the Brief Cope to develop an appropriate assessment tool for assessing coping, adaption, and resilience in adolescents in China. In this study, an assessment (the Brief Cope) that is well respected in the Western world was revised to address the Asian culture. Researchers reported that differences between the two cultures were significant, warranting revision of the assessment.

A study by Auigestad (2017) undertook a systematic review of articles published between January 1998 and July 2016, from 17 publications representing 13 countries, regarding the social-emotional development of children with visual impairment. The majority of the studies suggested that children and young adults with visual impairments had more emotional problems than did their sighted peers. In addition, more girls with visual impairments experienced serious symptoms of depression and anxiety than did boys with visual impairments, consistent with results from the general population. Two of the studies indicated that the emotional problems could decrease with maturation. Results of this review were inconsistent due to the age range, cultures, countries, small sample sizes, and varying methods of measurement and analysis. Nevertheless, the study results generally reported that children with visual impairment from birth or early childhood showed improved mental health as they aged, most likely due to early intervention services. The studies showed that family intervention, social support, friendship, and independence in mobility are important factors for enhancing the mental health of all children with visual impairment (Auigestad, 2017). The one certain conclusion of this review was that there is a need for more knowledge and high-quality experimental studies in this area.

Additional studies have been conducted in Australia. Cochrane et al. (2011) studied the development of a quality-of-life self-reporting assessment to further define the area of quality of life for children with visual impairment. The purpose of the study was to validate the Impact of Vision Impairment for Children (IVIC) assessment. The IVIC was given to both vision-impaired and sighted children ages 8 to 18 to determine reliability and validity. The IVIC was determined to be a valid and reliable assessment of the outcomes of interventions and needs in children with VI who have no additional disabilities.

In Australia, Frydenberg et al. (2015) discussed the concepts of resilience and hardiness in children, the development of positive parenting programs, and parental involvement in various aspects of life in Italy, Australia, and other countries. In Korea, in a study of adults who had visual impairment from birth, researchers conducted interviews regarding the subjects' experiences. Participants reported hurtful experiences and bullying, and noted that they felt anger and hurt due to negative societal views of their impairments. Parents also reported that they showed negative behavior toward their own children because of their visual impairment. As a result, the researchers determined that it is important to help parents support their children by reducing the stress, conflict, and anxiety associated with having a child with visual impairment. To do so, it is necessary to strengthen parental self-esteem and have parents receive early education, knowledge, and support so that the parents can, in turn, support their children's development of productive coping skills (Sim, 2020).

ESSENTIAL THINGS OCCUPATIONAL THERAPISTS NEED TO CONSIDER TO BUILD ADAPTATION, COPING, AND RESILIENCE

Essential considerations for work with children with visual impairment are described in this section. Table 10-2 describes issues that may affect coping styles and Table 10-3 provides specific assessment and intervention strategies that may be helpful for occupational therapists.

Table 10-2

Issues That Affect Coping Style		
Cognitive Problem Solving	**Personality Styles**	**Temperament/ Behavioral Style**
• Social bonds/ relationships interpersonal skills • Empathy • Problem solving • Self-regulation emotional awareness	• Positive school experiences • Educational support • Adaptability • Self efficacy • Variety of interests/hobbies • Self-esteem	• Niche picking • Realistic optimism • Parent/child relationships • Strong attachments

Table 10-3

Practical Assessment and Intervention Tips to Support Children With Visual Impairments		
Building Functional Cognition, Metacognition, and Executive Function		
Study	*Assessments*	*Practice Tips and Tools*
Compas et al. (2001)	Coping and Emotion Regulation: Domains, Factors, and Strategies Emotion Regulation Checklist Cognitive Emotion Regulation Questionnaire (CERQ)	Wellness, problem solving, emotional expression, emotional modulation, secondary control coping (acceptance, cognitive reappraisal, positive thinking, distraction) Strategies of coping and emotion regulation, including emotional expression, emotional suppression, problem solving, cognitive reappraisal, distraction, acceptance, avoidance, wishful thinking, denial, emotional modulation, unregulated release of emotions, and humor
Heyl & Hintermair (2015)	Behavior Rating Inventory of Executive Function (BRIEF-D)	Early focus on competencies, such as attention shifting and emotional understanding; reinforcing communicative competence
Building Adaptive Capacity, Coping, Resilience, and Skills for Life		
Sturrock et al. (2015)	Vision Impairment Questionnaire	Vision-related functioning and vision-related emotional well-being Quality of life

(continued)

Table 10-3 (continued)

Practical Assessment and Intervention Tips to Support Children With Visual Impairments		
Study	Assessment	Practice Tips and Tools
Oregon Project (2020)	The Oregon Project for Preschoolers with Visual Impairment	Compensatory strategies, self-help, fine/gross motor, mobility, cognition, and communication
Compas et al. (2001)	Responses to Stress Questionnaire (RSQ)-Children's Coping Strategies Checklist (CCSC)	Problem-focused coping, emotion-focused coping, engagement/approach coping, disengagement coping, primary control coping, secondary control coping, and social support coping
Cochrane et al. (2011)	The Impact of Vision Impairment for Children (IVI-C)	Awareness of quality of life and self-advocacy, self-concept; self-report
Building Mastery and Competence in Occupational Participation		
Cordier et al. (2016)	Canadian Occupational Performance Measurement AOTA Occupational Performance Template Functional Independence Measure for Children (WeeFIM) The Activities Scale for Kids (ASK) Pediatric Evaluation of Disability Inventory (PEDI) VIPP Intervention	Client-centered areas identified to increase occupational participation Focus on reducing barriers in context/environment Self-help, mobility, cognitive skills Participation in daily activities Self-help, mobility, cognitive skills Video-feedback intervention to promote positive parenting

Coping, resilience, and adaptability are the three aspects of personality that can most positively affect a person's outcome in life; this is especially true of children who have visual impairment. No matter what kind of family, economic status, or cultural complexity a person has, the influence of coping, resilience, and adaptability on outcomes is still difficult to determine. However, children who have the unconditional support of at least one parent, and the "just right" amount of stress in order to practice active strategies to learn to adapt, cope, and develop resilience tend to have positive outcomes.

Case Study 10-3
Alex

Review of Medical and Educational Records

Medical Information: Alex is a 7-year-old male child with a diagnosis of peri-ventricular leukomalacia (PVL), cortical visual impairment, and attention deficit disorder. His medical history includes parental gestational diabetes, meconium aspiration at birth, plagiocephaly, and torticollis. He had typical birth weight and was full term. He has a seizure disorder but recently has been seizure free. An electroencephalogram showed slowing in frontal/temporal regions of the brain suggestive of cerebral dysfunction; magnetic resonance imaging showed thinning of the corpus callosum and periventricular gliosis consistent with PVL. He has been diagnosed with global developmental delays and expressive language disorder. Alex currently has delays in self-help skills, vision, speech, fine and gross motor skills, cognition, and social development. He is a verbal communicator but uses a dedicated speech device to assist with speech and communication.

School Information: Alex attends first grade in a public school in a special education classroom. He participates in limited regular education activities, such as art and music. Due to an increase in maladaptive behaviors impeding his participation in the classroom, he will attend a self-contained program next year. He has a Functional Behavior Plan (FBP) addressing his maladaptive behaviors, which have increased since his transition to the public school. He previously attended a preschool and kindergarten at a school for children with visual impairment where there were typical peer role models in the classroom. There were fewer children in the room, trained paraprofessional support, consultative psychologist support, and a teacher who was a certified teacher of the visually impaired. All therapists had training in visual impairment. In this setting, Alex had fewer maladaptive behaviors, and his sensory processing, visual, and language needs were supported.

Cortical Visual Impairment Range

Alex scored 5-6.25 on the Cortical Visual Impairment (CVI) Range, which is in Phase 2: integrating vision with function. He was able to localize and fixate for 3 to 4 seconds on a target in near space. He was able to view objects with two to three colors with increased latency as the complexity increased. He viewed objects more easily than pictures or photographs. He responded best to lighted objects or the backlit screen of an iPad. He was attracted to movement of objects or pictures. He was able to view simple objects in near (8 to 15 inches) or middle (15 inches to 3 feet) space. Distance viewing (more than 3 feet away) was brief (a few seconds). He had difficulty using his lower visual fields initially but was able to attend to lower fields with movement or lighting of the object or picture. He initially performed reach and looking separately, but with movement of the object was able to look briefly while reaching. He tolerated low levels of

(continued)

Case Story 10-3 (continued)

auditory distraction during the assessment but became distracted with increased auditory input, such as sounds outside the window from traffic or talking. He became agitated if not allowed to touch objects and pictures or get closer to view them in his near space.

AOTA Occupational Profile Template

Parent/Child report: According to Alex's mother, they would like him to participate more in his home and community. She states that he is most successful in playing 1:1 with a friend with familiar activities. He is outgoing and seeks social situations but doesn't know how to interact appropriately. He participates with his family at home and in going to movies, community activities, and church. They try to limit him to only one type of activity each day due to his visual fatigue. With visual fatigue, Alex often becomes so tired that he falls asleep or becomes very agitated, has increased distractibility, lack of calming, or becomes sad. His mother feels that as he becomes more mature, he will be able to compensate or ask for help. He seems to understand his limitations more often than in the past and demonstrates more confidence in his abilities. He has had occupational therapy and vision services, along with psychological counseling and coaching by his parent on how to cope with changes and support his needs. Coping strategies involve decreasing or calming sensory input (visual and auditory), nature walks, relaxation tapes or music, a quiet space with a beanbag chair and a tent, lotion massage on arms, back rub, and redirection or support for motor or language needs.

Environment: Supports to Alex's occupational engagement include his good memory, which helps him recall information. He has a supportive family, sibling and family friends, and community. Barriers to his occupational engagement include going to unfamiliar settings that have increased visual complexity, which is difficult for him. Often people in the community do not understand his special needs, especially because he looks typical.

Context: Alex and his family are supported by their faith. Recently, Alex participated in summer camps and other social activities that were successful due to the ability to control visual inputs, which his mother finds helpful to expand his social opportunities. His use of assistive technology, especially his iPad, allows him to have success in several areas, which contributes to his self-esteem. His age and developmental level negatively affect his ability to engage in the community.

Goals: His mother reports that she would like Alex to have a good quality of life, to be happy, and be socially included in his community.

Parent/Child Report

Self-Care: Alex is currently able to complete self-care with some assistance. He is an independent ambulator and is able to navigate familiar environments such as his home but has difficulty in unfamiliar environments in the community. His

(continued)

Case Study 10-3 (continued)

mother reports that she holds his hand for safety when walking in parking lots or near the street because he does not always notice moving cars and people. She reports that he has difficulty with lower fields of vision and will trip on curbs or surface changes. On playgrounds, he often does not see obstacles, edges/drops, or surface changes. This results in safety issues with falling and tripping. He also does not always notice children on swings or other moving equipment. He has more difficulty when more people are on the playground, as visual complexity increases. His mother said, "If there are more kids he has a harder time and moves slower than when we are there by ourselves. He has a hard time looking and kids move quickly." As a result, he often stays in one place and plays less on the playground equipment or with peers. He is able to navigate a familiar playground at his neighborhood school. "He is proud that he has learned our playground and can play more independently," according to his mother. He asks what time it is, is learning to read a clock, and understands days of the week during calendar time at school.

Productivity/Play: In play opportunities, Alex usually plays in parallel with an-other child and needs facilitation by an adult due to difficulty with vision and communication. He is more successful with play in 1:1 situations than in the classroom or a group. He has developed a relationship with one other child who is supportive and able to verbally and physically assist him during play. His favorite thing to play with is his iPad, especially puzzles. He likes to play hide and seek. He watches movies over and over again, but only watches a new movie in sections until he learns the characters and what is happening. In school, he colors pictures vigorously but does not color inside the lines and fre-quently looks away from his paper. He does best when the paper is placed on a slant board instead of flat on a table. He learns sight words using "bubbling" or an outline of the word with a contrasting color (usually yellow or red). He is able to count to 100 using colored sticks in alternating colors. When the class is working on the smartboard, he has it "mirrored" on his iPad in closer proximity, 12 to 15 inches from his eyes. When he is looking at other pictures, instructors use red or yellow highlighting of salient features for learning vocabulary or concepts (Figure 10-3).

Leisure: At home, Alex enjoys talking on the phone and watching or sending videos for special occasions. He takes taekwondo in individual and group les-sons. He plays soccer, but is often overwhelmed by the sensory input with the group of children, which makes it difficult for him to participate in the game or socialize with other players. He likes to play outside in his backyard and jumps on the trampoline. During recreational pursuits, he has difficulty determining who people are from far away and will often misinterpret who is there unless the person talks. Even when up close, he relies on context, outline of the person, and voice to determine who it is. His mother reports that "there is so much he has to do even for play, when other kids can just play; it's so hard for him."

(continued)

Case Study 10-3 (continued)

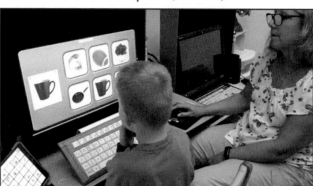

Figure 10-3. Alex using a smartboard.

The AOTA Occupational Performance Template

Parent/Child report: Alex's mother reports that she would like him to be able to participate more. With peers, he needs a familiar person to facilitate the interaction or task to make it easier. She sees him seeking social situations, but recognizes that he doesn't know how to maintain the social exchange. He participates with family, at church, movies, and community activities on a more limited basis due to his vision impairment. She sees him getting more mature as he gets older. He has more awareness and asks for help in order to complete difficult tasks. He continues to try to complete tasks, but understands his own limitations more.

Environment: His mother reports that Alex has a good memory, which helps him to recall his surroundings, but that he still has problems with motor tasks, unfamiliar settings, and the visual complexity in the world. She reports that they have supportive family, friends, and people in the community. There are barriers at his public school with some activities due to the unpredictability of the setting.

Context: In the community, it is difficult because sometimes people do not understand Alex's differences. His mother has found successful activities in the community where there is support for his needs and where he can practice coping strategies with support by knowledgeable adults, peers, or a parent. As he "practices," he develops his self-concept, resilience, and adaptability.

REFERENCES

American Foundation for the Blind. (2020). Low vision and legal blindness terms and descriptions. https://www.afb.org/blindness-and-low-vision/eye-conditions/low-vision-and-legal-blindness-terms-and-descriptions#Facts_about_LowVision

American Occupational Therapy Association. (2020). Occupational therapy practice framework: Domain and process (4th ed.). *American Journal of Occupational Therapy, 74*(Suppl. 2), 7412410010. https://doi.org/10.5014/ajot.2020.74S2001

Auigestad, L. B. (2017). Mental health among children and young adults with visual impairments: A systematic review. *Journal of Visual Impairment and Blindness, 111*(5), 411-425. https://doi.org/10.1177/0145482X1711100503

Bakke, H. A., Cavalcante, W. A., de Oliveira, I. S., Sarinho, S. W., & Cattuzzo, M. T. (2019). Assessment of motor skills in children with visual impairment: A systematic and integrative review. *Clinical Medicine Insights: Pediatrics, 13*, 1179556519838287. https://doi.org/10.1177/1179556519838287

Brémond-Gignac, D., Copin, H., Lapillonne, A., & Milazzo, S. (2011). Visual development in infants: Physiological and pathological mechanisms. *Current Opinion in Ophthalmology, 22*, S1-S8. https://doi.org/10.1097/01.icu.0000397180.37316.5d

Bruegger, T., Dickson, B., Moranville, E., Ryan, C., & Swisher, K. (2021). Correlation of visual impairment to sensory processing, coping, participation in and quality of life of children with visual impairment [unpublished paper]. Occupational Therapy Faculty, Rockhurst University.

Callier Center for Communication Disorders. (2020). Callier-Azusa scale. University of Texas at Dallas. https://calliercenter.utdallas.edu/evaluation-treatment/callier-azusa-scale

Centers for Disease Control and Prevention. (2017). Vision health initiative: Basics of vision and eye health. https://www.cdc.gov/visionhealth/basics/index.html

Chan, T., Friedman, D. S., Bradley, C., & Massof, R. (2017). Estimates of incidence and prevalence of visual impairment, low vision, and blindness in the United States. *JAMA Ophthalmology, 136*(1), 12-19. https://doi.org/10.1001/jamaophthalmol.2017.4655

Chien, C., Rodger, S., Copley, J., Branjerdporn, G., & Taggart, C. (2016). Sensory processing and its relationship with children's daily life participation. *Physical & Occupational Therapy in Pediatrics, 36*(1), 73-87. https://doi.org/10.3109/01942638.2015.1040573

Chokron, S., & Dutton, G. N. (2016). Impact of cerebral visual impairments on motor skills: Implications for developmental coordination disorders. *Frontiers in Psychology.* https://doi.org/10.3389/fpsyg.2016.01471

Cochrane, G., Marella, M., Keeffe, J., & Lamoureux, L. (2011). The Impact of Vision Impairment for Children (IVI_C): Validation of a vision-specific pediatric quality-of-life questionnaire using Rasch analysis. *Investigative Ophthalmology & Visual Science, 2011, 52*(3), 1632-1640. https://doi.org/10.1167/iovs.10-6079

Compas, B. E., Connor-Smith, J. K., Saltzman, H., Thomsen, A. H., & Wadsworth, M. E. (2001). Coping with stress during childhood and adolescence: Problems, progress, and potential in theory and research. *Psychological Bulletin, 127*(1), 87-127. https://pubmed.ncbi.nlm.nih.gov/11271757

Cordier, R., Chen, Y.-W., Speyer, R., Totino, R., Doma, K., Leicht, A., Brown, N., & Cuomo, B. (2016). Child-report measures of occupational performance: A systematic review. *PLoS ONE 11*(1): e0147751. https://doi.org/10.1371/journal.pone.0147751

Dandona, L., & Dandona, R. (2006). Revision of visual impairment definitions in the *International Statistical Classification of Diseases. BMC Medicine, 4*(7). https://doi.org/10.1186/1741-7015-4-7

Dean, E., Little, L., Tomchek, S., & Dunn, W. (2018). Sensory processing in the general population: Adaptability, resiliency, and challenging behavior. *American Journal of Occupational Therapy, 72*(1), 7201195060. https://doi.org/10.5014/ajot.2018.019919

Frydenberg, E., & Lewis, R. (2015). Teaching coping to adolescents: When and to whom? *American Educational Research Journal 2000, 37*(3): 727-745. https://doi.org/10.3102/00028312037003727

Grajo, L. (2019). Occupational adaptation as a normative and intervention process: Schkade and Schultz's legacy. In L. C. Grajo & A. Boisselle (Eds.), *Adaptation through occupation: Multidimensional perspectives.* SLACK Incorporated.

Grajo, L., Boisselle, A., & DaLomba, E. (2018). Occupational adaptation as a construct: A scoping review of literature. *The Open Journal of Occupational Therapy, 6*(1). https://doi.org/10.15453/2168-6408.1400

Hamed-Daher, S., & Engel-Yeger, B. (2019). The relationships between sensory processing abilities and participation patterns of children with visual or auditory sensory impairments. *The American Journal of Occupational Therapy, 73*(4), 1. https://doi.org/10.5014/ajot.2019.73S1-PO7021

Hatton, D. D., McWilliam, R. A., & Winton, P. J. (2013). *Family-centered practices: For infants and toddlers with visual impairments.* University of North Carolina, Chapel Hill.

Heyl, V., & Hintermair, M. (2015). Executive function and behavioral problems in students with visual impairments at mainstream and special schools. *Journal of Visual Impairment & Blindness, 109*(4), 251-263. https://eric.ed.gov/?id=EJ1114483

Kong, L., Fry, M., Al-Samarraie, M., Gilbert, C., & Steinkuller, P. G. (2012). An update on progress and the changing epidemiology of causes of childhood blindness worldwide. *Journal of American Association for Pediatric Ophthalmology and Strabismus 16*(6), 501-507. https://doi.org/10.1016/j.jaapos.2012.09.004

Lueck, A., & Dutton, G. (2015). *Vision and the brain: Understanding cerebral visual impairment in children.* AFB Press American Foundation for the Blind.

Merabet, L. B., Mayer, D. L., Bauer, C. M., Wright, D., & Kran, B. S. (2017). Disentangling how the brain is "wired" in cortical (cerebral) visual impairment. *Seminars in Pediatric Neurology, 24*(2), 83-91. https://doi.org/10.1016/j.spen.2017.04.005

National Sensory Impairment Partnership. (2012). *Promoting resilience and well being in children and young people with sensory impairment.* London, UK: Department for Education.

Oluonye, N., & Sargent, J. (2019). Severe visual impairment: Practical guidance for paediatricians. *Paediatrics and Child Health, 28*(8), 379-383. https://doi.org/10.1016/j.paed.2018.06.007

The Oregon Project for Children (6th ed.). (2020). http://www.soesd.k12.or.us/oregon-online

Pletcher, L., & Younggren, N. (2013). *The early intervention workbook: Essential practices for quality services.* Paul Brookes Publishing.

Prior, M. (2015). Resilience and coping: The role of individual temperament. Developing as a person in complex societies. In E. Frydenberg (Ed.), *Learning to cope: Developing as a person in complex societies* (p. 33). Oxford University Press. https://doi.org/10.1093/med:psych/9780198503187.003.0002

Project IDEAL. (2013). *Visual impairment.* Texas Council for Developmental Disabilities.

Roman-Lantzy, C. (2018). *Cortical visual impairment: An approach to assessment and intervention, 2^d edition.* AFB Press.

Sim, I. O. (2020). Analysis of the coping process among visually impaired individuals, using interpretative phenomenological analysis (IPA). *International Journal of Environmental Research and Public Health, 17*(8), 2819. https://doi.org/10.3390/ijerph17082819.

Sturrock, B., Xie, J., Holloway, H., Lamoureux, E., Keeffe, J., Fenwick, E., & Rees, G. (2015). The influence of coping on vision-related quality of life in patients with low vision: A prospective longitudinal study. *Investigative Ophthalmology & Visual Science, 56*(4), 2416-2422. https://doi.org/10.1167/iovs.14-16223

van den Broek, E., van Eijden, A., Overbeek, M., Kef, S., Sterkenburg, P., & Schuengel, C. (2017). A systematic review of the literature on parenting of young children with visual impairments and the adaptations for Video-Feedback Intervention to Promote Positive Parenting (VIPP). *Journal of Developmental Physical Disabilities, 29*, 503-545. https://doi.org/10.1007/s10882-016-9529-6

Varma, R., Tarczy-Hornoch, K., & Jiang, X. (2017). Visual impairment in preschool children in the United States: Demographic and geographic variations from 2015 to 2060. *Journal of the American Medical Association Ophthalmology, 135*(6), 610-616. https://doi.org/10.1001/jamaophthalmol.2017.1021

Varma, R., Vajaranant, T. S., Burkemper, B., Wu, S., Torres, M., Hsu, C., Choudhury, F., & McKean-Cowdin, R. (2016). Visual impairment and blindness in adults in the United States: Demographic and geographic variations from 2015 to 2050. *JAMA Ophthalmology, 134*(7), 802-809. https://doi.org/10.1001/jamaophthalmol.2016.1284

World Health Organization. (2019). Blindness and visual impairment. https://www.who.int/news-room/fact-sheets/detail/blindness-and-visual-impairment

Yuan, W., Zhang, L., & Li, B. (2017). Adapting the Brief COPE for Chinese adolescents with visual impairments. *Journal of Visual Impairment & Blindness, 111*(1), 20-32. https://doi.org/10.1177/0145482X1711100103

Personal Contexts and Lived Experience

11

Children and Youth Who Have Experienced Bullying

Christine Urish, PhD, OTR/L, BCMH, FAOTA, CCAP

CHAPTER OBJECTIVES By the end of the chapter, the reader will be able to:
- Discuss the impact of bullying on youth in all areas of occupation and the incidence/prevalence of bullying within the United States and globally.
- Describe the role of the occupational therapy practitioner in assessment and intervention regarding bullying in youth relative to coping, adaptation, and resilience.
- Critically evaluate bullying prevention, intervention, and school mental health programs and resources available in the United States and abroad.

OVERVIEW OF THE POPULATION

Bullying is defined as "any unwanted aggressive behavior(s) by another youth or group of youths who are not siblings or current dating partners that involves an observed or perceived power imbalance and is repeated multiple times or is highly likely to be repeated." Bullying may "inflict harm or distress on the targeted youth, including physical, psychological, social, or educational harm" (Gladden et al., 2014, p. 7). Bullying may occur in a direct or indirect manner. *Direct bullying* is aggressive behavior that occurs in the presence of the targeted youth and may include aggressive behavior such as pushing, or verbal or written communication that is harmful and directed toward the youth. *Indirect bullying* is behavior that is not directly communicated to the targeted youth. This can include the bully starting rumors or spreading inaccurate communication about the youth.

To be considered bullying, the behavior must be aggressive in nature and must demonstrate the following: (1) An imbalance of power (e.g., physical strength, access to embarrassing information about the individual, or the bully is considered more popular);

Grajo L. C., & Boisselle, A. K. (Eds.). *Adaptation, Coping, and Resilience in Children and Youth: A Comprehensive Occupational Therapy Approach* (pp. 263-287).
© 2022 Taylor & Francis Group.

and (2) Repetition. Behavior is considered bullying if the behavior has occurred more than once or has the potential to occur again (StopBullying.Gov, 2019a). This behavior is of concern for the profession of occupational therapy because the behavior often involves school-aged children, and a high percentage of occupational therapists (19.9%) and occupational therapy assistants (15%) work with this population (American Occupational Therapy Association [AOTA], 2015). The repetitive nature of bullying places youth at risk not only of being bullied, but also of becoming the perpetrator of bullying behavior. Youth who have been bullied have the potential to experience serious, lasting problems because of this behavior (StopBullying.Gov, 2019a).

There are three basic categories of bullying behavior: verbal bullying, social bullying, and physical bullying. *Verbal bullying* includes verbally saying or writing things to tease, insult, or harm another youth. This can include engaging in taunting, threatening to cause harm, making inappropriate sexual comments toward the youth, and name calling (StopBullying.Gov, 2019a). *Social bullying* influences an individual by negatively affecting social relationships or the person's reputation. This form of bullying can include leaving a youth out of a formal or informal conversation or activity on purpose, directing others not to engage or be friends with the individual being targeted, instigating rumors about the individual, and embarrassing the individual in public (StopBullying .Gov, 2019a), among other behaviors. The last type of bullying is *physical bullying*. This form of bullying involves physical harm to the person who is the target of the bully or to the bullied person's possessions. Examples of physical bullying include tripping, kicking, pinching, spitting on, and/or pushing the individual; harming the person's belongings (such as breaking or taking items [e.g., ripping up completed homework, taking a book bag]), and directing mean or rude hand gestures toward the individual.

Statistics regarding bullying of students in the United States are concerning. Data obtained from the 2017 United States Department of Justice (U.S. DOJ) School Crime Supplement (U.S. Department of Education, 2019) were used to examine survey results from 24,650,000 students. The sample included public and private schools throughout the United States from each region of the country. The study sample was comprised of 83.3% male and 76.2% female youth. Students who completed the survey represented grades 6 to 12. Of these, 20.2% (4,986,000) of students reported experiencing bullying during the 2016-2017 academic year. Bullying behaviors reported included being made fun of, called names, or insulted (13%); being the subject of rumors (13.3%); being threatened with harm (3.9%); being pushed, shoved, tripped, or spit on (5.3%); being made to do things they did not want to do (1.9%); being excluded from activities on purpose (5.2%); and having property destroyed on purpose (1.4%; U.S. Department of Education, 2019). These statistics are alarming considering the negative impact that bullying can have upon a young person. Location of bullying varied across a variety of environments, including classroom (42.2%), hallway or stairwell (43.3%), bathroom or locker room (11.8%), cafeteria at school (26.4%), outside on school grounds (21.5%); school bus (8.0%); and online or by text (15.5%). As to the frequency of bullying, the study reported variation from once per day to daily for more than 10 days. Further, 41.2% of youth were concerned that the bullying would happen again (U.S. Department of Education, 2019). The peak age of bullying is from ages 11 to 13, and per self-report, one in three students aged 12 to 18 were bullied in the past year (BullyPolice.org, 2017).

It is important to note that each of the 50 states in the United States as well as Puerto Rico have legislation related to bullying and how it is to be addressed (BullyPolice .org, 2017). Nevertheless, the challenge remains. Some legislation provides more information on the role of the school and jurisdiction, whereas other legislation is broader and does not address the full scope of bullying (including cyberbullying). The organization Bullypolice.org provides a "grade" for each state ranging from A++ to C- (Bullypolice .org, 2017).

DEFINING ADAPTATION, COPING, AND RESILIENCE IN CHILDREN WHO EXPERIENCE BULLYING

From an occupational therapy perspective, bullying must be considered in a multifaceted way. Although legislation exists at the state level for all 50 states, questions remain about how these laws and policies are being translated to and enforced in the individual communities and schools, community organizations, and clubs in which youth participate. Consider the documentary *BULLY* by Lee Hirsch, which was filmed during the 2009/2010 school year. Although the documentary was filmed more than a decade ago, the challenges presented therein continue to occur today. The film depicts the challenges in addressing bullying from the youth, family, and education system perspectives (The Bully Project, 2020). The documentary highlights the experiences of those who were being bullied and those who lost their lives due to the pain and anguish of not being able either to obtain help or to cope with the bullying situation they were experiencing.

The film portrayed bullying as a problem that does not have geographic, racial, ethnic, or economic boundaries. The film highlights the responses of school administrators to parents and students who are raising concerns about aggressive behaviors: many fell back on "kids will be kids" clichés, rather than taking action to address this significant and concerning problem that can negatively affect all aspects of occupational engagement and performance for a young person. Societal change regarding how persons react to and cope with individuals who are not like themselves is an ongoing challenge within the United States.

Resilience assists youth in building positive responses to cope with challenges that may be faced at any time. To assist youth in developing resilience, occupational therapy practitioners need to be aware of occupations that foster a sense of resilience. Social connections are important for support as well as coping. Assisting youth in development of social competence is key in the development of resilience (The Royal Children's Hospital Melbourne, 2012). Assisting youth to establish occupation-focused goals that are motivating and meaningful to them can help them develop positive coping skills as well as resilience and adaptation to the challenges presented. Providing youth opportunities for decision making within success-ensured activities or environments allows them to develop adaptation responses, as well as coping when occupations are challenging for them.

Assisting youth to realize that everything will not always go as they planned and that everyone will not always treat them as they anticipate they should be treated, and arming them with positive coping strategies to deal with life challenges, are important in developing youth who demonstrate resilience (The Royal Children's Hospital Melbourne, 2012). Assisting youth in learning from challenging situations can create opportunities to develop adaptive behavior as well as learning from direct experience.

Case Study 11-1

The occupational therapist is approached by a third-grade classroom teacher who asks the therapist to speak with some parents about their son's behavior during lunch and indoor recess. Students were required to have indoor recess because of the frigid temperatures in the Midwest in January. In prior weeks, the five students who were engaging in bullying behavior had made fun of the food one of their classmates brought to eat for lunch. The lunch staff redirected student conversation; however, the negative behavior continued. One day, during indoor recess, five students began using paper to create walls around the child's desk. The teacher redirected the boys' behavior and dismantled the "walls," but the bullying continued, with name-calling and alienation of the child who was being targeted.

Although the scenario from Case Study 11-1 is challenging, the more significant challenge arose when the teacher reached out to speak to the individual parents: the parents were confused as to why they were being "called" about their children's behavior, as they did not see anything wrong with it. Parents play a vital role in supporting and modeling appropriate behavior. Parents need to promote "upstander" behavior (standing up for oneself and others through assertive behaviors and communication with others) rather than "bystander" behavior (allowing whatever behavior is occurring to occur, though it may be negative in nature and harmful to others). Parents have a role in teaching appropriate social interaction and communication by teaching and modeling empathy within the home (The Bully Project, 2020). When this does not happen, negative behavior spills into the classroom and school environment. Occupational therapists have a role in supporting parents through providing education and resources on how to model assertive communication and how to maintain a calm, focused, and empathetic demeanor when faced with challenges, and affording parents the opportunity to assist their children with problem solving in complex social relationships.

In this scenario, the teacher reached out to the occupational therapist in a consultant role to devise social-emotional learning and coping strategies for all students within the classroom to address the bullying situation. Further, the occupational therapist supported the teacher in developing materials regarding the negative social, emotional, and educational impacts of bullying as well as being a bully; these materials were also shared electronically with parents. Occupational therapists are front-line service providers to youth in schools, outpatient clinics, afterschool youth programs, and outside of

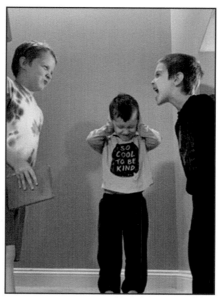

Figure 11-1. Youth being bullied with a bystander present.

professional settings in church groups and other youth organizations such as scouting or sports. In all these environments, occupational therapists are exposed to youth who have the potential to be bullied or may be experiencing bullying. The role of the occupational therapist is to identify and address bullying to maximize occupational performance in self-care, education, and leisure.

Bullying can negatively affect the youth from a multitude of occupational performance areas considered in the *Occupational Therapy Practice Framework: Domain and Process, Fourth Edition* (*OTPF-4*; Figure 11-1). See Table 11-1.

THE ROLE OF OCCUPATIONAL THERAPY: BEST AND EVIDENCE-BASED PRACTICES FOR ASSESSMENT AND INTERVENTIONS

An occupational therapist can assume several roles when addressing bullying from an individual or population perspective. First and foremost, the occupational therapy practitioner must have an awareness of what constitutes bullying (Figure 11-2). The Centers for Disease Control and Prevention (CDC) classify bullying information in the area of "injury prevention and control" (CDC, 2020). Although information regarding bullying is readily available, individuals are directed to seek information from reputable sources, as many resources available may not be grounded in or guided by research evidence. The occupational therapy practitioner can address bullying from an individual

Table 11-1

Challenges in Occupational Performance Due to Bullying	
Area of Occupation	Challenge
Activities of daily living (ADLs)	*Eating habits:* Could change due to others making fun of food choices or foods brought to school (e.g., loss of appetite). Not eating could also be attributed to feelings of depression or anxiety or overeating to try and cope with negative feelings. *Dressing/personal hygiene and grooming:* Problems may be reflected in change in appearance through change in personal hygiene habits, and/or lack of attention to hygiene or clothing selection due to feeling that they will be ostracized no matter what they look like.
Instrumental activities of daily living (IADLs)	*Communication management:* May be affected through sending or receiving information on smartphone. May demonstrate increased or decreased texting/chatting/video use due to being bullied.
Health management	*Social and emotional health promotion and maintenance:* Issues may manifest as withdrawal from engagement in activities that formerly supported social engagement and health and wellness. May be unable to identify personal strengths, which could negatively affect other areas of occupational performance and engagement.
Rest and sleep	*Rest:* May be negatively affected, as demonstrated by difficulty quieting mind and not being able to relax, always feeling "on edge." *Sleep preparation:* Problems may be seen, such as difficulty in engaging in structured routine to prepare for sleep due to feeling preoccupied by behavior of others outside of self. *Sleep participation:* Problems may be demonstrated by difficulty with falling asleep and/or staying asleep, awakening with feeling of not being rested.
Education	*Formal educational participation:* Can be negatively affected by school avoidance and not wanting to attend/participate due to challenges experienced within the school environment; difficulty with completion of school work due to feelings of depression and/or anxiety; poor concentration, challenges within the nonacademic environment (e.g., lunch, recess) due to fears of bullying; lack of, or decreased, engagement in extracurricular activities (e.g., sports, LEGO club, band, cheerleading) due to interactions with others or lack of feelings of personal capacity to meet activity challenge; decrease in grade performance; school avoidance; increased reporting of physical illness to avoid school environment, which results in absenteeism and decrease in academic performance.

(continued)

Table 11-1 (continued)

Challenges in Occupational Performance Due to Bullying	
Area of Occupation	Challenge
Work	*Job performance and maintenance:* Difficulty evidenced by not completing job tasks effectively due to poor concentration and anxiety; isolative behavior that can lead to absenteeism and decreased job performance.
	Volunteer participation: Suffers from lack of engagement due to low motivation, feelings of depression/anxiety; decreased self-efficacy; difficulty identifying positive contributions to volunteer organization/work.
Leisure	*Leisure exploration:* Issues demonstrated by potential unwillingness to explore new interests due to low self-esteem/self-efficacy.
	Leisure participation: Issues revealed by lack of participation or engagement in activities once previously enjoyed; isolation by participation only in activities of a solitary nature.
Social participation	*Community participation:* Problems evidenced by lack of engagement in extracurricular school activities or neighborhood or youth activities due to worries about potential bullying behavior of others; lack of self-efficacy regarding personal performance in activities; potential for feelings of depression and anxiety, which could negatively affect initiation of and engagement in activities.
	Family participation: Problems evidenced by noticeable change in behavior and communication toward family members as a result of being bullied; starting arguments with other family members or siblings or engaging in bullying behavior toward family members; withdrawal or isolation.
	Friendships: Evidenced by isolation or withdrawal from friends because of feeling inadequate due to being bullied, or being fearful of the potential bullying behavior of others. Research supports the contention that those who have been bullied have a high likelihood of bullying others, so this could also be a concern.
	Peer group participation: May withdraw from peers; wish to spend more time with adults or alone due to having experienced being bullied or fear of being bullied again in the future.

perspective by working with the youth who has experienced bullying or the perpetrator of the bullying behavior. Further, the occupational therapist may work with the teacher, school, or school district as a consultant on social-emotional learning, education, and prevention programming (AOTA, 2013b).

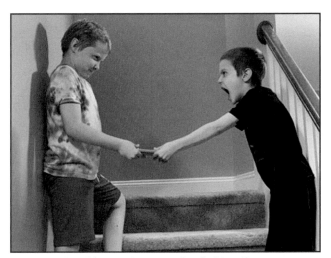

Figure 11-2. Youth attempting to stand up for himself.

Assessment

Occupational therapy practitioners engage in completion of an occupational profile, as well as analysis of occupational performance, when providing occupational therapy services to an individual or population (AOTA, 2020). Bullying is addressed as an individual concern, but it is also as a systemic or population-based concern. Thus, the occupational therapy practitioner must critically examine the impact of bullying on many areas of occupation as well as on performance skills and patterns. Some youth may engage in bullying behavior because a bully has victimized them. Other youth may engage in bullying due to lack of or underdevelopment of effective social skills; for these youth, bullying may serve as a defense mechanism to keep them protected from others.

The CDC's Division of Violence Prevention has developed a compendium of assessment tools that could be beneficial for the occupational therapy practitioner (Hamburger, Basile, & Vivolo, 2011). The compendium provides measures including bully-only scales, victim-only scales, bully and victim scales, and bystander, bully, and victim scales. Descriptions of the measures in the compendium are presented with characteristics of the assessment, target group, psychometrics, and developer contact information. Several assessments are reprinted with permission in the compendium and information regarding scoring and interpretation is provided for use (Hamburger, Basile, & Vivolo, 2011).

From an occupational therapy perspective, after completion of the occupational profile, an analysis of occupational performance will be conducted. Considering the areas in Table 11-1, which could be negatively impacted by bullying, the occupational therapist would select an assessment to identify specific areas of concern. One assessment that is well suited for use in occupational therapy is the Social Skills Improvement System by Gresham and Elliott (2008). This assessment is a self-report for the youth, and includes forms for completion by the teacher/educator as well as the parent so that information can be examined from multiple perspectives. The assessment measures social skills, including communication, cooperation, assertion, empathy, and self-control. Further problem behaviors, including bullying, hyperactivity, inattention, internalizing, and externalizing, are also addressed. Based upon the evaluation outcome information, the occupational therapist can target interventions within the home, school, and community environments to address any challenges the youth is experiencing in social skills and problematic behavior.

An occupational therapist would also address any area of occupation identified through the occupational profile process as being challenging for in the youth. For example, if the young person was being bullied during physical education class due to challenges with motor or social skills, the occupational therapist would engage in an assessment of gross/fine motor skills. Upon completion of the assessment, the occupational therapist would develop a treatment plan to address occupational performance deficits, while building coping skills and resilience with the young person to help them deal with challenging and possibly inappropriate behavior of others.

Intervention

The occupational therapist could address occupational performance, improvement, prevention, health and wellness, participation, role competence, well-being, and occupational justice when considering targeted outcomes as defined in *OTPF-4*. Researchers have identified bullying as a form of occupational injustice, so occupational therapists are directed to work toward systemic change at the school and community levels to combat the impact of bullying and engage in prevention of this behavior (Pereira, 2010).

StopBullying.Gov (2019b) developed specific guidance for occupational therapists to understand the specific roles of health and safety professionals in community-wide bullying prevention efforts. Professionals are directed to identify when bullying may be occurring (school avoidance; change in behavior/mood; be on alert for youth who are a higher risk of being bullied, such as youth with disabilities and LGBTQ+ youth) and provide effective, evidence-based intervention, as well as advocate for effective bullying prevention and response in a variety of environments in which youth find themselves (StopBullying.Gov, 2019b).

From an occupational therapy perspective, bullying should be addressed from a multi-tier perspective, as directed by the National Academies of Science, Engineering & Medicine (NASEM) public health prevention approach (2016). Services are identified within the tiers and are described in Table 11-2.

Considering the role of the occupational therapist through the lens of the NASEM multitiered prevention framework, one finds that in Tier 1, the implementation of social-emotional learning programs and mindfulness-based interventions that will benefit the entire school system are important considerations. Resilience, coping, and adaptation should be guiding concepts as occupational therapists examine youth interaction and formulate effective interventions for individual youth as well as for school-wide programming. There are a vast number of social-emotional learning (SEL) programs available. It

Table 11-2

NASEM Multitiered Prevention Framework	
Tier 1	Preventative interventions focused on social-emotional learning and behavioral expectations within the classroom and school environment delivered to all youth (most bullying prevention programs fall within this tier)
Tier 2	Selective preventative interventions focused on youth who are being bullied or are at risk of becoming a bully. These may include more intensive social-emotional learning programs than Tier 1, as well as coping skills and de-escalation strategies for students who are involved in bullying behavior. Tier 2 interventions are utilized for students who have not responded effectively to Tier 1 interventions of universal prevention.
Tier 3	Indicated preventative interventions that address the needs of the youth who has experienced bullying or the youth who is engaging in bullying behavior. Behavioral and mental health concerns are further assessed and addressed, along with family involvement and support from individuals who ecologically support the youth in their natural environment.

is important that the occupational therapy practitioner examine the research supporting each program. Evidence-based research supporting positive outcomes is important when considering a program for utilization, as well as in finding a program that can be readily implemented into the school/clinic environment. At times, implementation within a school environment becomes complex, as the emphasis must be on ongoing educational goals and "core curriculum." One SEL program that relates to educational outcomes and has research to support its effectiveness is the *MindUP* curriculum. This program includes components for assisting students in the development of positive coping skills through use of mindfulness-based interventions. Research conducted in Canada and the United States has yielded positive outcomes in the following areas: improved mindful awareness, improved social and emotional competencies in peer and teacher relationships, improved academic success and engagement, and overall positive improvement in individual well-being (Maloney et al., 2016). These positive changes foster increased resilience in students and improve student coping when faced with academic, peer, or life challenges or stressors. Further, the program curriculum is manualized and easily accessible through internet booksellers. The MindUP curriculum is organized developmentally according to grade level, with three modules (Pre-K to Grade 2, Grades 3 to 5, and Grades 6 to 8) being available at a reasonable cost of less than $20 per module.

Occupational therapists should also be actively involved in school-based social-emotional learning activities and programs, whether those are embedded programs or embedded strategies within the school and community environment (Every Moment Counts, 2016). These programs have been shown to yield positive outcomes in supporting youth in developing resilience and adaptive ability to cope with behavioral and environmental challenges of others (Arbesman et al., 2013).

In Tier 2, the occupational therapist can be involved in the provision of more focused social-emotional learning programming, either individually or within a group or classroom. Programs such as *Strong Kids, Strong Teens* have demonstrated positive

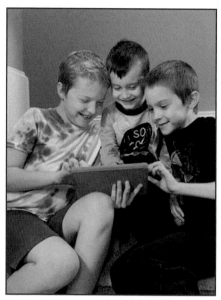

Figure 11-3. Youth demonstrating adaptive capacity following social challenges with peers.

outcomes and appear to have overcome common implementation challenges (Gueldner & Feurborn, 2016). The *Strong Kids, Strong Teens* program examines classroom lessons and incorporates mindfulness-based interventions that can be used to target the client's adaptive capacity and overcome occupational challenges in the areas of individual emotions, emotions of others, dealing with anger, clear thinking, problem solving, stress, and positive living. Research has supported student engagement in positive social-emotional learning experiences in order to decrease stress; students who have undertaken such learning experiences also demonstrate improved peer relationships, which could lead to decreased potential to bully or, if a victim, improved resilience and adaptation to the experience of being bullied. Resilience in a youth can be identified by increased engagement with a wide variety of peers (rather than withdrawal or retreat), demonstrating positive self-efficacy despite challenges, and a willingness to seek assistance from an adult authority figure early when youth become concerned about behavior they observe from others, rather than feeling guilty or avoiding bringing attention to a negative situation (Figure 11-3). Further, bystanders of bullying may be less affected and demonstrate improved ability to support peers, as well as seeking adult intervention for bullying they have observed. Countless social-emotional learning programs and approaches are available. Occupational therapy practitioners are encouraged to consider which programs will be the best match for the specific environment in which they are working, which have the greatest likelihood of success and consistent implementation, and—most importantly—which programs have been empirically validated.

Tier 3 interventions address youth who have experienced bullying directly or as bystanders. Byjos et al. (2016) reported personal factors that facilitate adaptive response: positive and close family connections, supportive relationship with peers and other adult authority figures such as a teacher or community leader (Scouts, sports, employer), and positive coping skills. Social support from peers and families is considered a protective factor. Knowing this, the occupational therapist could assist in providing intervention and classroom resources aimed at development of positive coping skills and adaptive response to school and peer stress. Byjos et al. (2016) found that even years after a bullying experience, the experience affected youths' self-esteem and motivated them to make improvements in the school mental health environment. This is just one study; imagine the countless number of youth who have experienced bullying and carry the long-lasting effects with them! It should be obvious from the research that occupational therapists play an *essential* role by having knowledge of the impact of bullying, knowing how to assess and appropriately intervene in bullying situations, and also developing programs and interventions that are effective for children and youth.

According to the findings of Walters (2020), programs delivered within the school environment should address bullying in a comprehensive fashion, and focus not only on perpetrators and victims of bullying, but also on bystanders within the context of the school environment. One of the most researched and utilized bullying prevention programs in the United States is the Olweus Bullying Prevention Program (OBPP; Walters, 2020). This evidence-based program has demonstrated ongoing effectiveness and viability that was attributable to the manner in which the program assists youth in managing thoughts, feelings, and behavior that "mark, motivate, and characterize victimization and perpetration" (Walters, 2020, p. 8). The OBPP program, developed in Norway by Dr. Dan Olweus, has been utilized and revised since its development in 1983. The program has been proven effective and includes the essential elements highlighted in Table 11-3.

Juvonen et al. (2016) examined the KiVa, an evidence-based program to prevent and address bullying within the school environment. This program is based upon extensive research conducted in Finland by the Ministry of Education and Culture (KiVa School, 2020). Although many anti-bullying programs are available, the KiVa program been rigorously researched, and has been modified and refined based upon research findings. Findings from the Juvonen et al. study (2016) indicated that the KiVa program was beneficial in facilitating the perception of a caring school climate by youth who were victimized prior to the intervention. Further, the program demonstrated benefits in the areas of depression and self-esteem in victimized youth. The KiVa program has materials for varying age levels. There is a unit for ages 6 to 9 years, 10 to 12 years, and 13 to 16 years. The program, which is available in several languages, offers materials that can be utilized by parents at home, a teachers' manual, and videos and online games for students. However, this program is a licensed program primarily being utilized in Europe, although a study is also being conducted in Chile (Gaete et al., 2017).

Table 11-3

Intervention Strategies for Adaptation, Coping, and Resilience Through Use of OBPP Essential Elements

Element	Description	Occupational Therapist's Role
School environment	The OBPP is a school-wide program that encompasses the entire school environment, including classroom activities, extracurricular school activities, and individual interventions. To reduce bullying, the school environment and climate, as well as social norms, must be critically examined and possibly changed.	School personnel (including occupational therapy practitioners) must increase awareness to observe and respond when a youth is being bullied or left out. Bullying prevention and intervention are not the sole responsibility of one individual within the school environment (e.g., principal or school counselor); rather, they are necessary for all school personnel (e.g., bus driver, nurse, resource officer, custodian, occupational therapist, physical therapist, speech-language pathologist, librarian), students, and parents to be able to respond effectively.
Bullying assessment	Olweus Bullying Questionnaire (OBQ), an anonymous, research-based assessment, is administered to students to ascertain the nature and degree of bullying in the school environment. This is essential, as adults' estimation of the prevalence of bullying within the school may not be accurate. Further, they may be surprised to learn of "hot spots" where bullying is most commonly happening, which may not have been considered or recognized.	School personnel (including occupational therapy practitioners) can be involved in administration of bullying assessment, as well as developing individual and school-wide interventions to address identified concerns.
Group support for bullying prevention	The program requires a group from the school to serve as a leader and guide implementation of the OBPP; this group should include an administrator, a teacher from each grade, non-teaching staff (could be an occupational therapy practitioner), a school counselor or other mental health professional, parents, and community persons.	The individuals in the group complete a 2-day training by an OBPP-certified trainer-consultant. The team is directed to meet twice a month to plan bullying-prevention events; train staff; and motivate students, parents, and staff over time to ensure program implementation and ongoing delivery of identified initiatives following the program. Occupational therapists,

(continued)

Table 11-3 (continued)

Intervention Strategies for Adaptation, Coping, and Resilience Through Use of OBPP Essential Elements

Element	Description	Occupational Therapist's Role
		with their focus on occupation, adaptation, coping, and development of student resilience, can be tremendously valuable when included in the training and implementation of the OBPP program.
All staff training	Staff are trained in a comprehensive fashion to gain insight into the nature of bullying, its effects, how to respond, and how to prevent bullying from occurring in the first place. Initial staff training is 6 hours. Ongoing monthly professional development is indicated.	Occupational therapy professionals can be involved in training other school professionals and assisting with the implementation of a school-wide intervention.
Establish and enforce school rules regarding bullying	The OBPP provides four straightforward rules about bullying that schools are recommended to adopt: 1. We will not bully others. 2. We will try to help students who are bullied. 3. We will try to include students who are left out. 4. If we know that somebody is being bullied, we will tell an adult at school and an adult at home. The rules are taught to students, posted throughout the school environment, and followed consistently.	The occupational therapist can provide positive, age-appropriate reinforcement for students and developmentally appropriate corrective consequences. Students learn that school personnel take bullying seriously in a consistent manner, and they are aware that school personnel will not tolerate bullying and will intervene.
Involve youth in discussions about bullying	Children and youth are actively engaged in the development and maintenance of a safe and humane school environment. Class meetings, student discussions, and content that is aligned with the core curriculum support the effectiveness of this program. Fidelity to the program	Occupational therapy professionals approach bullying from a coping and development-of-resilience perspective by engaging youth in the development of a positive coping toolkit, and by monitoring the fidelity of the program. Through utilizing effective social-emotional learning interventions such as those detailed in

	requires that time be dedicated to bullying discussion, peer relationships, and social and emotional student issues at a minimum of every other week; weekly is preferred. Student advisory group can provide insightful feedback to school personnel.	Every Moment Counts, occupational therapy professionals assist students in developing resilience to negative situations that may arise/occur, as well as motivating youth to speak up and speak out to foster ongoing change.
Increased adult supervision in locations where bullying occurs	The OBPP program examines where bullying is occurring and where it may occur within a specific school setting. As a result, the school is able to modify supervision, as research supports the contention that bullying will thrive in locations where adult authority figures are not present or are not vigilant about observation and behavior management.	
Intervene consistently and appropriately	When bullying is observed, suspected or reported staff need to be prepared to respond. The OBPP program prepares staff through a comprehensive six-step, on-the-spot intervention to address bullying observed first-hand.	Follow-up interventions offer school personnel (which could include occupational therapy practitioners) the opportunity to continue dialogue with students, staff, and parents to develop additional solutions for student safety, growth, and adaptation.
Parent support	Parents and caregivers should be involved from the development of the plan through implementation of the OBPP program.	Parents and caregivers are essential in providing insights to school personnel, including occupational therapy practitioners, regarding the effectiveness of the program through their observations of the young person and their peers.
Ongoing support	A specific support structure has been developed within the OBPP program to assist in implementation of the program with fidelity to the design through which it has achieved the results documented in a multitude of research studies.	Occupational therapy practitioners are consistently focused on the goals of the OBPP program. Delivery of the program with fidelity to the model is essential. Evaluation of outcomes is relative to the programmatic goals in developing youth who are able to adapt to challenges, cope with situations that are outside of their control, and demonstrate resilience in the face of challenges or potential adversity outside of themselves.
Ongoing, continued effort	OBPP is not a 1-year program. The program is designed to be an ongoing focus in the school environment. Systemic change and change in school climate are necessary to obtain the desired result of obtaining a safe and humane school environment.	Ongoing evaluation of changes made, and changes that continue to be required, can be included within the role of an occupational therapy professional.

Case Study 11-2

Lorenzo is just starting sixth grade. He is small for his age, with both weight and height being lower than those of his peers. He was being bullied because of his "scrawny" appearance and then became a bully himself. He was viewed by his teachers and parents as a sensitive, kind, and caring young person who would watch out for others younger than himself. His bullying experience began when a fellow student began bullying his friend. Words were exchanged and Lorenzo was jumped; due to limitations in strength and stature, he was physically and emotionally harmed. Since the incident, Lorenzo has become quiet, does not socialize with peers, and has been observed keeping to himself. His grades were mostly As and Bs, but now have dropped to Cs and below. The teacher approaches the occupational therapist to see what can be done.

Lorenzo is not on the occupational therapist's caseload; however, the teacher is reaching out for support. There is no comprehensive bullying prevention or intervention program within the school, or anywhere within the district that the occupational therapist is aware of. Individual schools have attempted to address bullying, some more effectively than others. The occupational therapist is seeing a child on the autism spectrum and another child with social anxiety disorder in Lorenzo's class; therefore, the teacher feels comfortable requesting assistance in this area.

From a macro perspective, the occupational therapy practitioner could examine the potential for bullying prevention and intervention programming to be implemented more consistently within the school environment. Unfortunately, this takes time and money, both which are in short supply in the school environment.

The occupational therapist could work with the teacher to implement social-emotional learning programming and increased social skill building, as well as coping and adaptive strategies, within the classroom environment. Within the classroom environment, the occupational therapist could work collaboratively with the teacher to implement the MindUP curriculum (Maloney et al., 2016). MindUP is a social-emotional learning program focused on the development of competencies such as self-awareness, self-management, social awareness, relationship skills, and decision making. The key components of this program focus on interactive activities (doing occupations) that are directed to promote executive function in youth to organize, sequence, and regulate behavior (adaptation). The program emphasizes stress regulation (coping), personal well-being, and prosocial behavior (developing and fostering a sense of resilience).

Further, the occupational therapist and teacher collaborate to support Lorenzo, because research supports positive relationships with adult authority figures as a positive factor. The occupational therapist and teacher engage in Tier 2 interventions according to the NASEM multi-tier categorization. Importantly, the occupational therapist and teacher need to assure student safety; demonstrate that bullying has consequences; and involve other teachers, parents, and all school personnel to support the safety of all students, while not specifically causing Lorenzo or the peer he was defending to feel targeted or specifically "called out."

Table 11-4

U.S. and International School Mental Health Resources	
Organization	URL
World Health Organization School Health Initiative; Preventing Youth Violence	https://www.who.int/publications/i/item/preventing-youth-violence-an-overview-of-the-evidence
Mental Health Technology Transfer Center	https://mhttcnetwork.org/centers/global-mhttc/school-mental-health-resources
National Center for School Mental Health (NCSMH)	http://www.schoolmentalhealth.org
Center for Mental Health in Schools at UCLA	http://smhp.psych.ucla.edu
Education Policy Institute (UK)	https://epi.org.uk

COLLABORATION WITH FAMILY AND CAREGIVERS OF YOUTH

The family has an integral role when a young family member has been bullied, is at risk of being bullied, or has engaged in bullying behavior. Youth learn social skills and norms from the home environment. If that environment is dysfunctional, the youth may not have a good foundation to build on. Thus, occupational therapists may need to provide support and resources to the family when developing effective communication skills, coping skills, and support for the youth. Countless resources are available online; however, information that is concise, action-oriented, and practical is strongly suggested for use with parents. Many resources exist for occupational therapists to deliver to families to strengthen communication, enhance relationships, and build resilience in coping with bullying, trauma, and bystander victimization. A list of suggested resources is provided in Table 11-4.

The occupational therapist should consider the family dynamic and coping strategies of the individual or individuals responsible for providing care to the youth. Literacy of the care provider is an essential consideration, as this could be a challenge if the practitioner wishes to provide written or printed information (Grajo & Gutman, 2019). Occupational therapists are encouraged to be innovative and utilize a variety of resources to provide information, such as photos and video as well as printed media. Encouraging open communication, time aside from technology, and family-focused activity will assist youth in developing the resilience and adaptive capacity necessary to formulate and integrate coping strategies to address the occupational challenges present in a variety of environments. Because coping is a dynamic process, parents and caregivers need to be encouraged not to view a specific intervention or communication with youth as a singular event to address an isolated issue or episode (Compas et al., 2001). Development of effective coping strategies occurs when the youth is able to engage in both problem-focused coping to address environmental challenges (bullying and bystander victimization) and effective expression of the negative emotions that arise as a result of stress exposure. Parents and caregivers can offer youth support, develop activities and present challenges to promote the youth's development and demonstration of adaptive strategies and competence. Occupational therapy practitioners can assist parents and caregivers in gaining insight into success-assured activities, building appropriate challenges, and offering appropriate but not excessive support (excessive support is at times observed in those described as "helicopter parents," who constantly hover over the youth and allow no or very few failure experiences). Challenges are always present within the variety of environments in which youth find themselves, thus affording multiple opportunities to develop the ability to cope through adaptation to a variety of experiences.

Caregivers may be hesitant or uncertain about how to talk to young persons regarding their current challenges related to the behavior of others. Providing conversation starters (Substance Abuse and Mental Health Services Administration [SAMHSA], 2003) can be a helpful strategy. SAMHSA has created conversation starter cards specifically on bullying, as well as more generic conversation starters, via the program *Make Time to Listen, Take Time to Talk*. These cards can be easily printed from this website: https://store.samhsa.gov/sites/default/files/d7/priv/sma08-4321.pdf. Further conversation starters are available that vary depending on the age of the youth, from elementary age ("Which kids were there, what happened, what did you see, experience, what did they say to you?"), to tweens ("Who did you sit with at lunch today, how was the bus ride home, are there cliques at school, what do you think about the kids in the cliques, what do your teachers tell you about bullying in school?"). Occupational therapists can provide support and assistance to caregivers by providing strategies to begin the conversation about the youths and their concerns. Encourage active listening by caregivers, as this demonstrates to the youths that they are being heard, that the ideas they are sharing matter, and that the caregiver is concerned. If, based on conversations with the youth, caregivers recognize that the youth is being bullied, they are encouraged to be brief in their communications. Keep it simple, be positive, convey that you heard the youth's message and that the youth does not deserve to be bullied (no one does), and encourage the youth not to bully back. Youths' feeling that they are heard and supported fosters resilience within them; assists them in being able to discuss, develop, and collaborate with their parent/caregiver on strategies for responding to situations that they may encounter in the school or other environment where the parent/caregiver is not present. Occupational therapists can support parents/caregivers by providing information on programming that is occurring within the school or clinic environment to develop coping and adaptive behavior, so that parents/caregivers can continue to provide the same support, encouragement, and reinforcement outside of the school/clinic environment.

Occupational therapy practitioners are directed to consider the significant impact the family has upon the behavior, engagement, and mood of a young person. Ttofi and Farrington's (2011) systematic review found a decrease in bullying and victimization when parent training and meetings were conducted; these provided an opportunity for sensitization regarding school bullying. Further, these researchers suggested that professionals from various disciplines should collaborate regarding anti-bullying efforts so as to draw from the expertise of all. Findings indicated that disciplinary cooperation yielded significant reduction in bullying and victimization (Ttofi & Farrington, 2011). Because occupational therapists are well versed in activity analysis (foundation of the occupational therapy process; AOTA, 2020) and health education and literacy (Grajo & Gutman, 2019), our role in the multidisciplinary team is obvious. Occupational therapy practitioners have the opportunity to collaborate with teachers, school-support personnel, school-district leaders, and youth community workers to provide safe and supportive environments that appropriately challenge and foster growth in youth.

BUILDING INTERPROFESSIONAL COLLABORATIONS

Occupational therapy professionals are an integral part of intra-, inter-, and multidisciplinary teams that assist youth in developing adaptive behavior and foster the use of effective coping skills and resilience. As such, occupational therapy professionals need to educate themselves on strategies to foster collaboration and effective team dynamics to address the needs of the youth first and foremost. At times, professionals can become territorial over who has what role and responsibility. As professionals, occupational therapy practitioners should consider the unique skills they can bring to the educational environment to address bullying through fostering resilience in youth. Working collaboratively as a model for behavior can be a significant benefit to youth who view professionals interacting effectively.

A GLOBAL PERSPECTIVE

Unfortunately, bullying is not unique to youth within the United States. The 2020 annual bullying survey in the UK reported a 25% increase in bullying in the past 12 months, with one in four young people having been physically attacked and one in three having experienced bullying on online platforms (Ditch the Label, 2020). In another UK study, school-based occupational therapists (n = 28) were surveyed regarding bullying (D'Elia & Brooks, 2017); a high percentage of the occupational therapists surveyed (82.1%) did not address bullying, but 64.3% identified that occupational therapists could assume a role in the prevention of bullying. These practitioners stated that occupational therapy intervention could address barriers that interfere with occupational performance, social skills, and environmental impact. The study also reported that interventions can be most beneficial when they begin with the individual and then expand to the classroom and the entire school environment (D'Elia & Brooks, 2017). Similar to information presented in the United States, the UK and Norway have recognized the positive outcomes of the empirically supported Olweus Bullying Prevention Program (Dupper, 2013).

Occupational therapy practitioners are encouraged to build adaptive capacity through becoming involved in communities of practice with other therapists who are focused on examining, intervening in, and enhancing the mental health and well-being of youth

(Bazyk et al., 2015). Practitioners who participate in a community of practice are positively challenged and supported to critically examine how they engage in occupational therapy practice, represent the profession to youth and others, and make positive changes in clinical practice (Bazyk et al., 2015). Occupational therapists are encouraged to examine the significant contributions of their profession toward anti-bullying efforts, and to contribute to the continual development of the profession by highlighting the unique role of occupational therapy in addressing engagement in occupation from a strength-based perspective, as well as targeted services to at-risk youth (Arbesman et al., 2013).

The contributions of various disciplines are desired, according to the systematic review by Ttofi and Farrington (2011). Practitioners need to clearly articulate occupational therapy's contributions to the multidisciplinary team in clinical-practice settings that serve youth. The American Occupational Therapy Association has developed a wide variety of resources for practitioners to access within the School Mental Health Toolkit (AOTA, 2013a). Although occupational therapy practitioners work with youth in a variety of clinical and non-clinical settings (outpatient pediatric and youth clinics, community programs such as after-school programming, vocational programming, and the like), youth spend a significant percentage of their time involved in educational pursuits—specifically, school. Thus, occupational therapy practitioners who work with youth in school settings could assume leadership roles in school mental health initiatives. School mental health initiatives offer occupational therapy practitioners the opportunity to be actively involved in school-wide approaches that focus on prevention, positive youth development, and comprehensive approaches to foster mental health and wellness in youth (Every Moment Counts, 2016). Links to school mental health initiative resources are provided in Table 11-4.

ESSENTIAL CONSIDERATIONS FOR OCCUPATIONAL THERAPISTS

In work with children and youth, use a comprehensive approach in developing and building positive social-emotional skills, and employ evidence-based resources consistently. Be aware of materials that are available and support educators, families, and youth workers to address bullying behavior from a perspective of developing positive social-emotional behavior and empathy, rather than just addressing bullying when an incident occurs or a problem arises. Bullying can occur in any environment, specific resources consulted should be comprehensive in nature. Refer to governmental agencies such as the CDC or U.S. Department of Education for guidance; their websites are locations to secure timely and research-based information (CDC, 2020; StopBullying.gov, 2020). Understanding the plethora of research available on bullying, cyberbullying, child trauma, and prevention and intervention programs can be daunting. Evidence-based intervention programs such as OBPP and KiVa should be considered the "gold standard" due to the rigorous research evidence supporting the positive outcomes available from fidelity-based intervention. Although occupational therapy research specifically addressing bullying is somewhat limited, research regarding school mental health prevention

Case Study 11-3

Sam is a seventh-grade student at a suburban public school. Sam's family is of Middle Eastern descent and is new to the area. At his previous school, Sam got straight A grades, and was considered a well-adjusted student. Sam is beginning at his new school this fall because his parents moved to live closer to where they are employed. Sam is having a hard time making friends in this school; he has been noticed to have withdrawn from group activities that he previously was very excited about and interested in (i.e., LEGO club). Sam frequently appears easily frustrated in class and demonstrates difficulty adapting to the change in his school environment. In the area of coping, Sam refers to himself negatively when he cannot perform to meet his self-imposed expectations. He makes disparaging statements about himself, the move, and his new school. It has been noted that Sam does not engage with peers during lunch or when passing between classes; when teachers/staff approach him, his eyes are downcast and he rarely offers a verbal response. During passing period between classes, Sam often hears other students talking about him and making snide remarks about his appearance. Sam tries to block out the teasing, but he is struggling to adjust to his new school environment and the social behavior of his peers is considered bullying. Because of the bullying behavior, Sam's grades have fallen below average and he is earning Cs and Ds in most of his classes. When walking through the halls, other seventh-grade boys are becoming more physical with him: they push past him as if he were not even there. In addition, countless notes have been left on his locker with messages such as "go back to where you came from" and "we don't want you here."

In this case, clearly bullying has already been occurring. Sam's social studies teacher has contacted you (the occupational therapist) because you are already seeing a student in Sam's class for occupational therapy services. The teacher reaches out to you because you have utilized effective social-emotional learning activities as a part of your intervention with youth in their classroom. The teacher alerts you to the concerns regarding Sam. You review with the teacher the guidelines of the school and district regarding bullying and then notify the principal and school counselor.

You and Sam's teacher complete the Social Skills Improvement Survey (SSIS) to identify Sam's skills and strengths in the areas of cooperation, assertion, empathy, and self-control (Gresham & Elliott, 2008). The survey results will assist you in providing support to the teacher and provide insight into what resources you can provide to address the teacher's identified concerns for her student. Results from the teacher indicate that Sam is struggling to cope with the changes he has been confronted with, and he lacks the coping and communication skills necessary to meet the challenges confronting him.

As an occupational therapist, you serve as a consultant to the teacher to provide information on evidence-based interventions, which can be utilized with the entire class to address the bullying behavior of other students within the classroom. Because Sam is not on your caseload, you provide the teacher with support and resources she can utilize to assist Sam; you also follow up

(continued)

Case Study 11-3 (continued)

at weekly intervals to assess and support the teacher and provide additional resources and guidance as necessary. One resource you introduce the teacher to is "Calm Moment Cards" that she can use not only with Sam, but also other class members. These cards and other materials available from Every Moment Counts can be used as embedded strategies to benefit not only Sam, but also all students within the classroom and school environment (Every Moment Counts, 2016). As the occupational therapist, you decide to collaborate and implement lessons from the MindUP curriculum that would benefit all students and assist in the development of positive coping skills and resilience. Research has identified the outcomes of this program as yielding benefits in prosocial behavior, overall well-being, improved stress physiology, and increased school success. These were identified areas of concern for Sam and could also benefit many other students within the classroom (Maloney et al., 2016).

---

and intervention in which bullying is included and addressed is readily available (AOTA, 2013a; Arbesman et al., 2013; Bazyk et al., 2015; Every Moment Counts, 2016).

The type of behavior described in Case Study 11-3 can be disturbing to the occupational therapy practitioner. As a result, the practitioner can be motivated into advocacy and action, such as using the anti-bullying programs and resources described in this chapter to work with the school and possibly the entire school district on broad approaches to address the identified concern. Materials from the American Occupational Therapy Association (2013a) within the School Mental Health Toolkit, and all materials on the Every Moment Counts (2016) website, are exceptional resources.

Individual schools and districts may already have anti-bullying programs in place; however, if this behavior is continuing to be present in the school environment, something is awry. Research regarding effective and ineffective elements of bullying prevention efforts, as well as the involvement of occupational therapy through utilization of evidence-based school mental health interventions, can continue to validate the necessity of occupational therapy for addressing occupational challenges such as bullying present for youth.

Addressing the challenging and traumatic experiences that youth encounter may take an emotional toll on the occupational therapy practitioner. Practitioners are encouraged to identify components of compassion fatigue, vicarious trauma, and burnout; take steps to engage in regular professional self-care; and seek supervision to support professional and personal well-being. If an occupational therapist is unable to engage in or neglects professional self-care, the challenge of addressing the complex needs of youth who have experienced bullying or who are perpetrators of bullying could become overwhelming, and the occupational therapist may be tempted to focus narrowly on issues of motor skills, handwriting, and other performance skills or patterns. As the profession of occupational therapist is holistic and person-centered, the occupational therapy practitioner is directed to engage in regular self-care to address all identified needs observed and expressed by youth, parents, schools, and the community at large.

A quick-reference tip sheet for bullying resources appears in Table 11-5.

Table 11-5

Quick Reference Bullying Resources	
Resource	**URL**
Every Moment Counts—Comfortable Cafeteria, Refreshing Recess, Embedded Programs, Embedded Strategies, School Mental Health	www.everymomentcounts.org
Olweus Bully Prevention Program (OBPP)	http://www.violencepreventionworks.org/public/bullying.page
KiVa	http://www.kivaprogram.net
Victoria State Government Bullying, Cyberbullying, Racist Bullying Advice Sheets for Parents, Teachers and Students	https://www.education.vic.gov.au/about/programs/bullystoppers/Pages/default.aspx
NASEM Preventing Bullying through Science, Policy and Practice	http://nap.edu/23482
Stop Bullying.gov Specialized information addressing youth with disabilities, military connected youth, and LGBTQ	https://www.stopbullying.gov/bullying/what-is-bullying
Best Practices in Bullying Prevention and Intervention	https://www.cde.state.co.us/mtss/bullying/bestpractices
Parent Action Toolkit	https://rb.gy/wbcdd1

REFERENCES

American Occupational Therapy Association. (2013a). Bullying prevention and friendship promotion. https://www.aota.org/-/media/Corporate/Files/Practice/Children/SchoolMHToolkit/BullyingPreventionInfoSheet.pdf

American Occupational Therapy Association (2013b). How to use AOTA mental health information sheets. https://www.aota.org/-/media/Corporate/Files/Practice/Children/SchoolMHToolkit/How%20To%20Use%20Mental%20Health.PDF

American Occupational Therapy Association (2015). Salary and workforce survey executive summary. https://www.aota.org/-/media/Corporate/Files/Secure/Educations-Careers/Salary-Survey/2015-AOTA-Workforce-Salary-Survey-LOW-RES.pdf

American Occupational Therapy Association. (2020). Occupational therapy practice framework: Domain and process (4th ed.). *American Journal of Occupational Therapy, 74*(Suppl. 2), 7412410010. https://doi.org/10.5014/ajot.2020.74S2001

Arbesman, M., Bazyk, S., & Nochajski, S. M. (2013). Systematic review of occupational therapy and mental health promotion, prevention, and intervention for children and youth. *American Journal of Occupational Therapy, 67*(6), e120-e130. https://doi.org/10.5014/ajot.2013.008359

Bazyk, S., Demirjian, L., LaGuardia, T., Thompson-Repas, K., Conway, C., & Michaud, P. (2015). Building capacity of occupational therapy practitioners to address the mental health needs of children and youth: A mixed-methods study of knowledge translation. *American Journal of Occupational Therapy, 69*(6), 6906180060p1-6906180060p10. https://doi.org/10.5014/ajot.2015.019182

BullyPolice.org (2017). A watch-dog organization—Advocating for bullied children & reporting on state anti bullying laws. http://bullypolice.org

The Bully Project. (2020). *Bully* (film). http://www.thebullyproject.com

Byjos, O., Dusing, J., Zartman, C., & Cahill, S. M. (2016). Perspectives of individuals who experienced bullying during childhood. *The Open Journal of Occupational Therapy, 4*(4). https://doi.org/10.15453/2168-6408.1249

Centers for Disease Control and Prevention. (2020). Injury prevention and control: #StopBullying. https://www.cdc.gov/injury/features/stop-bullying/index.html

Compas, B. E., Connor-Smith, J. K., Saltzman, H., Thomsen, A., & Wadsworth, M. E. (2001). Coping with stress during childhood and adolescence: Problems, progress, and potential in theory and research. *Psychological Bulletin, 127*(1), 87-127. https://doi.org/10.1037//0033-2909.127.1.87

D'Elia, M., & Brooks, R. (2017). Bullying prevention: A survey of school-based occupational therapists. *Children, Young People and Families Occupational Therapy Journal* (Autumn), 12-18. https://www.researchgate.net/publication/321168052_Bullying_Prevention_A_Survey_of_School-based_Occupational_Therapists

Ditch the Label. (2020). *The annual bullying survey 2020.* https://www.ditchthelabel.org/wp-content/uploads/2020/11/The-Annual-Bullying-Survey-2020-2.pdf

Dupper, D. R. (2013). *School bullying: New perspectives on a growing problem.* Oxford University Press.

Every Moment Counts. (2016). Calm moment cards. https://everymomentcounts.org/view.php?nav_id=227

Gaete, J., Valenzuela, D., Rojas-Barahona, C., Valenzuela, E., Araya, R., & Salmivalli, C. (2017). The KiVa antibullying program in primary schools in Chile, with and without the digital game component: Study protocol for a randomized controlled trial. *Trials, 18*(1), 75. https://doi.org/10.1186/s13063-017-1810-1

Gladden, R. M., Vivolo-Kantor, A. M., Hamburger, M. E., & Lumpkin, C. D. (2014). *Bullying surveillance among youths: Uniform definitions for public health and recommended data elements, version 1.0.* National Center for Injury Prevention and Control, Centers for Disease Control and Prevention and U.S. Department of Education.https://www.cdc.gov/violenceprevention/pdf/Bullying-Definitions-FINAL-a.pdf

Grajo, L. C., & Gutman, S. A. (2019). The role of occupational therapy in functional literacy. *The Open Journal of Occupational Therapy, 7*(1). https://doi.org/10.15453/2168-6408.1511

Gresham, F., & Elliott, S. N. (2008). Social skills improvement system: SSIS rating scales. https://www.pearsonassessments.com/store/usassessments/en/Store/Professional-Assessments/Behavior/Social-Skills-Improvement-System-SSIS-Rating-Scales/p/100000322.html?tab=product-details

Gueldner, B. A., & Feuerborn, L. L. (2016). Integrating mindfulness-based practices into social and emotional learning: A case application. *Mindfulness, 7,* 164-175. https://doi.org/10.1007/s12671-015-0423-6

Hamburger, M. E., Basile, K. C., & Vivolo, A. M. (2011). *Measuring bullying victimization, perpetration, and bystander experiences: A compendium of assessment tools.* Centers for Disease Control and Prevention, National Center for Injury Prevention and Control. https://www.cdc.gov/violenceprevention/pdf/bullycompendium-a.pdf

Juvonen, J., Schacter, H. L., Sainio, M., & Salmivalli, C. (2016). Can a school-wide bullying prevention program improve the plight of victims? Evidence for risk × intervention effects. *Journal of Consulting and Clinical Psychology, 84*(4), 334-344. https://doi.org/10.1037/ccp0000078

KiVa School. (2020). Welcome to KiVa school. http://www.kivaprogram.net

Maloney, J. E., Lawlor, M. S., Schonert-Reichl, K. A., & Whitehead, J. (2016). A mindfulness-based social and emotional learning curriculum for school-aged children: The MindUP Program. In K. Schonert-Reichl & R.W. Roeser (Eds.), *Handbook of mindfulness in education, mindfulness in behavioral health* (pp. 313-334). https://doi.org/10.1007/978-1-4939-3506-2_20

National Academies of Sciences, Engineering, and Medicine. (2016). Preventing bullying through science, policy, and practice. The National Academies Press. https://doi.org/10.17226/23482

Pereira, R. (2010). What are occupational therapists doing about bullying? *British Journal of Occupational Therapy, 73*(2), 47. https://doi.org/10.4276/030802210X12658062793681

The Royal Children's Hospital Melbourne. (2012). Developing resilience and dealing with bullying fact sheet. https://www.rch.org.au/uploadedFiles/Main/Content/transition/Developing_Resilience.pdf

StopBullying.gov. (2019a). *What is bullying.* https://www.stopbullying.gov/bullying/what-is-bullying

Stop Bullying.gov. (2019b). Understanding the roles of health and safety professionals in community-wide bullying prevention efforts. https://www.stopbullying.gov/sites/default/files/2017-09/hrsa_guide_health-and-safety-professionals_508v2.pdf

StopBullying.gov. (2020). *Research resources.* https://www.stopbullying.gov/resources/research-resources

Substance Abuse and Mental Health Services Administration. (2003). Make time to listen, take time to talk conversation starter cards. https://store.samhsa.gov/sites/default/files/d7/priv/sma08-4321.pdf

Ttofi, M. M., & Farrington, D. P. (2011). Effectiveness of school-based programs to reduce bullying: A systematic and meta-analytic review. *Journal of Experimental Criminology, 7*, 27-56. https://doi.org/10.1007/s11292-010-9109-1

U.S. Department of Education. (2019). Student reports of bullying: Results from the 2017 School Crime Supplement (SCS) to the National Crime Victimization Survey. https://nces.ed.gov/pubs2019/2019054.pdf

Walters, G. D. (2020). School-age bullying victimization and perpetration: A meta-analysis of prospective studies and research. *Trauma, Violence and Abuse,* 1-11, https://doi.org/10.1177/1524838020906513

12

LGBTQ and Gender Expansive Children and Youth

Karrie L. Kingsley, OTD, OTR/L

CHAPTER OBJECTIVES By the end of this chapter, the reader will be able to:
- Differentiate between sexual orientation, sex assigned at birth, gender identity, gender expression, and gender attribution.
- Summarize the impact of societal, school, familial, and individual factors on the health, well-being, and occupational participation of LGBTQ and gender expansive youth.
- Evaluate clinical environments and clinical reasoning practices in terms of inclusivity and best practices supporting coping, adaptation, and resilience in LGBTQ and gender expansive children and youth.
- Modify clinical environments and reasoning to incorporate best practices supporting the coping, adaptation, and resilience of LGBTQ and gender expansive youth

OVERVIEW OF LGBTQ AND GENDER EXPANSIVE CHILDREN AND YOUTH

Many identities are captured by the acronym *LGBTQ* and the term *gender expansive* (GE). Most typically, the acronym LGBTQ is thought of as standing for lesbian, gay, bisexual, transgender, and queer (although the "Q" is sometimes used for questioning). It is important to think of each of these identities as spectrums of experiences and expressions of identities. It is also important to recognize that the acronym itself is often used

Grajo L. C., & Boisselle, A. K. (Eds.). *Adaptation, Coping, and Resilience in Children and Youth: A Comprehensive Occupational Therapy Approach* (pp. 289-312). © 2022 Taylor & Francis Group.

by and applied to individuals who represent a variety of non-heterosexual and gender non-conforming ways. Often sub-identifiers are used within these communities to further refine and explicate one's identity. *Gender expansive* is an umbrella term that may be seen in the literature as gender variant. The term *gender expansive* has a less negative connotation than gender variant and it captures all identities that are non-cisgender (see definition in the next sections). In the research literature, LGBTQ and GE youth are sometimes referred to as sexual and gender minority youth. Language in these communities is constantly evolving. It is important to periodically revisit and update language and understanding.

Sexual Orientation

Sexual orientation describes an individual's romantic, physical, or sexual attraction toward another individual. Sexual orientations include identities such as gay, lesbian, bisexual, pansexual, and asexual. *Gay* refers to men (including trans and cis men) experiencing attraction toward men. *Lesbian* refers to women (including trans and cis women) who experience attraction toward women. *Bisexual* refers to a person who experiences attraction toward individuals belonging to two different gender identities. *Pansexual* refers to someone attracted to all genders. Finally, *asexual* refers to someone who does not experience sexual attraction. Sexual orientation is not the same as gender identity, and gender presentation does not correspond to particular sexual orientations.

Sex Versus Gender

It is important to recognize the difference and correctly differentiate between the terms *sex* and *gender*. *Sex* is assigned to an individual at birth or prior to birth by medical doctors. Typically, doctors assign female, male, or intersex as an infant's sex. Sex assigned to an individual refers to chromosomes, external genitalia, reproductive organs, and hormone profiles (National Institutes of Health [NIH], 2019). Sex assigned may or may not align with a person's gender identity. *Gender* refers to socially constructed and enacted roles and behaviors that occur in a historical and cultural context and vary across societies and over time (NIH, 2019).

Gender Identity

Gender identity is a person's inner understanding of their gender. To oversimplify, gender identity is how one personally thinks of oneself—as feminine, masculine, both, or neither. An individual's gender identity may or may not match their sex assigned at birth or their gender expression. When a person's gender identity and sex assigned at birth do not match, the person may use one of a variety of terms that best describe their experience, including *transgender, trans, gender fluid, non-binary, genderqueer, agender, bigender*, or *gender non-conforming*. When someone's gender identity and sex assigned at birth match, the person is *cisgender*.

Gender Expression

Gender expression is how an individual chooses to outwardly present their gender. This may include things like behavior, clothing, haircut, make-up, and voice. An individual's gender expression may or may not align with society's concepts of masculine or feminine, the individual's sex assigned at birth, or the individual's gender identity.

Gender Attribution

Gender attribution is the assignment of a gender label to another person. Often we attribute gender to an individual based on our perception of their sex assigned at birth or their gender presentation. When the attribution of one's gender by others conflicts with one's gender identity, this is called *misgendering*. Being misgendered causes distress and is harmful to a youth's well-being (Pollitt et al., 2019). At its worst, misgendering is intentional and, therefore, poses a safety risk for gender expansive and particularly trans youth who experience higher rates of victimization and bullying (Baum et al., n.d.).

Queer

Historically, the term *queer* was a term of oppression used to marginalize individuals who identified as sexual and gender minorities. However, the term is re-appropriated language for the LGBTQ and GE communities. It is used as an umbrella term applied to those who do not align with heterosexual and cisgender expectations of society. Many youth today use the term to label their identity, and it may refer to their gender identity, sexual orientation, or both.

BIPOC

The acronym *BIPOC* stands for Black, Indigenous, and People (or Persons) of Color. Many cultural communities reject the Eurocentric language used in the LGBTQ umbrella. It is important when working with BIPOC communities to learn the terms they use to identify gender identities and sexual orientations—while recognizing that not all languages offer translations. Among North American Indigenous communities, *Two Spirit* is an umbrella term that may refer to gender identity, gender expression, sexual orientation, or a spiritual identity. In Black and African American communities, the term *same gender loving* may be utilized to indicate a non-heterosexual orientation.

Prevalence of LGBTQ and Gender Expansive Identities

Thirty percent of 18- to 24-year-old respondents to the 2017 Gallup poll were LGBT, compared to 8% of adults 65 and older (The Williams Institute, 2019). The Centers for Disease Control (CDC) Youth Risk Behavior Surveillance report found that

14.6% of youth surveyed in grades 9 to 12 are non-heterosexual (Kahn et al., 2018). In California, 27% of youth aged 12 to 17 are gender non-conforming (Wilson et al., 2017). A national survey reported that 12% of youth aged 14 to 18 identify as gender expansive (Gill & Frazer, 2016). Many surveys are defining terms differently; therefore, it is difficult to identify stable statistical estimations of the number of gender expansive children and youth.

Being LGBTQ or GE is not a medical diagnosis or condition and, therefore, clients will not be referred to occupational therapists specifically because of these identities. Occupational therapists working in acute and rehabilitation hospital settings, school districts, community-based clinics, outpatient clinics, juvenile justice, and mental health settings will encounter clients who are LGBTQ or gender expansive. There are no specific occupational therapy interventions designed for these communities or identities. However, there are best practices that have been shown to foster coping, resilience, and adaptation in LGBTQ and GE youth.

BARRIERS TO ADAPTATION, COPING, AND RESILIENCE: CHALLENGES FACED BY LGBTQ AND GENDER EXPANSIVE YOUTH

The number of challenges LGBTQ and GE youth face is daunting. There are challenges at the societal, school, family, and individual levels. At the societal level, LGBTQ and GE youth face systemic discrimination and oppression contributing to health disparities, homelessness, and incarceration (Abramovich, 2016; Dank et al., 2015). At the school level, LGBTQ and GE youth experience more bullying, violence, and exclusionary discipline, and have poorer educational outcomes, than their cisgender counterparts (Baum et al., n.d.; Kahn et al., 2018). At the family level, LGBTQ and GE youth are more likely to experience family rejection, violence, and subsequent home removal because of their identities (Tobin et al., 2018). Individually, as a result of their exposure to stigma, discrimination and violence, LGBTQ and GE youth are more likely to experience health disparities and mental health problems, and are at higher risk for completing suicide (Johns et al., 2019; Kahn et al., 2018).

Homelessness and Incarceration

Currently, up to 40% of unaccompanied homeless youth are LGBTQ nationally, with higher numbers in major cities (Choi et al., 2015). Often several factors intersect, such as family rejection, abuse, and lack of adequate social services, leading to LGBTQ and GE youth experiencing homelessness (Abramovich, 2016). Transgender youth of color are disproportionately represented in the homeless youth population and are more likely to experience intersecting and complex forms of systemic discrimination and oppression such as racism, transphobia, and homophobia (Abramovich, 2016).

Homelessness is associated with higher risk of depression, post-traumatic stress disorder (PTSD), sex trafficking, physical and sexual assault, substance use, crimes of survival, and incarceration for LGBTQ and GE youth (Kelly & Ratliff, 2017). LGBTQ homeless individuals report higher rates of profiling, false arrest, and abusive police encounters than non-LGBTQ individuals experiencing homelessness (Dank et al., 2015).

Several factors contribute to LGBTQ and GE youths' having a higher likelihood of interaction with the justice system, including higher experiences of violence, homelessness, and family disruption (Dank et al., 2015). LGBTQ and GE youth are overrepresented in the juvenile justice system. Several studies examining the number of LGBTQ and GE identified youth incarcerated in the United States have found ranges of at least twice the representation than in the general youth population, with more severe disproportionality in girls (Wilson et al., 2017). For example, authors found that 40% of girls in pretrial detention in New York were lesbian, bisexual, or gay (Irvine & Canfield, 2016).

School Environments

LGBTQ and GE youth face harsher school environments than their non-LGBTQ and GE peers. As students, youth hear the majority of negative messaging regarding LGBTQ and GE identities at school (Baum et al., n.d.). LGBTQ and GE youth who are victimized at school have poorer educational outcomes and mental health (Kosciw et al., 2018). During the 2017 school year, 60% of LGBTQ students reported feeling unsafe, 70% experienced verbal harassment, 57% were sexually harassed, 29% were physically harassed, and 12% were physically assaulted because of their orientation or gender expression (Kosciw et al., 2018). Additionally, there are many reports of unfair and discriminatory use of discipline by schools that targeted LGBTQ and GE youth, such as differential enforcement of dress codes, rules about public displays of affection, and the lack of access to restrooms that reflect students' gender expression and identity (Abramovich, 2016; Kosciw et al., 2018). For youth with intersecting identities (e.g., both LGBTQ and a racial or ethnic minority), there is a higher prevalence of exclusionary school discipline such as suspension and expulsion (Kosciw et al., 2018).

Family

Many LGBTQ and GE youth experience family rejection, violence, and removal from their parents' care. Youth who were gender non-conforming by 11 years of age are at the highest risk for sexual, physical, and psychological abuse by their parents (Tobin et al., 2018). Although they may enter the system for a variety of reasons, LGBTQ and GE youth are disproportionately represented in foster care. In studies examining the foster youth population in Los Angeles, authors found that 19% were LGBTQ (Wilson et al., 2014) and 5.6% were transgender (Wilson & Kastanis, 2015). Once in the foster system, LGBTQ and GE youth experience more change in placements due to foster family rejection of their identities, more violence secondary to their identity, and are more likely to be placed in group homes (Wilson et al., 2014).

Mental Health Challenges

First, it is important to recognize that mental health challenges are not inherent to LGBTQ and GE identities. Rather, they are often a byproduct of stigma, discrimination, and negative experiences otherwise known as *minority stressors*. Minority stress theory proposes that individuals from marginalized communities are subjected to chronic and unique stressors related to their identity, which over time adversely affects mental health (McManama O'Brien et al., 2016). Minority stress theory is commonly applied to better understand the mechanisms of anxiety, depression, and suicidality in LGBTQ and GE youth. Mental health support is critical for LGBTQ and GE youth, as they are four times more likely to attempt suicide than heterosexual and cisgender youth (Kahn et al., 2018). A 2018 study examined the relationship of sexual-minority youth, a thwarted sense of belonging, a sense of being a burden to others, and mental health. The authors found that youth with a higher sense of perceived burden and higher minority stress had higher depressive symptoms (Baams et al., 2018). The pervasiveness of minority stress during childhood and adolescence is as impactful as adverse childhood events and may have lasting impacts on the development of LGBTQ and GE youth (Tobin et al., 2018). There is a general lack of research differentiating identities, but professionals should consider that the experiences of gender expansive children and youth are very different from those of LGBTQ children and youth. In a study surveying transgender and gender nonconforming youth, 59% reported long-standing mental health problems as compared to 17% of cisgender youth (Rider et al., 2020).

Impact on Occupational Participation

Given the challenges these youth face, it is not surprising that there would be documented adverse impacts on occupational participation and access. Students who identify as LGBTQ (including GE youth) without supportive school environments are more likely to have skipped school because of perceived lack of safety, to have lower grade-point averages, and to drop out of high school, and are less likely to pursue higher education (Kosciw et al., 2018). About 70% to 75% of LGBTQ youth surveyed report avoiding school functions and extracurricular activities, citing lack of safety and feeling uncomfortable (Kosciw et al., 2018). More than 50% of GE youth report never participating in organized sports, church communities, LGB organizations, and other service organizations (e.g., Scouts of America; Baum et al., n.d.). The lack of participation is directly related to feeling a thwarted sense of belonging, lack of safety, and a lack of supportive adults and environments (Baams et al., 2018; Kulick et al., 2019). For GE youth, the need for safe access to bathrooms (Figure 12-1) and locker rooms, combined with a lack of gender-neutral bathrooms and locker rooms, presents an additional barrier to participation in sports and school extracurricular programs (Kulick et al., 2019).

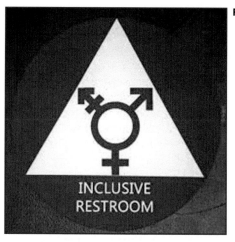

Figure 12-1. Inclusive restroom sign.

Another area with a huge impact on participation is health care. Many LGBTQ and GE children and youth report negative encounters with health care providers, and adolescents in particular may frequently change providers or avoid routine care rather than address conflicts (Tobin et al., 2018). Additionally, transgender and gender nonconforming youth rated their health as poorer and reported fewer visits to the doctor and dentist than their cisgender peers (Rider et al., 2020). These disparities are established early and are further experienced in adulthood: LGBTQ adults report that negative care experiences with providers lead to their avoiding important screenings such as prostate, breast, and pelvic exams, resulting in increased prevalence and cancer mortality (Lambda Legal, 2010).

There are many ways LGBTQ and GE youth are able to participate in occupations, but many are not accessing the same occupations as their cisgender and heterosexual peers. Barriers such as homophobia and transphobia contribute to LGBTQ and GE youth not feeling like they belong and feeling unsafe. As occupational therapists, we are keenly aware of the value of occupation and should be concerned about the impacts of occupational deprivation on the health and well-being of LGBTQ and GE youth. While occupational therapy best practices for LGBTQ and GE youth are nonexistent, there are many identified best practices supporting resilience, adaptation, and coping for these youth from a variety of key professions, including social work, nursing, and medicine. Case Study 12-1 illustrates the occupational impacts of a child identifying as transgender.

> ## Case Study 12-1
> ## Xander
>
> Xander is an 8-year-old transgender boy referred to an outpatient pediatric mental health clinic with diagnoses of post-traumatic stress disorder, anxiety, and depression. The state Department of Family Services removed Xander from his parental home 6 months ago after he was brought to the emergency department with injuries consistent with a severe beating. In sessions with his psychologist, Xander revealed there was a pattern of physical punishment for not conforming to expected female behaviors in his biological parental home. Xander's foster parents are supportive of his gender identity and social transition. Two months ago, Xander received his first gender-affirming haircut, changed his name to Xander, began dressing in masculine clothing, and began using he/him/his pronouns. Since his social transition, his foster parents report a decrease in self-harm behaviors and depression, stating that "when he saw himself in the mirror after getting his haircut, his smile was huge. It was the first time we saw him genuinely smile." His foster parents are concerned with Xander's disrupted sleep, periods of withdrawal, and behavioral meltdowns. Xander experiences increased anxiety around new or unfamiliar environments, which reduces his comfort in trying new activities. He wants to play Little League baseball, but has a meltdown when his foster parents talk about signing up. When extended family visits, Xander withdraws to his room and will have more disrupted sleep for the duration of their visit. Xander is independent with eating, dressing, bathing, and most grooming tasks. He has been asking for assistance with styling his hair from his foster parents since his recent haircut. Xander has a 504 plan in place at school to accommodate for his anxiety.

BEST PRACTICES IN ADDRESSING ADAPTATION, COPING, AND RESILIENCE FOR LGBTQ AND GENDER EXPANSIVE YOUTH

In recognition of the systemic issues of stigma, discrimination, and oppression impacting LGBTQ and GE youth, there are suggested best practices to support these communities at the individual and environmental/societal levels. Practices to support LGBTQ and GE youth include a variety of programs and interventions that range from supporting gender transition of the youth to tackling school climate and discipline. When supporting coping in LGBTQ and GE youth, it is important to help them develop adaptive coping skills, including help seeking, joining community, and navigating their safety across environments (Asakura, 2016; Colvin et al., 2019; Johns et al., 2019). Adaptation for these youth include gender transition and locating "chosen" family in the face of family rejection (Fredriksen-Goldsen et al., 2014). Facilitating resilience includes asserting one's agency, self-acceptance, outness/being out, transition, and activism including Gay Straight Alliances (GSAs; Asakura, 2016; Johns et al., 2019). Protective factors for LGBTQ and GE youth include supportive families, educators, and peers; adult role models; and inclusive schools and communities; these are critical in offsetting the impact of discrimination and stigma (Johns et al., 2019). There are best practices for trans and GE identified youth that are distinct from those for cisgender lesbian, gay, and bisexual youth. For transgender and GE youth, accepting educators, school staff, and trans role models all serve as protective factors (Johns et al., 2018). It is important to recognize that although trans and GE youth are often included in studies, when data are disaggregated, they are revealed to experience significant differences in prevalence of violence, barriers in contexts, mental health, and health disparities.

Gender-Affirming Care

The American Academy of Pediatrics recommends that professionals use gender-affirming practices (Rafferty, 2018). Best practice for trans and GE youth is to treat any gender dysphoria. *Gender dysphoria* is the emotional response to the dissonance between one's sex assigned at birth and gender identity, and, in its most severe presentation, can lead to self-harm in young children (Durwood et al., 2017). The treatment for gender dysphoria includes *gender transition,* a process in which an individual may change aspects of their gender expression to better align with their gender identity. The transition may be social or medical. In a social transition, an individual makes changes to their gender expression via names, pronouns, clothing, haircut, and behavior, and lives as their true gender. Current best medical practices include suppressing puberty at onset for trans and GE youth, to allow the youth time to explore their gender identity and should they decide to do so, begin gender-affirming hormone treatment at 16 years of age (Levine & the Committee on Adolescence, 2013). Timely and responsive care for transgender youth can be the key to offsetting negative mental health impacts and risk behaviors and is necessary for them to achieve health and wellness (Olson-Kennedy, 2016).

Gender-affirming practices further include validating the youth's gender identity by normalizing variations in gender identity as part of human diversity and destigmatizing by acknowledging that GE and trans identities are not mental health disorders, and that any associated anxiety and depression are related to societal stigma and negative experience (Rafferty, 2018). Children whose gender identity is affirmed (Figure 12-2) demonstrate positive mental health, and prepubescent children who socially transition show depression levels commensurate with those of their cisgender peers (Durwood et al., 2017; Olson-Kennedy, 2016).

Acceptance

One of the most powerful protective factors for LGBTQ and GE youth is the acceptance and support of their identities. Supportive family, educators, and peers are key to these youth developing resilience (Johns et al., 2019). Parental acceptance mitigates suicide in LGB and trans youth and promotes positive mental health in trans youth

Figure 12-2. Gender expansive toddler.

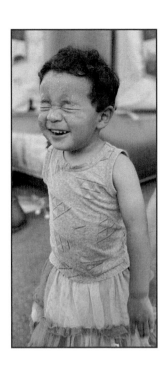

(Asakura, 2016). Professionals who provide accepting and affirming care are reducing the risks of depression and suicidal ideation (Hunt et al., 2018). For trans and GE youth, acceptance includes using names and pronouns best reflecting their identity. Research has shown that the use of one's chosen name across home, school, and work environments can positively affect mental health. For youth using their chosen name at home and work, there was a decrease in depressive symptoms, less negative suicidal ideation, and improved self-esteem (Pollitt et al., 2019).

School Climate and Inclusivity

All children and youth benefit from fair and inclusive policies at school. From the school-to-prison pipeline to the individual student's mental health, attendance, and safety, school policies can make or break outcomes for LGBTQ and GE youth. School connectedness, fair and inclusive policies regarding gender norms and public displays of affection, and access to bathrooms that reflect a student's gender identity, all contribute to reducing the suicide risk for LGBTQ and GE youth (Colvin et al., 2019). Schools with anti-bullying programs and inclusive curricula with LGBTQ and GE representation act as protective factors for LGBTQ and GE youth (Asakura, 2016; Johns et al., 2019). School environments have the potential to provide protective factors to facilitate adaptation and resilience in LGBTQ and GE youth.

Gay and Straight Alliances

One of the features of inclusive school environments is the presence of a gay and straight alliance (GSA). GSAs are student-run clubs focusing on support, advocacy, and climate for LGBTQ students and their allies. There are three types of GSAs: social, support, and activist; each GSA is encouraged to establish its own mission and goals based on needs of its specific school (GSA Network, n.d.). Support and socialization from their GSA was shown to increase LGBTQ youth's sense of agency more significantly than family support and to promote a positive LGBT school climate (Poteat et al., 2016). Based on research, it appears that GSAs benefit LGBT and GE youth more than straight allies who also participate, and may not be as beneficial for LGBTQ and GE youth of color (Poteat et al., 2016). GSAs were found to reduce suicide risk for LGB students but not trans or GE youth, and to reduce bullying of LGBT students (Asakura, 2016). In their systematic review, authors found that GSAs were associated with trans youth reporting higher levels of self-advocacy, less absenteeism, and a more positive school climate (Johns et al., 2018). GSAs are nationally recognized as important programs in educational environments, acting as protective opportunities that support resilience in LGBTQ and GE youth.

Trauma-Informed Care

Much of the research and literature about LGBTQ and GE youth focuses on adverse experiences and risks associated with these identities. Use of a trauma-informed care approach is needed to move the conversation from risk to resilience (McCormick et al., 2018). It is important for providers to expand their knowledge and training to achieve a trauma-informed approach tailored to the unique needs of LGBTQ and GE youth.

Safety, connections, and emotional regulation are the three core priorities when addressing complex trauma (Kelly & Ratliff, 2017). To prioritize safety, it is important to design spaces and environments that communicate to LGBTQ and GE youth that they will be protected physically, psychologically, and emotionally (Kelly & Ratliff, 2017). Specific strategies facilitating safety include nondiscrimination policies inclusive of sexual orientation, gender identity, and gender expression and zero tolerance policies for homophobia, biphobia, and transphobia (Kelly & Ratliff, 2017; McCormick et al., 2018). Further, it is important to signal your inclusiveness of LGBTQ and GE youth in the environment through signs, symbols, banners, and books, because these youth engage in additional assessments of the environment looking for signs that they will be safe (McCormick et al., 2018). Expanding connections and support may be accomplished by honoring names, pronouns, and identities during your interactions; referring LGBTQ and GE youth to GSAs at their schools, and collaborating with supporting teachers, parents, peers, and caregivers (Kelly & Ratliff, 2017; McCormick et al., 2018). Supporting emotional regulation includes addressing environmental stressors, addressing high levels of arousal preceding emotional deregulation, and intentionally responding to outbursts by validating the trigger and the emotions related to it (Kelly & Ratliff, 2017; McCormick et al., 2018).

Specific Needs of LGBTQ and Gender Expansive Youth

For LGBTQ and GE youth, the path to resilience comes with additional barriers requiring them to adapt and cope in hostile social climates. Coming out is a developmental milestone that, while it reflects a youth's sense of self and resilience, comes with a price. Outness in LGBTQ and GE youth was found to relate to higher victimization, higher self-esteem, and lower depression (Kosciw et al., 2015). LGBTQ and GE youth have to learn to navigate a variety of environments while maintaining their safety (Asakura, 2016). For some youth, this may include remaining "in the closet" by not disclosing an identity or changing their expressed behavior when faced with an unsafe environment. Other youth may not have this privilege, because the very nature of their appearance places them at risk. In addition to navigating their safety and being out, youth who assert their agency can find and develop relationships with LGBTQ and GE peers or adults, feel safe and included, and seek positive change for themselves and others, thereby demonstrating their resilience (Asakura, 2016; Johns et al., 2019).

THE ROLE OF OCCUPATIONAL THERAPY: PRACTICES TO MEET THE NEEDS OF LGBTQ AND GENDER EXPANSIVE YOUTH

To meet the needs of their LGBTQ and GE clients, occupational therapy professionals can make some adjustments to their current practices. Changes must be made at the therapist/individual, clinical environment, and professional levels.

What Occupational Therapists Should Do

As individuals, occupational therapy professionals can learn about, support, validate, and affirm LGBTQ and GE identities. Importantly, occupational therapy professionals should stop assuming that all children and youth are heterosexual and cisgender. The use of a trauma-informed approach is strongly recommended.

1. **Use inclusive language.** According to the American Academy of Pediatrics, providers should learn inclusive language and validate identities as part of normal human sexuality and gender expression (Kelly & Ratliff, 2017). This includes using the names and the gender pronouns clients choose to reflect their gender identity. Using a youth's chosen name and gender-affirming pronouns mitigates suicide risk (Pollitt et al., 2019). There is a large number of gender pronouns from which an individual may select; however, the most commonly used pronouns are *they, she,* or *he*. Using novel pronouns requires practice. It is acceptable to make mistakes, but in order to maintain rapport it is imperative that occupational therapists acknowledge their mistakes by apologizing quickly, correcting the mistake, and moving on. When encountering an unfamiliar gender identity or orientation, it is the occupational therapy professional's responsibility to educate themselves (see Table 12-3).

2. **Protect your LGBTQ and GE clients' rights to confidentiality.** Occupational therapists may encounter complicated scenarios when their clients are "out" in some spaces but not in others. It is important that occupational therapists have a conversation with clients about how they would like to have their identities honored in therapy sessions and how that might differ across interactions with caregivers, family members, peers, and teachers. It is not acceptable to disclose a client's LGBTQ or GE identity to anyone else without explicit permission, and doing so can lead to direct harm to your client. Make sure to check with the client about who will read documentation and if any requirements for reimbursement will contradict the client's identity in documentation. For example, even if a child has socially transitioned, their insurance company may require the documentation to reflect the client's sex assigned at birth; or a high school student may not be out to their family and, therefore, Individualized Education Plan (IEP) documentation may not reflect the youth's gender identity or chosen name.

3. **Be inclusive within the occupational therapy process.** There are specific strategies occupational therapists can utilize during the evaluation process to be more inclusive. When working with GE youth, it would be best to select standardized assessment tools that offer mixed gender norms or non-gendered norms. Be mindful about cover pages of scoring sheets, which often have "male" or "female" as the only gender identifiers. When clients disclose a LGBTQ or GE identity and your evaluation includes activities of daily living, ask additional open-ended questions regarding dressing, grooming, and hygiene routines, as there may be additional garments and routines supporting gender expression and sexual health.

4. **Tailor interventions to be trauma informed.** To be trauma-informed and responsive interventionists with LGBTQ and GE youth, occupational therapists should address safety, connections, and emotional regulation in their treatment plans. Facilitating LGBTQ and GE youths' safety includes incorporating inclusive practices to ensure that LGBTQ and GE clients feel safe interacting with their provider and safe in the clinical care environment, and advocating for change when there are identified barriers to youth safety. Facilitating connections includes identifying safe adults, peers, and programs where LGBTQ and GE youth and their families can find support, affirmation, and access to safe educational and health care opportunities. LGBTQ and GE may need to be taught how to seek help after identifying safe adults and peers.

The final principle to address is emotional regulation. There is scant evidence in the occupational therapy literature regarding the use of trauma-informed interventions for children and youth. However, occupational therapy professionals working with children and youth can find many intervention approaches that can be reframed to address self-regulation and emotional regulation for LGBTQ and GE youth. Traditionally, when addressing self-regulation or emotional regulation through direct intervention, occupational therapists utilize sensory or cognitive approaches. Using a sensory approach to support self-regulation and emotional regulation from a trauma-responsive perspective may involve providing strategies to downregulate an over-alerted nervous system. A qualitative study, surveying adults during an inpatient psychiatric stay, found that patients exclusively reported using a sensory room for downregulation to support their emotional regulation (Barbic et al., 2019). In their systematic review, authors found strong evidence for the use of Qigong massage with children to improve emotional regulation (Bodison & Parham, 2018). When working with a population who has experienced complex trauma, occupational therapists should work with clients, families, and care teams to determine if a touch-based sensory strategy is appropriate. Yoga is another sensory-based intervention used by occupational therapists to address self-regulation. Children aged 5 to 12, who participated in The Get Ready to Learn yoga program, showed statistically significant improvement in overall behavior and specifically a reduction in irritable behaviors postintervention compared to controls (Koenig et al., 2012). Another study found a statistically significant increase in emotional regulation in high school students who participated in a yoga class postintervention, as compared to their peers who participated in traditional physical education (Daly et al., 2015). Although literature is scant, the use of practice-based evidence in identifying specific sensory strategies to support self-regulation and emotional regulation with clear data collection may also be utilized when supporting the emotional regulation of LGBTQ and GE youth.

Several cognitive approaches have evidence supporting outcomes related to self-regulation and emotional regulation. There is strong evidence supporting use of the Alert Program® with children aged 6 to 12 years diagnosed with fetal alcohol spectrum disorder. Children demonstrated statistically significant improvements in executive functioning and emotional problem solving compared to controls (Wells et al., 2012); increased gray matter in the frontal lobe with associated improvements in emotional and inhibitory control compared to controls (Soh et al., 2015); and improved inhibitory control, social cognition, parent-reported behavior and emotional regulation, and a reduction in externalized behaviors compared to controls (Nash et al., 2015). Mindfulness has a wealth of evidence supporting its use in early childhood and school settings. The use of a mindfulness intervention with at-risk preschool populations yielded statistically significant improvements in attention, behavior, social-emotional development, self-regulation, and behavioral control (Flook et al., 2015; Lemberger-Truelove et al., 2018; Moreno-Gómez & Cejudo, 2018). When using a mindfulness intervention with 9- to 12-year-olds, authors found large-effect sizes with a reduction in anxiety postintervention (Malboeuf-Hurtubise et al., 2017). Other programs of intervention and cognitive approaches that are available to occupational therapists have variable levels of evidence. Once again, the use of practice-based evidence may serve occupational therapy providers on a case-by-case basis when using cognitive approaches with LGBTQ and GE expansive youth to address emotional regulation and self-regulation. Table 12-1 summarizes inclusive occupational therapy interventions according to the core priorities for addressing complex trauma.

Table 12-1

Trauma-Informed Occupational Therapy Interventions for LGBTQ and GE Youth	
Core Priorities for Trauma-Informed Care	Inclusive Occupational Therapy Practice Strategies/Interventions
Safety	• Obtain training regarding identities and inclusive practices for LGBTQ and GE youth. • Post symbols indicating your acceptance of LGBTQ and GE youth (e.g., SafeZone stickers, badge pin, lanyard); place representational and inclusive books and reading material in waiting rooms. • Introduce yourself using your gender pronouns, which invites your client to share theirs. • Protect your LGBTQ and GE clients (see Table 12-2).
Connections	• Refer LGBTQ and GE youth to GSAs at their school, and collaborate with supporting teachers, parents, peers, and caregivers. • Refer LGBTQ and GE youth and their families to local community organizations, such as LGBTQ centers and PFLAG chapters. • Assist LGBTQ and GE youth to identify safe adults and help-seeking behaviors/strategies.

Emotional regulation	• Emotional regulation includes addressing environmental stressors, such as through environmental modification (e.g., sensory qualities, predictability of environment, interpersonal aspects, safe areas for regulation).
	• Address high levels of arousal preceding emotional dysregulation.
	• Interventions supporting regulation:
	  ▪ Alert Program
	  ▪ Mindfulness
	  ▪ Sensory strategies
	    ♦ Yoga
	    ♦ Massage
	    ♦ Other
	• Intentional response to outbursts, validating the trigger and its related emotions.
	  ▪ Therapeutic use of self
	  ▪ Reflective listening
	  ▪ Co-regulation

Fostering Inclusive Practice Settings

Occupational therapists work across a broad number of environments. Many of these environments have barriers that make accessing care difficult for LGBTQ and GE youth and their families. Barriers include lack of trained professionals, leading to homophobia, biphobia, and transphobia; lack of materials and environmental indicators of acceptance; lack of gender-neutral bathrooms and locker rooms; and in some spaces, no protections from discrimination. Posting symbols in the environment indicating trained staff and safety for LGBT and GE youth is a simple way to communicate inclusiveness (Hunt et al., 2018). Equipping waiting-room spaces with reading materials and books depicting diversity including LGBT and GE youth is another simple strategy. By making representation and symbols available within the clinical environment, occupational therapists are using a trauma-informed approach to address the extra assessment of environments for safety that LGBTQ and GE youth engage in (McCormick et al., 2018). Request the availability of gender-neutral restrooms in clinical environments. Ensure that all forms and electronic medical records include adequate options for gender identity, chosen names, orientation, and diverse family structures (e.g., boy, girl, non-binary; "parents" instead of mother and father). Advocate for nondiscrimination policies that include sexual orientation, gender identity, and gender expression, and set out clear disciplinary actions for those who fail to comply. Another way to protect clients is to step in and shut down homophobic, biphobic, gender-biased, and transphobic language and actions in your work environment. If a direct statement or action is made toward a client, the occupational therapist needs to address it immediately in order to protect and promote the safety of the client (Kelly & Ratliff, 2017).

Change at the Profession Level

As a profession, occupational therapy has scant literature examining the needs of LGBTQ and GE people across the lifespan. Other professions advocate for tailoring clinical practices to meet the unique needs and facilitate resilience of LGBTQ and GE youth (Kelly & Ratliff, 2017). More research is needed exploring occupational engagement, unique occupational aspects, and occupational therapy interventions supporting coping, adaptation, and resilience for LGBTQ and GE youth. Despite the fact that many professional organizations (e.g., the American Academy of Pediatrics, the American Medical Association, the American Psychological Association, and the National Association of Social Workers) have developed practice guidelines and position statements regarding LGBTQ and GE individuals, the American Occupational Therapy Association does not currently have any position statements or practice guidelines supporting LGBTQ and GE individuals. This reinforces a professional climate that dismisses these communities and their needs.

Occupational therapy curricula need to expand to include addressing the specific and unique aspects of LGBTQ and GE people across the lifespan. Partnering with local LGBTQ+ organizations would be a valuable and authentic way to increase student engagement with the LGBTQ+ community through unique service learning, fieldwork,

Table 12-2

Inclusive Practices Summary

- Obtain training regarding identities and inclusive practices for LGBTQ and GE youth.
- Post symbols indicating your acceptance of LGBTQ and GE youth (e.g., SafeZone stickers, badge pin, lanyard); place representational and inclusive books and reading material in waiting rooms.
- Introduce yourself using your gender pronouns, which invites your client to share theirs.
- Ask open-ended questions.
- Obtain/confirm the name the client uses.
- Avoid gender policing (e.g., boys don't/can't; girls don't/can't).
- Select assessment tools that offer non-gendered or mixed-gender norms when scoring.
- Protect your LGBTQ and GE pediatric clients:
  - Honor chosen names and pronouns.
  - Model affirming behavior for others.
  - Protect confidentiality; don't disclose a client's orientation or gender identity without their explicit consent.
  - Advocate and educate others.

and residency experiences. Occupational therapy educational programs should prioritize supporting the work of LGBTQ+ students and faculty in generating specific intervention programs designed to meet the needs of LGBTQ and GE people across the lifespan through financial and resource commitment. Table 12-2 summarizes some suggested inclusive practices.

KEY COLLABORATIONS (PARENTS, CAREGIVERS, TEACHERS, HEALTH CARE TEAMS, AND THE COMMUNITY)

As part of a trauma-informed treatment plan, occupational therapists should assist clients to form connections and access supports. When working with LGBTQ and GE youth, it is important to specifically locate resources that are explicitly designed to support the unique needs of LGBTQ and GE youth. These resources include local LGBTQ centers; Parents, Family and Friends of Lesbians and Gays (PFLAG) chapters (Figure 12-3); psychologists who are trained to work with LGBTQ and GE clients; accepting and inclusive medical providers; local gender clinics; GSA programs at schools; and

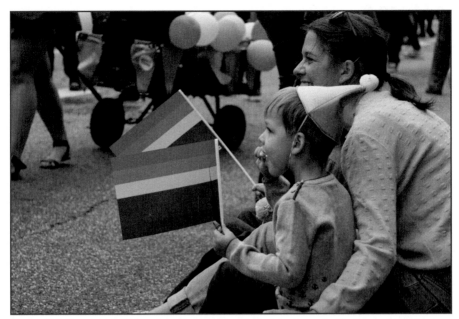

Figure 12-3. Parent and child participating in Pride parade. (oleschwander/shutterstock.com.)

inclusive and accepting extracurricular activities. Establishing partnerships and support networks with resources can be critical in maintaining safety and facilitating adaptation, coping, and resilience in LGBTQ and GE youth.

The need for and types of connections will vary across LGBTQ and GE clients. An example for an occupational therapist working in a school-based setting is working with school-site administration to perform environmental scans for signs of inclusiveness, including accessibility of gender-neutral restrooms and locker rooms, LGBTQ and GE representation in instructional materials, and the existence of GSAs and safe space indicators. For occupational therapists working in hospital settings, this may include consulting with a surgeon who completed top surgery for an adolescent client regarding contraindications, impact on upper extremity range of motion, and connecting the client to outpatient care for scar management.

Table 12-3

Adaptation, Coping, Resilience, and Best Practices		
	Adaptation/Coping	Resilience

Positive signs in LGBTQ and GE youth	• Help seeking
	  ▪ Locating safe peers and adults
	  ▪ Connecting to support services
	• Joining community
	• "Chosen" family
	• Navigating personal safety across environments (Colvin et al., 2019)
		• Gender transition
		• Outness
		• LGBTQ and GE friends
		• Self-acceptance
		• Sense of safety
		• Asserting agency
		• Activism
		(Asakura, 2016: Johns et al., 2019; Kosciw et al., 2015)

Best practices must facilitate:	• Trauma-informed care • School inclusion • Acceptance	• Gender-affirming care • Gay–straight alliances

Occupational therapy-specific interventions	• Use inclusive and accepting practices (see Table 12-1)
	• Facilitate self-regulation and coping skills
	  ▪ Sensory and cognitive strategies
	  ▪ The Alert Program
	  ▪ Mindfulness
	  ▪ Yoga	

ESSENTIAL CONSIDERATIONS FOR OCCUPATIONAL THERAPISTS

In conclusion, occupational therapy professionals should be knowledgeable about LGBTQ and GE identities. They should have an in-depth understanding of the barriers facing LGBTQ and GE youth, the impact on occupational access and participation, and the means of supporting adaptation, coping, and resilience for their LGBTQ and GE clients. Although LGBTQ and GE expansive youth may be referred to occupational therapists for a variety of developmental, mental health, social-emotional, and physical reasons, it is important to evaluate the safety and appropriateness of occupational therapy interventions for these vulnerable populations. Table 12-3 summarizes these best practices and essential considerations for occupational therapy. Table 12-4 lists some additional resources for assisting LGBTQ and GE expansive youth.

Table 12-4

Additional Resources	
Organization/Resource	**Supports Provided**
The Fenway Institute: https://fenwayhealth.org/the-fenway-institute	Online health care provider training, LGBTQ health care research
Family Equality: https://www.familyequality.org	Supports for LGBTQ families; advocacy, legal supports, podcasts, resource library, Open Door training for employers and providers
Gay and Lesbian Medical Association (GLMA): http://www.glma.org	Provides webinar trainings, list of national LGBTQ health care providers
Gay, Lesbian & Straight Educators Network (GLSEN): https://www.glsen.org	Provider/educator training, resources for K–12 education, GSA supports, school climate surveys, national campaigns (e.g., No Name Calling Week, Ally Week, Day of Silence)
Parents, Family and Friends of Lesbians and Gays (PFLAG): https://pflag.org	Education and advocacy, peer support, family support, resources, regional chapters

---

Case Study 12-1 Continuation

Xander

The occupational therapist used record review, caregiver interviews, and the Child Sensory Profile 2 (Dunn, 2014) to construct an occupational profile and identify Xander's areas of strength and concern.

Occupational Profile

Xander is an 8-year-old boy who enjoys riding his bicycle and playing Minecraft. Since being allowed to wear gender-affirming swim trunks, he loves going to swim at his community pool. His foster parents report that Xander's strengths include his sense of humor, curious nature, and honesty. Additional supports include a private psychologist, a supportive school environment (including access to a gender-neutral restroom), and a stable foster home. Caregivers are concerned about Xander's meltdowns and difficulty sleeping.

Evaluation

Results indicate that Xander has an irregular pre-bedtime routine; demonstrates over-responsiveness to tactile, auditory, and olfactory sensory inputs; and frequently engages in activities that provide proprioceptive input (e.g., jumping, pushing, and hitting objects) during meltdowns.

(continued)

Case Study 12-1 Continuation (continued)

Treatment Plan

The occupational therapist prioritized a trauma-informed approach when designing Xander's intervention plan. Therapeutic priorities were sensory modulation and working with caregivers to identify ways to support Xander's self-regulation in the home environment. Outcomes were improved sleep latency and reduced meltdowns. The Alert Program was selected for use, as it has been shown to improve executive functioning and self-regulation and reduce impulsivity (Soh et al., 2015). Additionally, the occupational therapist is supporting the family in establishing pre-bedtime routines, improving sleep hygiene, and investigating sensory experiences in the environment that affect Xander's ability to reduce arousal level for sleep. As the family indicated being supported by a psychologist, a pediatrician, and an inclusive school environment, no other referrals were made.

Session

Initial session with Xander was informed by the manualized first session of the Alert Program. Collaboration with his foster parents on incorporating calming and organizing strategies throughout Xander's day and specifically leading into the bedtime routine.

REFERENCES

Abramovich, A. (2016). Preventing, reducing and ending LGBTQ2S youth homelessness: The need for targeted strategies. *Social Inclusion, 4*(4), 86-96. https://doi.org/10.17645/si.v4i4.669

Asakura, K. (2016). It takes a village: Applying a social ecological framework of resilience in working with LGBTQ youth. *Families in Society, 97*(1), 15-22. https://doi.org/10.1606/1044-3894.2016.97.4

Baams, L., Dubas, J. S., Russell, S. T., Buikema, R. L., & van Aken, M. A. G. (2018). Minority stress, perceived burdensomeness, and depressive symptoms among sexual minority youth. *Journal of Adolescence, 66,* 9-18. https://doi.org/10.1016/j.adolescence.2018.03.015

Barbic, S. P., Chan, N., Rangi, A., Bradley, J., Pattison, R., Brockmeyer, K., Leznoff, S., Smolski, Y., Toor, G., Bray, B., Leon, A., Jenkins, M., & Mathias, S. (2019). Health provider and service-user experiences of sensory modulation rooms in an acute inpatient psychiatry setting. *PLoS ONE 14*(11): e0225238. https://doi.org/10.1371/journal.pone.0225238

Baum, J., Brill, S., Brown, J., Delpercio, A., Kahn, E., Kenney, L., & Nicoll, A. (n.d.). Gender-expansive youth report: Lessons from the Human Rights Campaign's youth survey. https://www.hrc.org/resources/2018-gender-expansive-youth-reportBodison, S. C., & Parham, L. D. (2018). Specific sensory techniques and sensory environmental modifications for children and youth with sensory integration difficulties: A systematic review. *American Journal of Occupational Therapy, 72*(1), 7201190040. https://doi.org/10.5014/ajot.2018.029413

Choi, S. K., Wilson, B. D. M., Shelton, J., & Gates, G. (2015). *Serving our youth 2015: The needs and experiences of lesbian, gay, bisexual, transgender, and questioning youth experiencing homelessness.* The Williams Institute with True Colors Fund.

Colvin, S., Egan, J. E., & Coulter, R. W. S. (2019). School climate & sexual and gender minority adolescent mental health. *Journal of Youth and Adolescence, 48,* 1938-1951. https://doi.org/10.1007/s10964-019-01108-w

Daly, L. A., Haden, S. C., Hagins, M., Papouchis, N., & Ramirez, P. M. (2015). Yoga and emotion regulation in high school students: A randomized controlled trial. *Evidence-Based Complementary and Alternative Medicine Volume 2015,* Article ID 794928, 1-8. https://doi.org/10.1155/2015/794928

Dank, M., Yu, L., Yahner, J., Pelletier, E., Mora, M., & Conner, B. (2015). Locked in: Interactions with the criminal justice and child welfare systems for LGBTQ youth, YMSM, and YWSW who engage in survival sex. Urban Institute. https://doi.org/10.15496/publikation-8607

Dunn, W. (2014). *Sensory profile 2 manual* (2nd ed.). Pearson.

Durwood, L., McLaughlin, K. A., & Olson, K. R. (2017). Mental health and self-worth in socially transitioned transgender youth. *Journal of the American Academy of Child & Adolescent Psychiatry, 56*(2), 116-123. https://doi.org/10.1016/j.jaac.2016.10.016

Flook, L., Goldberg, S. B., Pinger, L., & Davidson, R. J. (2015). Promoting prosocial behavior and self-regulatory skills in preschool children through a mindfulness-based kindness curriculum. *Developmental Psychology, 51*(1), 44-51. https://doi.org/10.1037/a0038256

Fredriksen-Goldsen, K. I., Simoni, J. M., Kim, H., Lehavot, K., Walters, K. L., Yang, J., Hoy-Ellis, C. P., & Muraco, A. (2014). The health equity promotion model: Reconceptualization of lesbian, gay, bisexual, and transgender (LGBT) health disparities. *American Journal of Orthopsychiatry, 84*(6), 653-663. https://doi.org/10.1037/ort0000030

Gill, A. M., & Frazer, M. S. (2016). *Health risk behaviors among gender expansive students: Making the case for including a measure of gender expression in population-based surveys.* Advocates for Youth.

GSA Network. (n.d.). What is a GSA club? www.gsanetwork.org/what-is-a-gsa

Hunt, L., Vennat, M., & Waters, J. H. (2018). Health and wellness for LGBTQ. *Advances in Pediatrics, 65*(1), 41-54. https://doi.org/10.1016/j.yapd.2018.04.002

Irvine, A., & Canfield (2016). The overrepresentation of lesbian, gay, bisexual, questioning, gender nonconforming and transgender youth within the child welfare to juvenile justice crossover population. *Journal of Gender, Social Policy & the Law, 24*(2), 243-261. https://digitalcommons.wcl.american.edu/cgi/viewcontent.cgi?article=1679&context=jgspl

Johns, M. M., Beltran, O., Armstrong, H. L., Janye, P. E., & Barrios, L. C. (2018). Protective factors among transgender and gender variant youth: A systematic review by socioecological level. *Journal of Primary Prevention, 39*(3), 263-301. https://doi.org/10.1007/s10935-018-0508-9

Johns, M. M., Poteat, P., Horn, S. S., & Kosciw, J. (2019). Strengthening our schools to promote resilience and health among LGBTQ youth: Emerging evidence and research priorities from the state of LGBTQ youth health and wellbeing symposium. *LGBT Health, 6*(4), 146-155. https://doi.org/10.1089/lgbt.2018.0109

Kann, L., McManus, T., Harris, W. A., Shanklin, S. L., Flint, K. H., Queen, B., Lowry, R., Chyen, D., Whittle, L., Thornton, J., Lim, C., Bradford, D., Yamakawa, Y., Leon, M., Brener, N., & Ethier, K. A. (2018). Youth risk behavior surveillance—United States, 2017. *MMWR Surveillance Summaries, 67*(8), 1-114. https://www.cdc.gov/mmwr/volumes/67/ss/ss6708a1.htm

Kelly, B. L., & Ratliff, G. A. (2017). Strengths-affirming practice with LGBTQ youth. In M. P. Dentato (Ed.), *Social work practice with the LGBTQ community: The intersection of history, health, mental health, and policy factors.* Oxford University Press.

Koenig, K. P., Buckley-Reen, A., & Garg, S. (2012). Efficacy of the Get Ready to Learn yoga program among children with autism spectrum disorders: A pretest–posttest control group design. *American Journal of Occupational Therapy, 66*(5), 538-546. https://doi.org/10.5014/ajot.2012.004390

Kosciw, J. G., Greytak, E. A., Zongrone, A. D., Clark, C. M., & Truong, N. L. (2018). *The 2017 National School Climate Survey: The experiences of lesbian, gay, bisexual, transgender, and queer youth in our nation's schools.* GLSEN.

Kosciw, J. G., Palmer, N. A., & Kull, R. M. (2015). Reflecting resiliency: Openness about sexual orientation and/or gender identity and its relationship to well-being and educational outcomes for LGBT students. *American Journal of Community Psychology, 55*(1-2), 167-178. https://doi.org/10.1007/s10464-014-9642-6

Kulick, A., Wernick, L. J, Espinoza, M. A. V., Newman, T. J, & Dessel, A. B. (2019). Three strikes and you're out: Culture, facilities, and participation among LGBTQ youth in sports. *Sport, Education and Society, 24*(9), 939-953. https://doi.org/10.1080/13573322.2018.1532406

Lambda Legal. (2010). *When health care isn't caring: Lambda Legal's survey of discrimination against LGBT people and people with HIV.* Lambda Legal.

Lemberger-Truelove, M. E., Carbonneau, K. J., Atencio, D. J., Zieher, A. K., & Palacios, A. F. (2018). Self-regulatory growth effects for young children participating in a combined social and emotional learning and mindfulness-based intervention. *Journal of Counseling & Development, 96*(3), 289-302. https://doi.org/10.1002/jcad.12203

Levine, D. A., & the Committee on Adolescence. (2013). Office-based care for lesbian, gay, bisexual, transgender, and questioning youth. *Pediatrics, 132*(1), e297-e313. https://doi.org/10.1542/peds.2013-1283

Malboeuf-Hurtubise, C., Lacourse, E., Taylor, G., Joussemet, M., & Ben Amor, L. (2017). Mindfulness-based intervention pilot feasibility study for elementary school students with severe learning difficulties: Effects on internalized and externalized symptoms from an emotional regulation perspective. *Journal of Evidence-Based Complementary & Alternative Medicine, 22*(3), 473-481. https://doi.org/10.1177/2156587216683886

McCormick, A., Scheyd, K., & Terrazas, S. (2018). Trauma-informed care and LGBTQ youth: Considerations for advancing practice with youth with trauma experiences. *Families in Society: The Journal of Contemporary Social Services, 99*(2), 160-169. https://doi.org/10.1177/1044389418768550

McManama O'Brien, K. H., Putney, J. M., Hebert, N. W., Falk, A. M., & Aquinaldo, L. D. (2016). Sexual and gender minority youth suicide: Understanding subgroup differences to inform interventions. *LGBT Health, 3*(4), 248-251. https://doi.org/10.1089/lgbt.2016.0031

Moreno-Gómez, A.-J., & Cejudo, J. (2018). Effectiveness of a mindfulness-based social-emotional learning program on psychosocial adjustment and neuropsychological maturity in kindergarten children. *Mindfulness, 10,* 111-121. https://doi.org/10.1007/s12671-018-0956-6

Nash, K., Stevens, S., Greenbaum, R., Weiner, J., Koren, G., & Rovet, J. (2015). Improving executive functioning in children with fetal alcohol spectrum disorders. *Child Neuropsychology: A Journal on Normal and Abnormal Development in Childhood and Adolescence, 21*(2), 191-209. https://doi.org/10.1080/09297049.2014.889110

National Institutes of Health. (2019). Sex & gender. https://orwh.od.nih.gov/sex-gender

Olson-Kennedy, J. (2016). Adolescent and young health: Mental health disparities among transgender youth: Rethinking the role of professionals. *JAMA Pediatrics, 170*(5), 423-424. https://doi.org/10.1001/jamapediatrics.2016.0155

Pollitt, A. M., Ioverno, S., Russell, S. T., Li, G., & Grossman, A. H. (2019). Predictors and mental health benefits of chosen name use among transgender youth. *Youth & Society, 53*(2), 320-341. https://doi.org/10.1177/0044118X19855898

Poteat, V. P., Calzo, J. P., & Yoshikawa, H. (2016). Promoting youth agency through dimensions of gay-straight alliance involvement and conditions that maximize associations. *Journal of Youth Adolescence, 45,* 1438-1451. https://doi.org/10.1007/s10964-016-0421-6

Rafferty, J., AAP Committee on Psychosocial Aspects of Child and Family Health, AAP Committee on Adolescence, AAP Section on Lesbian, Gay, Bisexual, and Transgender Health and Wellness. (2018). Ensuring comprehensive care and support for transgender and gender diverse children and adolescents. *Pediatrics, 142*(4), e20182162. https://doi.org/10.1542/peds.2018-2162

Rider, N. G., McMorris, B. J., Gower, A. L., Coleman, E., & Eisenberg, M. E. (2020). Health and care utilization of transgender and gender nonconforming youth: A population-based study. *Pediatrics, 141*(3), e20171683. https://doi.org/10.1542/peds.2017-1683

Soh, D. W., Skocic, J., Nash, K., Stevens, S., Turner, G. R., & Rovet, J. (2015). Self-regulation therapy increases frontal gray matter in children with fetal alcohol spectrum disorder: Evaluation by voxel-based morphometry. *Frontiers in Human Neuroscience, 9*(108), 1-12. http://doi.org/10.3389/fnhum.2015.00108

The Williams Institute. (2019). LGBT demographic data interactive. UCLA School of Law.

Tobin, V., Bockting, W. O., & Hughes, T. L. (2018). Mental health promotion for gender minority adolescents. *Journal of Psychosocial Nursing, 56*(12), 22-30. https://doi.org/10.3928/02793695-20180601-02

Wells, A. M., Chasnoff, I. J., Schmidt, C. A., Telford, E., & Schwartz, L. D. (2012). Neurocognitive habilitation therapy for children with fetal alcohol spectrum disorders: An adaptation of the Alert Program®. *American Journal of Occupational Therapy, 66*(1), 24-34. https://doi.org/10.5014/ajot.2012.002691

Wilson, B. D. M., Choi, S. K., Herman, J. L., Becker, T., & Conron, K. J. (2017). *Characteristics and mental health of gender nonconforming adolescents in California: Findings from the 2015-2016 California health interview survey.* The Williams Institute and UCLA Center for Health Policy Research. https://williamsinstitute.law.ucla.edu/publications/gnc-youth-ca

Wilson, B. D. M., Cooper, K., Kastanis, A., & Nezhad, S. (2014). *Sexual and gender minority youth in foster care: Assessing disproportionality and disparities in Los Angeles.* The Williams Institute.

Wilson, B. D. M., & Kastanis, A. A. (2015). Sexual and gender minority disproportionality and disparities in child welfare: A population-based study. *Children and Youth Services Review, 58,* 11-17. https://doi.org/10.1016/j.childyouth.2015.08.016

13

Children and Youth Who Have Encountered Adverse Childhood Experiences*

Jennifer S. Pitonyak, PhD, OTR/L, SCFES and
Lauren E. Milton, OTD, OTR/L

CHAPTER OBJECTIVES By the end of this chapter, the reader will be able to:

- Define adaptation, coping, and resilience in relation to children and youth who have encountered adverse childhood experiences.
- Describe the assumptions and principles of a trauma-informed approach to working with children and youth who have encountered adverse life experiences.
- Identify evidence-informed and occupation-based intervention approaches for fostering adaptation, coping, and resilience in children and youth who have encountered adverse life experiences.

---

*Authors' Note

This chapter is dedicated to the memory of Dr. Dianna T. Derigo, occupational therapist and world changer.

OVERVIEW OF THE POPULATION

Trauma has been called an unaddressed societal health crisis (Carter et al., 2016). The National Child Abuse and Neglect Data System (NCANDS) of the U.S. Department of Health and Human Services (HHS) reported an 8.4% increase from 2014 to 2018 in the number of children who received a protective services investigation

Grajo L. C., & Boisselle, A. K. (Eds.). *Adaptation, Coping, and Resilience in Children and Youth: A Comprehensive Occupational Therapy Approach* (pp. 313-336).
© 2022 Taylor & Francis Group.

response or alternative response. In 2018, HHS reported a national rounded number of victims totaling 678,000, with more than 84.5% of victims suffering a single type of maltreatment (15.5% were victims of two or more maltreatment types). Of that population, 60.8% were neglected, 10.7% were physically abused, and 7% were sexually abused (HHS, 2020). The effects of trauma, including child abuse and neglect and collectively known as adverse childhood experiences (ACEs), are linked to a plethora of subsequent negative emotional, physiological, and cognitive effects (Edwards et al., 2005; Felitti et al., 1998; National Child Traumatic Stress Network Schools Committee [NCTSN], 2008; Substance Abuse and Mental Health Services Administration [SAMHSA], 2014). In a 2016 study by Jimenez et al., researchers found an association between ACEs and poor foundational skills in areas such as literacy and language, which are known to "predispose individuals to low education attainment and adult literacy" (p. 6). The higher the number of ACEs, the worse the outcomes (Jimenez et al., 2016). Ultimately, these negative effects can affect participation in meaningful occupations across all environments, including the formation of healthy attachments with others, sex and intimacy, sleep, and social participation (Carter et al., 2016).

According to SAMHSA (SAMHSA, 2014), "[t]rauma results from an event, series of events, or set of circumstances that is experienced by an individual as physically or emotionally harmful or threatening and that has lasting adverse effects on the individual's functioning and physical, social, emotional, or spiritual well-being" (p. 7). The *Diagnostic and Statistical Manual of Mental Disorders, Fifth Edition* (*DSM-5*), defines *trauma* as an occurrence when an individual person experiences "actual or threatened death, serious injury, or sexual violence" (American Psychiatric Association [APA], 2013, p. 271). Trauma can also be categorized into three main types: acute, chronic, and complex. Whereas *acute trauma* results from a single incident, *chronic trauma*, which includes abuse or neglect, is repeated and prolonged. *Complex trauma* involves exposure to multiple, varied, invasive, and interpersonal events, including but not limited to environmental stressors, school/community/domestic violence, crime, natural disasters, sexual or physical abuse, neglect such as malnutrition, medical trauma, and traumatic loss (Centers for Disease Control and Prevention [CDC], 2020). The term *developmental trauma* (van der Kolk, 2005), also known as *reactive attachment disorder*, is recognized due to the long-term detrimental impact of ACEs on the neurological system (Child Welfare Information Gateway, 2015).

In the pivotal CDC study by Felitti et al. (1998), known as the Adverse Childhood Experiences Study, researchers examined the effects of ACEs on the health of adults and found long-term detrimental health outcomes. This study was hailed as one of the largest investigations ever conducted to explore relationships between childhood maltreatment and long-term health and well-being. The ACEs recognized in the study included physical, emotional, and sexual abuse; substance abuse within the household during childhood; an incarcerated, mentally ill, or suicidal household member; spousal abuse between parents; and divorce or separation that resulted in one parent being absent during childhood (Felitti et al., 1998). Green et al. (2010) built on the ACEs study and further defined *childhood adversities* as parental death, parental divorce/separation, life-threatening illness, or extreme economic hardship, in addition to the childhood experiences included in the Adverse Childhood Experiences Study. Trauma-informed care

(TIC) was introduced to respond to the needs of trauma survivors. Hopper et al. (2010) conducted a review of literature and used themes to formulate a collective definition for trauma-informed care:

> A strengths-based service delivery approach that is grounded in an understanding of and responsiveness to the impact of trauma, that emphasizes physical, psychological, and emotional safety for both providers and survivors, and that creates opportunities for survivors to rebuild a sense of control and empowerment (p. 82).

Those who conduct research in the area of trauma assert that all providers and staff working with individuals at any age level must employ trauma-informed interventions in practice (Soleimanpour et al., 2017; Perfect et al., 2016). Although various fields are adopting a trauma-informed approach, trauma often goes undetected, leaving most patients without appropriate supports; thus, interventions can result in retraumatization. The estimated cost of the effects of trauma to the health care industry is between 333 to 750 billion dollars annually, or nearly 17% to 37.5% of the total health care expenditures in the United States (Carter et al., 2016). Many professionals, including occupational therapy practitioners, underestimate the prevalence of trauma (Marsac et al., 2016) or do not address trauma (Chung et al., 2016) in practice. Bright et al. (2015) found that professionals may not feel they are equipped to address trauma appropriately, thus increasing the risk of client retraumatization. Occupational therapy practitioners are uniquely qualified to evaluate and address universal, targeted, and intensive levels of intervention to address trauma across environments, including home and school (American Occupational Therapy Association [AOTA], 2019). Occupational therapy practitioners are critical members of any interdisciplinary team, making significant contributions in addressing trauma because of their extensive knowledge of evidence-based assessment and intervention, focus on client-centeredness, and contribution of the environment to performance and participation in meaningful, everyday activity (Gronski et al., 2013). Hence, it is critical for occupational therapy practitioners to understand the mechanism of adaptation and strategies for fostering coping and resilience in client populations who have experienced ACEs.

DEFINING ADAPTATION, COPING, AND RESILIENCE FOR CHILDREN WHO HAVE ENCOUNTERED ADVERSE CHILDHOOD EXPERIENCES

Fostering adaptation, coping, and resilience among children and youth who have encountered ACEs is an important focus for this population, particularly given the strong evidence associating ACEs with poor health behaviors, such as substance misuse, which in turn increase the risk for chronic health conditions that can lead to premature mortality (Bethell et al., 2017; Felitti, 2009; Felitti et al., 1998). Given the repeated exposure to adversity that comes from situations of intergenerational poverty and trauma, children and youth who have encountered ACEs, and subsequently have developmental trauma, may have few opportunities to develop their adaptive capacity. This section applies the overarching definitions of adaptation, coping, and resilience to the occupational situations of children and youth who have encountered ACEs, and considers how the strengths and challenges of this population may influence adaptation, coping, and resilience through occupation. A case study illustrates how adaptation, coping, and resilience manifest in the everyday life of a young woman who experienced human trafficking, among other ACEs.

Adaptation and Adaptive Capacity

Adaptation through occupation is an internal human process that is a product of engagement in occupation, and it is the process by which individuals overcome contextual challenges during participation in occupation (Grajo, 2019). Facilitating adaptation is key for children and youth who have encountered ACEs, as the adversities they experienced likely contributed to inconsistent adult responses to their expressed needs and exposure to impoverished contexts that lacked options for healthy, occupational engagement. Across areas of occupation, children and youth who have encountered ACEs may demonstrate impaired social skills, diminished motivation to complete daily routines, impaired executive function, and difficulty in managing emotions to successfully handle complicated situations—among other challenges at home, school, work, and in the community (AOTA, 2019). Therefore, children and youth who have encountered ACEs need opportunities to engage in consistent, healthy, and supportive routines-based occupation to establish the internal processes of adaptation and a desired sense of self. Because children and youth who have encountered ACEs face contextual barriers to adaptation in their everyday lives, they may benefit from interventions that support their adaptive capacity, defined by Schkade and Schultz (2003) and expanded by Grajo (2019) as the ability to plan, execute, revise as needed, and integrate new and old responses to overcome occupational challenges.

Coping

Coping is an essential adaptive response to adversity, and is, therefore, critical for children and youth who have encountered ACEs and their engagement in healthy, meaningful occupation. Coping is an ongoing dynamic process that changes in response to the demands of a stressful situation (Compas et al., 2001). For example, a teen who maintains a consistent bedtime and waking schedule to support school attendance despite a parent who is absent from the home due to substance misuse is an example of coping. Furthermore, coping is conceptualized as purposeful responses that are directed toward resolving the stressful relationship between the self and the environment or toward palliating negative emotions that arise as a result of stress (Compas et al., 2001). That same teen, while experiencing prolonged exposure to parental neglect due to parental substance misuse, is able to cope by identifying their negative emotions and managing them through cognitive awareness of the difference between the teen's actions and those of the parent. Unfortunately, many children and youth who have encountered ACEs have not developed the ability to cope, due to developmental trauma. Children and youth with developmental trauma often function in a state of hyperarousal and high alert, with high amounts of cortisol in their systems. They may not be able to cope, even in safe environments, relying on fight, flight, or freeze to dictate their responses (Purvis et al., 2013; Swinth & Pitonyak, 2021). Children and youth with developmental trauma benefit from occupation-based interventions that focus on relational attachment, trust, and safety as a means for developing coping. For example, occupational therapists can support parents of infants with developmental trauma and a history of neonatal abstinence syndrome in the co-occupation of feeding by coaching them to feed on demand, rather than on a timed schedule, in order to build the self-regulation skills necessary for coping (Oostlander et al., 2019; Swinth & Pitonyak, 2021).

Resilience

Resilience is an outcome of the adaptive capacity to respond to adversity (National Scientific Council on the Developing Child, 2015); in other words, coping is a process of adaptation, whereas resilience is reflected in outcomes for which coping has occurred in response to adversity (Compas et al., 2001). Therefore, in response to growing awareness of the burden of ACEs on life course health, health- and social-welfare advocates generally support widespread screening of children for ACEs. The overall goal is to provide services that build coping processes and foster resilience outcomes among children and youth who have encountered ACEs, and particularly those who present with developmental trauma. Many states and local communities have created policy and community-infrastructure initiatives to foster resilience that create opportunities for occupational therapy practitioners to offer services from a health promotion approach or potentially integrate services into primary care settings. For example, California was the first state to implement a formal process of screening for ACEs through the Medi-Cal program available to both adults and children (Feder Ostrov, 2020). Through this initiative, parents or caregivers are asked to voluntarily complete a screening questionnaire about ACEs during well-child visits. The questionnaire assesses risk of exposure to a variety of adverse experiences. Primary providers in California are working to identify the next step of the screening process: referral to services and resources that best meet the needs of children and youth who require supports due to ACEs. Occupational therapy providers can advocate to increase awareness among pediatricians about the role of occupational therapy in providing services to children and youth who have encountered ACEs.

Although the screening program in California continues to expand and develop (Feder Ostrov, 2020), experts across the country have expressed concerns about universal screening that quantifies the risk from ACEs and potentially assigns labels, such as toxic stress, and how this labeling may affect resilience outcomes in children and youth who have encountered ACEs. Therefore, organizations such as the Community Resilience Initiative (CRI) have taken a different resilience-building approach, and embrace the

Figure 13-1. Middle school student demonstrating resilience during the COVID-19 pandemic through participation in a learning pod. (Photo credit: Michele Schneidler.)

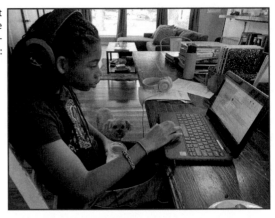

Figure 13-2. Middle school students demonstrating resilience during the COVID-19 pandemic through participation in a learning pod. (Photo credit: Michele Schneidler.)

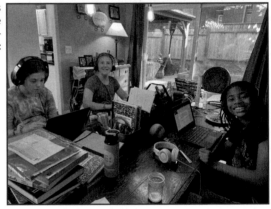

principle that individuals who have experienced ACEs can learn effective coping processes that foster the resilience to overcome ACEs. Community practices that foster resilience include access to healthy foods and safe, outdoor spaces for exercising, as well as integration of a trauma-informed approach into health care, school, and other community settings (CRI, 2017). Occupational therapy practitioners can provide universal health promotion programs in community settings to build resilience and mitigate the impact of ACEs on occupation and health, and those providers with advanced training in trauma-informed interventions can support children and youth with developmental trauma (AOTA, 2019; Swinth & Pitonyak, 2021). See Figures 13-1 to 13-5 for examples of supporting resilience.

So, while the practice of screening for ACEs in order to better identify and treat those with developmental trauma is important, awareness of the need for societal effort to prevent ACEs and the resulting complex impact on health and well-being is also growing (Srivastav et al., 2019; Swinth & Pitonyak, 2021). Srivastav et al. (2019) developed the Empower Action Model, a framework for preventing ACEs through health promotion approaches; the CDC also identified additional resilience initiatives, such as

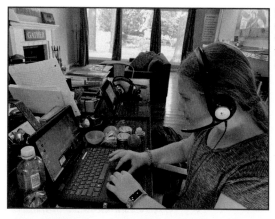

Figure 13-3. Middle school student demonstrating resilience during the COVID-19 pandemic through participation in a learning pod. (Photo credit: Michele Schneidler.)

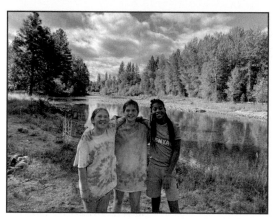

Figure 13-4. Youth engaging in time in nature as an essential adaptive response to stressors in their lives. (Photo credit: Michele Schneidler.)

access to quality care and education in early childhood and enhancing parenting skills, as important for promoting healthy child development (CDC, 2020) and fostering adaptation, coping, and resilience. Resilience initiatives seek to break the cycle of ACEs by mediating upstream exposure to social determinants such as poverty, and by fostering adaptive capacity for protective factors such as self-regulation, problem solving, and relational skills (Srivastav et al., 2019). The Empower Action Model synthesizes concepts from socio-ecological and life course perspectives with race, equity, and inclusion work to create a framework of protective factors and a map for action at individual, family, organization, community, and policy levels (Srivastav et al., 2019). Occupational therapy providers can expand their thinking about how policy and other contextual factors may affect participation in occupation for certain populations and subsequently contribute to the health disparities that are linked with ACEs (Pitonyak et al., 2020).

Figure 13-5. Youth engaging in time in nature as an essential adaptive response to stressors in their lives. (Photo credit: Michele Schneidler.)

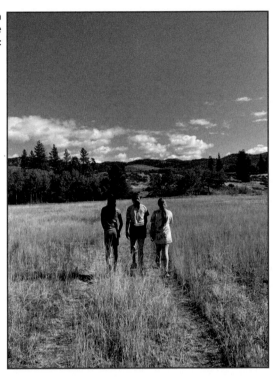

Case Study 13-1
Resilience in Children of Hope

Ana is a 23-year-old Venezuelan female who currently resides in a family shelter in a mid-sized urban area in the Pacific Northwest region of the United States. Ana and her now 5-year-old son, Issac, fled Venezuela 3 years ago to escape the economic and political chaos of their home country. In Venezuela, Ana was living with her uncle's family in the slum of Las Mayas in Caracas in a small, hillside house. Ana came to live with her uncle's family when she was 2 years old, following the death of both of her parents in the 1999 natural disaster of torrential rains, flooding, and mudslides that occurred in Vargas State. A relief worker rescued Ana from the wreckage of her parents' home and brought her to Caracas, where she was temporarily sheltered in La Casona, the presidential residence, until she was able to be reunited with relatives. Ana's uncle and aunt, though poor, were able to meet Ana's basic needs as a child, along with those of their own three children, and fostered her adaptive capacity and coping through their attentiveness to her needs. Ana also coped through her interactions with her three cousins who were all younger than her, as she spent hours making rag dolls and entertaining them with stories about the dolls. Ana attended school

(continued)

Case Study 13-1 (continued)

until the age of 15 and was a bright, engaged student; although she could have pursued 2 more years of non-compulsory secondary school, her uncle and aunt asked her to leave school to find work. Ana had continued to make rag dolls from scraps of fabric, and she began selling her dolls on a street corner. She enjoyed interacting socially with the people whom she met on the streets, and this social participation contributed to her resilience despite her life of poverty and past ACEs. She began an intimate relationship with a young man who often sat with her on the streets while she sold her dolls, to protect her from the street violence endemic in Caracas. Eventually, Ana became pregnant and she and her partner talked about getting married in the future after they saved up some money. However, one evening when Ana was gathering up her unsold dolls from the street corner, a robber held her at knife point and demanded her money. When her partner tried to intervene, he was murdered by the robber. Soon thereafter, Ana gave birth to Issac, and because she was fearful about leaving him at home with her aunt while she worked, she rarely left the house and was no longer able to contribute to her extended family's income. Although her uncle and aunt continued to try to provide for her and Issac, economic conditions and violence in Venezuela worsened, and eventually, they encouraged Ana to emigrate to the United States to join a distant cousin who was living in California and employed as a migrant farm worker. Ana applied for asylum with U.S. Citizenship and Immigration Services and eventually, she and Issac were granted asylum. However, when Ana arrived in California, she discovered that her cousin had deceived and trafficked her, against her will, to join a prostitution ring. Without other family to turn to, and fearful for Issac's safety, Ana was forced into prostitution. However, she continued to be hopeful that she could escape this current environment, and focused on caring for Issac as best as possible—bathing and reading to him each night, focusing on her sense of self as a parent rather than her exploitation to perform sex work. Because of her qualified status as an immigrant, Ana was able to receive childcare benefits for Issac. She eventually confided in a teacher at the daycare center, who helped connect her with a nonprofit organization that was able to support Ana in safely leaving the trafficking situation and relocating to Washington State. Ana found housing at a family shelter, which she is able to maintain as long as she meets requirements for education and/or work. Given Ana's strong sense of self as a parent, and her love of children, she enrolled in a certificate program to study child development that would eventually enable her to be employed by a childcare facility. Although both Ana and Issac experienced repeated exposures to adverse experiences, including poverty, violence, and other trauma, Ana's constant ability to cope with external challenges and separate her own sense of self from her surroundings and experiences helped to foster her resilience. After completing her certificate program and finding a part-time job in a childcare facility, Ana continued to seek opportunities to further her knowledge of child development and grow her bond with Issac. She participated in a family mental health program that was led by an occupational therapist at her neighborhood community health center. She attended the program regularly, demonstrating her adaptive capacity, and showing that hope and resilience can overcome ACEs.

THE ROLE OF OCCUPATIONAL THERAPY: BEST AND EVIDENCE-BASED PRACTICES FOR ASSESSMENT AND INTERVENTION

Carter et al. (2016) asserted that a trauma-informed approach to practice across disciplines could reap numerous substantial benefits for clients, and ultimately lead to a reduction in medical costs and improved health care overall. Research shows that implementation of trauma-informed care leads to better outcomes for both clients and families, and reduces the risk of retraumatization (Marsac et al., 2016). Berg (2016) called on professionals in diverse fields to act. Awareness of the need to implement a trauma-informed approach throughout the occupational therapy process has increased in recent years. Doing so requires occupational therapy practitioners to integrate principles of trauma-informed care with disciplinary conceptual models guiding evaluation and intervention.

Although a variety of frameworks for trauma-informed care exist, SAMHSA published "SAMHSA's Concept of Trauma and Guidance for a Trauma-Informed Approach," which addresses the importance of creating trauma-informed social environments within organizations (2014). SAMHSA's trauma-informed approach is grounded in a set of four assumptions and six principles and is a broad framework that encompasses trauma-specific interventions (2014). The assumptions of this approach, *The Four Rs,* are:

1. Realization: All members of the organization have a basic realization about trauma and how it may affect individuals and families.

2. Recognize: Members of the organization recognize the signs of trauma and use screenings or assessments to assist in identifying needs of children and youth and their families.

3. Respond: All members of the organization respond to the needs of children and youth who have experienced adverse life experiences and their families by changing language, policies, and behaviors to take into consideration the history of trauma experiences.

4. Resist retraumatization: Organizational members are aware of how certain policies or practices may trigger stressful memories and retraumatize individuals (2014).

Providers and organizations that uphold these assumptions are able to support the adaptive capacity of individuals who have encountered ACEs.

In addition to these assumptions of a trauma-informed approach, the SAMHSA (2014, p. 10) framework names six principles of trauma-informed care that are intended to guide practices across settings and situations of ACEs, rather than prescribing specific interventions.

1. Safety: Organizations and providers should understand safety as defined by the client to be essential; this includes feeling physically and psychologically safe.

2. Trustworthiness and transparency: Organizations and providers should assure transparency in the delivery of services as a means of building and maintaining trust with clients.

3. Peer support: Clients benefit from support from other individuals with lived experiences of ACEs; for children, their own family members or key caregivers may provide this peer support.

4. Collaboration and mutuality: Organizations and providers must be aware of power differences between clients, providers, and other organizational staff and strive to create open environments that are free of harm from structural power.

5. Empowerment, voice, and choice: Organizations and providers should support clients in shared decision making, choice, and goal setting throughout the treatment process.

6. Cultural, historical, and gender issues: Organizations and providers must work to dismantle cultural stereotypes, racism, and other biases; services should be gender responsive, culturally relevant, and acknowledge and address past historical trauma.

Given these assumptions and principles of trauma-informed care as a foundation, occupational therapy theorists Derigo, Russell, and Berg (2018) proposed an evidence-informed approach to assessment and intervention distinct to occupational therapy, the *Trauma-Informed Care in Occupational Therapy (TIC-OT) Model*. In the model, Derigo et al. (2018) provided a visual representation of dynamic factors to consider when viewing any client through a trauma lens: Guiding Values of Occupational Therapy (Table 13-1), Client-Environment Interaction (Table 13-2), Foundational Principles of Trauma-Informed Care (Table 13-3), and the "4 Rs" (Table 13-4), which are expanded upon later in this chapter to describe a guided approach. Derigo et al. (2018) challenged occupational therapy practitioners to change their perspective to a trauma-informed lens when considering all people, shifting from a traditional paradigm to a trauma-informed one (Table 13-5). The model focuses on an application-based approach, highlighting realistic strategies to be used in various settings.

Guiding Values of Occupational Therapy are standards of practice within occupational therapy that are specifically highlighted when using a trauma-informed approach. These values include therapeutic use of self; evidence-based practice; cultural competence; and holistic, humanistic, and client-centered care. The Client-Environment Interaction is based on the understanding that aspects of the environment can affect an individual's ability to engage in occupations and highlights appreciation of the bidirectional relationship between the client and their environment. The factors in the model include the client and community/extended social system, the client and home/family system, and the client and school/work environment. Foundational Principles of Trauma-Informed Care are universal principles of trauma-informed care that promote resiliency and recovery. These principles include safety, collaboration, trust, empowerment, and choice. The *Four Rs* (Realize, Recognize, Respond, and Resist), as previously described, are a process that outlines trauma identification, developed by SAMHSA (2014), to properly respond to trauma and limit retraumatization.

To address trauma adequately, an appropriate assessment battery must be administered. The example assessments listed in Table 13-6 may help to identify how trauma affects specific person factors, how environmental factors affect the client, and how the dynamic interaction of the two types of factors affect occupational performance and engagement.

Table 13-1

Application of a TIC-OT Model Principle: Guiding Values of Occupational Therapy	
TIC-OT Model Principle	**Occupational Therapy Applications and Examples of Use to Support Adaptation, Coping, and Resilience of Children Who Have Encountered ACEs**
Guiding Values of Occupational Therapy	
Therapeutic use of self	• Use empathy when working with the client/family/team • Collaborate with the client/family/team • Build hope when the client/family/team seem discouraged • Build therapeutic alliance and trust • Be aware of your own verbal and nonverbal cues • Grow the client's image of self-worth • Respond to crisis points appropriately (e.g., provide empathy break, grade down task)
Evidence-based practice	• Use of effective evidence-based assessment • Use of effective evidence-based intervention to optimize outcomes
Cultural respect	• Respect cultural differences • Be aware of cultural considerations when working with families • Know that clients of different cultures may require different therapeutic styles • Recognize internal cultural biases and understand how they can affect your relationship with your client
Holistic	• Include all domains of an individual in assessment and intervention (physical, cognitive, social, emotional, and spiritual) • Allow flexibility in intervention to work on varying client needs
Humanistic	• Support advocacy for current unmet services and referrals for survivors of trauma
Client-centered	• Consider the client to be an expert when determining goals and planning interventions • Encourage the client to problem-solve new ways of thinking • Collaborate and offer choices whenever possible • Make intervention reflective of the client's beliefs

Adapted from Derigo, D., Russell, D., & Berg, C. (2018). *A trauma-informed approach distinct to occupational therapy: The TIC-OT model* [Webinar]. American Occupational Therapy Association (Producer). https://myaota.aota.org/shop_aota/product/OL5140

Table 13-2

Application of a TIC-OT Model Principle: Client-Environment Interaction	
TIC-OT Model Principle	Occupational Therapy Applications and Examples of Use to Support Adaptation, Coping, and Resilience of Children Who Have Encountered ACEs
Client-Environment Interaction	
The dynamic interaction of person factors and environmental factors and impact on occupational performance and participation (Person-Environment-Occupation-Performance [PEOP] model; Christiansen et al., 2015)	• Consideration of all person factors (physiological, cognitive, spiritual, neurobehavioral, and psychological). • Consideration of the client within all contexts, which can include school, work, the home and family system, and the community. Additionally, extrinsic factors must be included, such as social support, social system, culture, values, and physical environment.
Client and community	• Help the client connect with community supports to improve social and financial supports. • Reduce environmental triggers within the community as much as possible. • Refer the client to other supports in the community to assist in trauma treatment (e.g., psychologist, social worker). • Assist in the prevention of future trauma by providing referrals to community supports or connecting with a caseworker to meet these needs (e.g., food stamps, housing assistance, legal services).
Client and home/family	• Educate members of the household about the effects of trauma and how to limit future trauma. • Include siblings/caregivers in therapy. • Train/educate parents on effective parenting styles.
Client and school/work	• Educate teachers and/or employers about the effects of trauma. • Support teachers and/or employers in adapting the environment to best meet client's needs.

Adapted from Derigo, D., Russell, D., & Berg, C. (2018). *A trauma-informed approach distinct to occupational therapy: The TIC-OT model* [Webinar]. American Occupational Therapy Association (Producer). https://myaota.aota.org/shop_aota/product/OL5140

Table 13-3

Application of a TIC-OT Model Principle: Universal Principles of Trauma-Informed Care	
TIC-OT Model Principle	OT Applications and Examples of Use to Support Adaptation, Coping, and Resilience of Children Who Have Encountered ACEs
Based on the Universal Principles of Trauma Informed Care (SAMHSA, 2014)	
Safety	• Provide therapy in a safe and secure setting. • Ensure patient confidentiality. • If possible, offer to address physiological needs (e.g., drink of water, snack) • Avoid shame-inducing conversations/situations. • Ask before touching a client.
Collaboration	• Work with the client and family to set goals. • Work with the client and family to problem-solve challenges. • View the client as the expert in their understanding of themselves. • Encourage client feedback before, during, and after intervention.
Trust	• Use of therapeutic use of self. • Follow through with what is said/promised in therapy. • Be transparent in therapy expectations and assessment results. • Provide a vivid explanation of assessment and intervention.
Empowerment	• Encourage clients to advocate for themselves. • Identify and acknowledge strengths of the client. • Praise the client for success in therapy. • Set realistic and obtainable goals for the client and acknowledge it when they are met or need to be adapted.
Choice	• Have the client choose where, how, and when they will receive services, if possible. • Offer choices of interventions to complete during therapy. • Offer choices of the order of activities during therapy.

Adapted from Derigo, D., Russell, D., & Berg, C. (2018). *A trauma-informed approach distinct to occupational therapy: The TIC-OT model* [Webinar]. American Occupational Therapy Association (Producer). https://myaota.aota.org/shop_aota/product/OL5140

Table 13-4

Application of a TIC-OT Model Principle: The 4 Rs	
TIC-OT Model Principle	OT Applications and Examples of Use to Support Adaptation, Coping, and Resilience of Children Who Have Encountered ACEs
The 4 Rs (SAMHSA, 2014)	
Realize	• Observe escalated emotions/behaviors through a trauma-informed lens, leading to deeper empathy and understanding and identification of the source of the behavior. • Attend trainings on trauma-informed care in your practice setting or community.
Recognize	• Advocate for the health care team to routinely screen/assess clients for trauma. • Interpret assessment results with a trauma-informed lens (may explain seemingly "unexplainable" results; may have increased anxiety, distractibility, which could lead to a decreased performance).
Respond	• Provide emotional support and coping resources to the family. • Emphasize continuity of care and collaboration among providers. • Refer to appropriate services (e.g., psychologist, social worker). • Provide intervention as appropriate if trauma is affecting ability to participate in occupations.
Resist	• Work to minimize potential triggers, such as self-care activities (e.g., showering, dressing, toileting/diapering), touching the client without asking, standing in close proximity to the client. • Respond to trauma disclosures appropriately (avoid invasive questions, actively listen, and provide emotional support and resources).

Adapted from Derigo, D., Russell, D., & Berg, C. (2018). *A trauma-informed approach distinct to occupational therapy: The TIC-OT model* [Webinar]. American Occupational Therapy Association (Producer). https://myaota.aota.org/shop_aota/product/OL5140

COLLABORATIVE APPROACH WITH FAMILIES AND THE SOCIAL ENVIRONMENT

It is essential that occupational therapy providers working with children and youth who have encountered ACEs use a trauma-informed approach to guide the occupational

Table 13-5

TIC-OT Model: A Shift in Perspective	
Traditional Paradigm Perspective	Trauma-Informed Paradigm Perspective
The client is not compliant with the home program.	I wonder what challenges the client is facing that prevent follow-through with the home program.
That child's behavior is terrible.	I wonder what is going on that is triggering these challenging behaviors.
The client seems lazy.	What can I do to motivate the client?
The client is in this position because of poor choices.	What barriers has the client faced throughout life?

therapy process and foster collaboration with clients and their families. Although occupational therapy is grounded in principles of client-centeredness, there are challenges with applying existing models of client-centeredness to children and youth who have encountered ACEs and their families (Pitonyak et al., 2015). Specifically, dominant theories guiding the occupational therapy process are rooted in predominantly Western, white, middle-class values and may not fully foster collaboration with individuals with diverse identities and experiences (Hammell, 2013; Pitonyak et al., 2015), nor take into consideration how policy and other contextual factors perpetuate disparities in access to services and occupational participation (Pitonyak et al., 2020). Therefore, a trauma-informed approach seeks to establish a social environment for service delivery that integrates trauma-informed principles into the organizational culture, building adaptation, coping, and resilience for clients and their families.

As previously introduced, the occupational therapy approach to assessment and intervention should reflect the assumptions and principles of trauma-informed care established by SAMHSA (2014). When collaborating with families, the occupational therapy practitioner must create a safe social environment constructed according to the six key principles of a trauma-informed approach: safety; trustworthiness and transparency; peer support; collaboration and mutuality; empowerment, voice, and choice; and cultural, historical, and gender issues (SAMHSA, 2014). Occupational therapy providers can use these principles to enhance client-centered care and collaboration with families. The principles, when integrated into practice, provide a pathway to adaptation, coping, and resilience. For example, the principle of safety may help guide professional reasoning about how to set up an intervention environment, by taking into consideration that the occupational therapy provider does not position themselves between the client and the door, which could be misperceived as blocking the exit. Further, the principle of attending to cultural, historical, and gender issues, when applied by occupational therapy providers, may include clarifying relationships of family members to the client (e.g., grandparent or foster parent), and addressing all present with names and pronouns that reflect their identity.

Table 13-6

Example Assessments for Measuring the Impact of Trauma on Performance		
Measure	Population	Description
Perceived Stress Scale (PSS; Cohen & Williamson, 1988)	Adult	A short measure used to identify perceived stress within the past month
NIH Toolbox Cognition Battery (Health Measures, 2020)	Persons 3+ years of age	Battery of cognitive assessments measuring attention, memory, etc.
The Sensory Profile 2 (Dunn, 2014)	Persons birth to 15 years of age	Assessment of sensory processing patterns in children
Peabody Developmental Motor Scales, Second Edition (PDMS-2; Folio & Fewell, 2000)	Persons birth to 5 years of age	Assessment of motor function
Bruininks-Oseretsky Test of Motor Proficiency, Second Edition (BOT-2; Bruininks & Bruininks, 2005)	Persons 4 to 21 years of age	Assessment of motor function
The Paediatric Activity Card Sort (PACS; Mandich et al., 2004)	Persons 5 to 14 years of age	Assessment of occupational performance and participation in typical childhood routines
Canadian Occupational Performance Measure (COPM; Law & Canadian Association of Occupational Therapists, 2017)	Adult	Assesses occupational profile
NIH Toolbox: Adult Social Relationship Scales (Cyranowski et al., 2013)	Adult	Used to measure various types of social support (e.g., emotional, information) companionship, and satisfaction
Iowa Cultural Understanding Assessment (SAMHSA, 2014)	Adult	A measure given to clients that rates their perception of culturally responsive care within an organization

BUILDING INTERPROFESSIONAL COLLABORATIONS

Children and youth who have experienced adverse life experiences may receive health and/or social services from a variety of providers. They also want to participate in occupations similar to those of their same-aged peers across school, civic, religious, and other community settings, which means that teachers, coaches, scouting leaders, and other adults in the lives of children and youth who have had adverse life experiences need an awareness and understanding of trauma and how it affects adaptation and coping.

Occupational therapy providers can assist with prioritizing consistency in approaches across settings through consultation and other interventions (Swinth & Pitonyak, 2021).

Knowing the importance of a trauma-informed approach in fostering collaboration with children and youth who have had adverse experiences and their families, occupational therapy providers can engage in interprofessional collaborations to provide trauma-informed care. Team collaboration, whether in a health care, school, or other community setting, ensures that children and youth who have had adverse experiences receive consistent, trauma-informed care across providers and environments.

Occupational therapy providers may take on varied roles and use various approaches— *promotion, prevention,* and *intensive intervention*—depending on the setting and individual, group, or population-level needs related to trauma (AOTA, 2019). For example, evidence-informed programs and curricula that occupational therapy providers may use to support the needs of children and youth who have had adverse experiences include intervention approaches such as education and advocacy. Every Moment Counts (EMC) is a mental health promotion initiative focused on child and youth mental health in schools and the community. Occupational therapy providers serve as consultants to key school personnel, providing embedded programs and strategies that promote child and youth mental health. Occupational therapy providers may consult with the school personnel who staff the playground and cafeteria to educate them about strategies that children and youth can use to cope with challenging social situations in these settings. Resources for implementing EMC are available to practitioners via the EMC website (EMC, n.d.) Other programs and interventions for interprofessional collaboration require continuing education or advanced training prior to use in practice. Promoting First Relationships (PFR) is a curriculum that can be used by occupational therapy providers collaborating with caregivers and other interdisciplinary team members to enhance their awareness of their responses to the behaviors of children and youth who have had adverse experiences (Kelly et al., 2008). Trust-based Relational Intervention® (TBRI) is an attachment-based, trauma-informed intervention that is designed to meet the complex needs of children who have experienced ACEs (Purvis et al., 2013) and requires intensive, advanced training for safe and effective practitioner use.

A GLOBAL PERSPECTIVE

Poverty is a global adverse childhood experience that may place children and youth in a life trajectory of exposures to other forms of adversity, trauma, and abuse. Worldwide, approximately 1.2 billion people live in extreme poverty, which the World Health Organization (WHO) defines as income of less than one dollar per day (WHO, 2021). Situations of poverty and related adversity vary widely from country to country depending on the sociopolitical climate and whether children and youth are exposed to conflict and war, human trafficking, or other factors that may lead to displacement. Several seminal works have brought attention to the potential roles of occupational therapy worldwide with children and youth who have experienced trauma, violence, abuse, and other adverse experiences, and provide a foundation for establishing occupational therapy approaches that build adaptation, coping, and resilience.

The text, titled *Occupational Therapy Without Borders: Learning from the Spirit of Survivors,* was first published in 2005 and shares international examples of the role of occupational therapy with people who endure chronic adversity which leads to marginalization and social exclusion (Kronenberg et al., 2005). In the first edition of this text, Kronenberg (2005) shared his experiences working with street children in Mexico and Guatemala. The occupational therapy approach that Kronenberg (2005, p. 264) described aligns well with theoretical principles for building adaptation, coping, and resilience, and included building a sense of belonging; listening, in order to enable the client to express feelings and share experiences; and collaborating with the client to establish new routines related to their goals. Specific intervention activities for these approaches included dance, graffiti, puppetry, journalism, photography, toy-making, and public performances—among other activities of personal meaning to the street children. A global perspective on the role of occupational therapy with children and youth who have encountered ACEs should reflect the principles of trauma-informed care (SAMHSA, 2014) by incorporating assessments and creating interventions that honor voice and choice and reflect cultural and historical contexts.

ESSENTIAL CONSIDERATIONS FOR OCCUPATIONAL THERAPISTS

Occupational therapy practitioners are uniquely qualified to address the occupational disruption caused by trauma, be it acute, chronic, or complex in nature. To best equip occupational therapy practitioners to address trauma, practitioners must seek advanced practice content and continued professional development on the topic through conferences, journal clubs, book studies, professional discussions, and other specialized training opportunities. Although occupational therapy practitioners may, by the nature of their profession, be equipped to provide promotion-level intervention (such as raising awareness about the impact of trauma) or prevention-level intervention (such as recognizing trauma or implementing positive behavior supports), best-practice guidelines suggest that for intensive-level intervention (such as specific intervention programs that collaborate with additional mental health professionals), advanced-level supplemental training should be obtained (Petrenchik & Weiss, 2015). In addition, examining one's own biases and abilities is an important step in preparing for the ongoing use of a trauma-informed lens. An occupational therapist might benefit from taking the Ethnic Sensitivity Inventory (SAMHSA, 2014), which is a measure that therapists can self-administer to assess their own cultural awareness. Ongoing self-assessment and reflection, combined with advanced-level professional development and mentored occupational therapy practice, supports one's commitment to the lifelong learning that is required for trauma-informed occupational therapy practice. Utilizing resources provided through membership in the American Occupational Therapy Association, as well as state-level associations, can enhance practice and provide evidence-based information and communities of support as practitioners seek continued training to address trauma in clients across the lifespan. See Table 13-7 for key considerations for occupational therapy practitioners.

Table 13-7

Key Considerations for Occupational Therapy Practitioners	
General Considerations for Occupational Therapy Practice	• Recognize signs of trauma • Create safe environments that support learning and development • Minimize traumatic experiences of the client • Support client engagement in therapy • Build a stronger therapeutic relationship • Help reduce effects of trauma • Provide compassion and care for clients (Derigo et al., 2018)
Advanced-Training Considerations for Occupational Therapy Practice	• Treat children who have experienced trauma • Collaborate to model and facilitate skills for managing emotions for the adults who serve children who are survivors of trauma • Collaborate with children who are survivors of trauma and the adults who serve them to develop skills and techniques to safely and proactively avoid crises • Develop reactive strategies to safely work through crisis situations to minimize additional trauma (Petrenchik & Weiss, 2015)

Although the notion of ACEs focuses on trauma during childhood, it is important to note that the manifestation of trauma may not surface until adulthood. As noted in the description of Ana's case earlier in this chapter, the experience of trauma throughout Ana's childhood and into early adulthood may induce occupational disruption well into her middle to late adulthood, thus also affecting her child, Issac. Occupational therapy practice through a trauma-informed lens that is mutually beneficial through the lifespan may include, but is not limited to:

- Establishing predictability in routine and environment
- Allowing choice in activities
- Pairing sensory-based activities with cognitive behavioral activities for calming
- Implementing stress-management strategies
- Empowering clients and families through collaborative goals and activities (Petrenchik & Weiss, 2015)

Implementation of the occupational therapy process, across environments, through a trauma-informed lens advances the occupational therapy profession while mutually benefiting the clients served.

Case Study 13-1 Continuation
Resilience in Children of Hope

Ana's own experience with ACEs and the resilience she found by focusing on the occupation of rearing Isaac fostered her continued adaptive capacity in her new life. She continued to participate in a family mental health program led by an occupational therapist at her neighborhood community health center. The organizational culture of the community health center and the approach of the occupational therapy practitioner reflected essential considerations of best practices with children and youth who have encountered ACEs. The occupational therapy program for family mental health was embedded in a neighborhood community health center that worked to create a physical and social environment that respected and represented the Hispanic and Latinx ethnicity and culture of the majority population in the neighborhood. Spanish-language interpretation was available for all services and occupational therapy intervention activities incorporated cultural traditions and celebrations. When Ana first began attending the family mental health program, the occupational therapy practitioner confirmed how to pronounce Ana's and Issac's names and invited them to create a name plate with their pronouns. The group activities often included developmental play on the floor, so the name plate could be set up in front of each parent–child dyad, thereby avoiding the use of nametags that adhere to the chest and could trigger uncomfortable interactions due to gazing at the chest to read participant names. The occupational therapy practitioner further set up the environment with safety in mind given the participants' history of ACEs. The participants were always positioned to allow them full view of the door in order to see who entered the room, and the door was left open. Ana appreciated that the occupational therapy practitioner was always clear and transparent about the plan for each group session and asked participants to suggest topics for discussion. Although the occupational therapy practitioner provided a variety of resources and strategies for child-rearing, Ana loved the opportunity to share her parenting experiences with other participants and developed supportive peer relationships with two other women who had experienced trafficking in their pasts. Continued participation in the family mental health program further supported Ana's resilience by adding to her identity as a caring parent and knowledgeable childcare provider.

REFERENCES

American Occupational Therapy Association. (2019). School mental health toolkit. https://www.aota.org/Practice/Children-Youth/Mental%20Health/School-Mental-Health.aspx

American Psychiatric Association. (2013). *Diagnostic and statistical manual of mental disorders* (5th ed.). Author. https://dsm.psychiatryonline.org/doi/book/10.1176/appi.books.9780890425596

Berg, A. (2016). The importance of the first 1,000 days of life. *Journal of Child and Adolescent Mental Health, 28*(2), 4. https://doi.org/10.2989/17280583.2016.1223803

Bethell, C. D., Solloway, M. R., Guinosso, S., Hassink, S., Srivastav, A., Ford, D., & Simpson, L. A. (2017). Prioritizing possibilities for child and family health: An agenda to address adverse childhood experiences and foster the social and emotional roots of well-being in pediatrics. *Academic Pediatrics, 17*(7 Suppl.), S36-S50. https://doi.org/10.1016/j.acap.2017.06.002

Bright, M. A., Thompson, L., Esernio-Jenssen, D., Alford, S., & Shenkman, E. (2015). Primary care pediatricians' perceived prevalence and surveillance of adverse childhood experiences in low-income children. *Journal of Health Care for the Poor and Underserved, 26*(3), 686-700. https://doi.org/10.1353/hpu.2015.0080

Bruininks, R. H., & Bruininks, B. D. (2005). *Bruininks–Oseretsky test of motor proficiency* (2nd ed.). Pearson Assessment.

Carter, P., Boustead, R., & Joseph, G. (2016). *Creating a trauma responsive Missouri.* Missouri Department of Mental Health.

Centers for Disease Control and Prevention. (2020). Preventing adverse childhood experiences. https://www.cdc.gov/violenceprevention/childabuseandneglect/aces/fastfact.html

Child Welfare Information Gateway. (2015). Understanding the effects of maltreatment on brain development. https://www.childwelfare.gov/pubPDFs/brain_development.pdf

Christiansen, C. H., Baum, C. M., & Bass, J. (2015). *Occupational therapy: Performance, participation and well-being, 4rd edition.* SLACK Incorporated.

Chung, E. K., Siegel, B. S., Garg, A., Conroy, K., Gross, R. S., Long, D. A., Lewis, G., Osman, C. J., Messito, M. J., Wade Jr., R., Yin, H. S., Cox, J., & Fierman, A. H. (2016). Screening for social determinants of health among children and families living in poverty: A guide for clinicians. *Current Problems in Pediatrics and Adolescent Health Care, 46*(5), 135-153. https://doi.org/10.1016/j.cppeds.2016.02.004

Cohen, S., & Williamson, G. (1988). Perceived stress in a probability sample of the United States. In S. Spacapam & S. Oskamp (Eds.), *The social psychology of health* (pp. 31-67). Sage.

Community Resilience Initiative. (2017). Community Resilience Initiative. https://criresilient.org

Compas, B. E., Connor-Smith, J. K., Saltzman, H., Thomsen, A. H., & Wadsworth, M. E. (2001). Coping with stress during childhood and adolescence: Problems, progress, and potential in theory and research. *Psychological Bulletin, 127*(1), 87-127. https://doi.org/10.1037//0033-2909.127.1.87

Cyranowski, J. M., Zill, N., Bode, R., Butt, Z., Kelly, M. A., Pilkonis, P. A., Salsman, J. M., & Cella, D. (2013). Assessing social support, companionship, and distress: National Institute of Health (NIH) Toolbox Adult Social Relationship Scales. *Health Psychology, 32*(3), 293-301. https://doi.org/10.1037/a0028586

Derigo, D., Russell, D., & Berg, C. (2018). *A trauma-informed approach distinct to occupational therapy: The TIC-OT model* [Webinar]. American Occupational Therapy Association (Producer). https://myaota.aota.org/shop_aota/product/OL5140

Dunn, W. (2014). *Sensory Profile 2 manual.* Pearson.

Edwards, V. J., Anda, R. F., Dube, S. R., Dong, M., Chapman, D. F., & Felitti, V. J. (2005). The wide-ranging health consequences of adverse childhood experiences. In K. A. Kendall-Tackett & S. M. Giacomoni (Eds.), *Child victimization: Maltreatment, bullying, and dating violence prevention and intervention* (pp. 8-1-8-12). Civic Research Institute.

Every Moment Counts. (n. d.). Model programs and toolkits. https://everymomentcounts.org

Feder Ostrov, B. (2020, January 7). 5 things to know as California starts screening children for toxic stress. https://californiahealthline.org/news/5-things-to-know-as-california-starts-screening-children-for-toxic-stress

Felitti, V. J. (2009). Adverse childhood experiences and adult health. *Academic Pediatrics, 9*(3), 131-132. https://doi.org/10.1016/j.acap.2009.03.001

Felitti, V. J., Anda, R. F., Nordenberg, D., Williamson, D. F., Spitz, A. M., Edwards, V., Koss, M. P., & Marks, J. S. (1998). Relationship of childhood abuse and household dysfunction to many of the leading causes of death in adults: The Adverse Childhood Experiences (ACE) study. *American Journal of Preventive Medicine, 14*(4), 245-258. https://doi.org/10.1016/s0749-3797(98)00017-8

Folio, M., & Fewell, R. (2000). *Peabody Developmental Motor Scales—Second Edition (PDMS-2): Examiner's manual.* Pro-Ed.

Grajo, L. (2019). Occupational adaptation as a normative and intervention process: Schkade and Schultz's legacy. In L. C. Grajo & A. Boisselle (Eds.), *Adaptation through occupation: Multidimensional perspectives.* SLACK Incorporated.

Green, J. G., McLaughlin, K. A., Berglund, P. A., Gruber, M. J., Sampson, N. A., Zaslavsky, A. M., & Kessler, R. C. (2010). Childhood adversities and adult psychiatric disorders in the national comorbidity survey replication I: Associations with first onset of DSM-IV disorders. *Archives of General Psychiatry, 67*(2), 113-123. https://doi.org/10.1001/archgenpsychiatry.2009.186

Gronski, M. P., Bogan, K. E., Kloeckner, J., Russell-Thomas, D., Taff, S. D., Walker, K. A., & Berg, C. (2013). Childhood toxic stress: A community role in health promotion for occupational therapists. *American Journal of Occupational Therapy, 67*(6), e148-e153. https://doi.org/10.5014/ajot.2013.008755

Hammell, K. R. W. (2013). Client-centred practice in occupational therapy: Critical reflections. *Scandinavian Journal of Occupational Therapy, 20*(3), 174-81. https://doi.org/10.3109/11038128.2012.752032

Health Measures. (2020). NIH toolbox cognition batteries. http://www.healthmeasures.net/explore-measurement-systems/nih-toolbox/intro-to-nih-toolbox/cognition

Hopper, E. K., Bassuk, E. L., & Olivet, J. (2010). Shelter from the storm: Trauma-informed care in homelessness services settings. *The Open Health Services and Policy Journal, 3*(2), 80-100. https://doi.org/10.2174/1874924001003020080

Jimenez, M. E., Wade, R., Lin, Y., Morrow, L. M., Reichman, N. E. (2016). Adverse experiences in early childhood and kindergarten outcomes. *Pediatrics, 137*(2): e20151839. https://doi.org/10.1542/peds.2015-1839

Kelly, J. F., Zuckerman, T., Sandoval, D., & Buehlman, K. (2008). *Promoting first relationships* (2nd ed.). NCAST-AVENUW Publications.

Kronenberg, F. (2005). Occupational therapy with street children. In F. Kronenberg, S. S. Algado, & N. Pollard (Eds.), *Occupational therapy without borders: Learning from the spirit of survivors* (pp. 261-276). Elsevier.

Kronenberg, F., Algado, S. S., & Pollard, N. (Eds.). (2005). *Occupational therapy without borders: Learning from the spirit of survivors.* Elsevier.

Law, M., & Canadian Association of Occupational Therapists. (1991). *Canadian occupational performance measure.* CAOT = ACE.

Mandich, A., Polatajko, H. J., Miller, L., & Baum, C. (2004). *The paediatric activity card sort.* The Canadian Association of Occupational Therapists. CAOT = ACE.

Marsac, M. L., Kassam-Adams, N., Hildenbrand, A. K., Nicholls, E., Winston, F. K., Leff, S. S., & Fein, J. (2016). Implementing a trauma-informed approach in pediatric health care networks. *JAMA Pediatrics, 170*(1), 70-77. https://doi.org/10.1001/jamapediatrics.2015.2206

National Child Traumatic Stress Network Schools Committee. (2008). *Child trauma toolkit for educators.* National Center for Child Traumatic Stress.

National Scientific Council on the Developing Child. (2015). Supportive relationships and active skill-building strengthen the foundations of resilience: working paper 13. http://www.developingchild.harvard.edu

Oostlander, S. A., Falla, J. A., Dow, K., & Fucile, S. (2019). Occupational therapy management strategies for infants with neonatal abstinence syndrome: Scoping review. *Occupational Therapy in Health Care, 33*(2), 197-226. https://doi.org/10.1080/07380577.2019.1594485

Perfect, M., Turley, M., Carlson, J. S., Yohanna, J., & Saint Gilles, M. P. (2016). School-related outcomes of traumatic event exposure and traumatic stress symptoms in students: A systematic review of research from 1990 to 2015. *School Mental Health, 8*, 7-43.. https://doi.org/10.1007/s12310-016-9175-2

Petrenchik, T., & Weiss, D. (2015). Childhood trauma. American Occupational Therapy Association. https://www.aota.org/~/media/Corporate/Files/Practice/Children/Childhood-Trauma-Info-Sheet-2015.pdf

Pitonyak, J. S., Gupta, J., & Pergolotti, M. (2020). Health policy perspectives—Understanding policy influences on health and occupation through the use of the life course health development (LCHD) framework. *American Journal of Occupational Therapy, 74*(2), 7402090010. https://doi.org/10.5014/ajot.2020.742002

Pitonyak, J. S., Mroz, T. M., & Fogelberg, D. (2015). Expanding client-centred thinking to include social determinants: A practical scenario based on the occupation of breastfeeding. *Scandinavian Journal of Occupational Therapy, 22*(4), 277-282. https://doi.org/10.3109/11038128.2015.1020865

Purvis, K. B., Cross, D. R., Dansereau, D. F., & Parris, S. R. (2013). Trust-Based Relational Intervention (TBRI): A systemic approach to complex developmental trauma. *Child & Youth Services, 34*(4), 360-386. http://doi.org/10.1080/0145935X.2013.859906

Schkade, J., & Schultz, S. (2003). Occupational adaptation. In J. Hinojosa & P. Kramer (Eds.), *Perspectives in human occupation*. Lippincott Williams & Wilkins.

Soleimanpour, S., Geierstanger, S., & Brindis, C. D. (2017). Adverse childhood experiences and resilience: Addressing the unique needs of adolescents. *Academic Pediatrics, 17*(7), S108-S114. https://doi.org/10.1016/j.acap.2017.01.008

Srivastav, A., Strompolis, M., Moseley, A., & Daniels, K. (2019). The Empower Action Model: A framework for preventing adverse childhood experiences by promoting health, equity, and well-being across the life span. *Health Promotion Practice, 21*(4), 525-534. https://doi.org/10.1177/1524839919889355

Substance Abuse and Mental Health Services Administration. (2014). SAMHSA's concept of trauma and guidance for a trauma-informed approach (HHS Publication No. (SMA) 14-4884). Substance Abuse and Mental Health Services Administration.

Swinth, Y., & Pitonyak, J. S. (2021). Children with prenatal substance exposure and post-natal trauma. In G. F. Clark & S. Parks (Eds.), *Best practices for occupational therapy in early childhood*. AOTA Press.

U.S. Department of Health & Human Services (HHS), Administration for Children and Families, Administration on Children, Youth and Families, & Children's Bureau. (2020). Child maltreatment 2018. https://www.acf.hhs.gov/cb/research-data-technology/statistics-research/child-maltreatment

van der Kolk, B. A. (2005). Developmental trauma disorder: Toward a rational diagnosis for children with complex trauma histories. *Psychiatric Annals, 35*(5), 401-408. https://doi.org/10.3928/00485713-20050501-06

World Health Organization. (2021).Social determinants of health. https://www.who.int/teams/social-determinants-of-health

14

Children of Migrant Farmworkers

Debra Rybski, MSHCA, PhD, OTR/L and
Kathleen Kauper, MOT, OTR/L

CHAPTER OBJECTIVES By the end of this chapter the reader will be able to understand:
- The sociocultural experience of children of migrant farmworkers.
- The occupational performance strengths and challenges of children of migrant farmworkers.
- The occupational therapy assessment and intervention strategies to address occupational performance adaptation, coping, and resilience in children of migrant farmworkers.

OVERVIEW OF THE POPULATION

Migrant farmworkers do essential work in many regions across the United States. A majority of migrant farmworkers work in southern and coastal regions (Free & Križ, 2016). Migrant farmworkers leave their permanent places of residence such as Mexico and or Central America and move to a country or state where they provide seasonal work (Kupersmidt & Martin, 1997). Most migrant work is agricultural; thus, most migrant farmworkers are referred to as *agricultural workers* or *mobile workers* (Migrant Clinician Network [MCN], 2020). Migrant farmworkers may move across international borders or between states within the United States' borders. The U.S. Department of Agriculture estimates that there are between 1 and 2.7 million hired farmworkers in the United States, which includes migrant farmworkers (Markowitz & Cosminsky, 2005).

It is estimated that approximately half of all farmworkers are parents with minor children (MCN, 2020). Many farmworkers travel year-round as they move back and

Grajo L. C., & Boisselle, A. K. (Eds.). *Adaptation, Coping,*
and Resilience in Children and Youth: A Comprehensive
Occupational Therapy Approach (pp. 337-359).

forth across the border or from state to state (Kupersmidt & Martin, 1997). Many farm-workers bring their families, including children, with them when they travel from state to state or region to region (Kupersmidt & Martin, 1997). Some migrant farmworkers may be unaccompanied minors (MCN, 2020) who travel across the border for work and to escape violence and gang persecution in their country of origin.

There are an estimated 1 million migrant/mobile children in the United States (Kim, 2020). Despite the desire of families to provide a good education for their children, many families must have high-school and even middle-school children work in the fields in the fall, spring, and summer. This farm work keeps children from attending school. Migrant children typically start farm work at age 14 and may work year-round. Middle-school-age children start work in the summer and are less likely to work year-round. Elementary-school children will likely attend school in the community where their families work. Children must attend multiple schools in different geographic locations as their parents travel seasonally for work throughout the year. They attend school in northern locations in late spring, summer, and early fall, and will attend school in southern locations in the winter. A parent's frequent moves for work require children to change schools frequently, making it difficult to maintain the health and vaccination records necessary for ongoing health checks (Kroening & Dawson-Hahn, 2019). Missing health records may interfere with access to education. Migrant students' school records may not be complete or may be lost during seasonal travel.

Despite parents' desire for their children to get a good education, many families may need middle- and high-school children to work in the fields during the planting or harvest seasons; this keeps their children from attending school. Many children strug-gle to complete school when families move from state to state to do seasonal work, as this requires students to attend different schools throughout the year. Infants and young children are cared for by mothers, grandmothers, or local community childcare (which is usually scarce, if it is available at all; MCN, 2020). In recent years, more landowners have begun to provide childcare for the infants and young children of those who work on their farms (American Academy of Pediatrics, 2005). This provides opportunities for mothers as well as fathers and age-appropriate children to work in the fields; this may be financially necessary but may not be advantageous for child development.

Social determinants of health are critical components of everyday life that support healthy living and are necessary for all children's health (Shonkoff, 2019). Such essential determinants include nutritious food, steady housing, clean water, sanitation, a safe sur-rounding environment, access to health care, childcare, education, and economic stabil-ity. These health-related social determinants can be difficult to access for many migrant working families (Lu, 2015), resulting in critical health risks for children of farmworkers who are mobile and even worse for school-age child workers. Migrant children expe-rience health risks as a result of food insecurity, poor and or crowded housing, and environmental and occupational exposures such as pesticides, heat and sun, dust, and zoonosis (American Academy of Pediatrics, 2005).

In addition, children also face health risks when living in farm environments, as numerous pieces of equipment are dangerous to child farmworkers. Farms typically do not offer many safe areas where children can engage in outdoor play and gross motor activities. The chances of injury and even death increase significantly when children play on and with unsafe farm tools and equipment, on unsafe outdoor structures, and in ponds (Sandra et al., 1995). Violence in farm-working communities is also a risk for children—not only for them to observe but also to experience. These traumatic experiences can leave young children with post-traumatic stress disorder (PTSD) and difficulty coping in home, school, and migrant farm-work environments (Sandra et al., 1995).

Parents' need to move for work makes it difficult to maintain children's health and vaccination records, which are necessary for ongoing health checks (Kroening & Dawson-Hahn, 2019). Access to education may be difficult. School records may not be complete or may have been lost in seasonal travel. As noted earlier, many families have middle- and high-school-age children work in the fields in the fall and spring rather than attend school. Many children, thus, struggle with disruptive or incomplete schooling when families move from region to region and state to state to work. Table 14-1 presents an occupational profile highlighting migrant children's strengths and challenges and highlights important physical, social, emotional, and educational factors affecting children and families.

Occupational therapy addresses occupational performance across multiple aspects of children's lives. With migrant children, occupational performance addresses daily living self-care, eating/feeding, sleeping, school, work across seasons in fields, chores, play, and religious and other community activities. It includes moves from one seasonal work site to another. Disruptions in any area of occupational performance can be addressed by an occupational therapist in the requisite environment, whether that is home, school, worksite, play areas, or places of worship in the community. Occupational therapy in schools can help children adjust to new schools. Occupational therapists can identify learning, social skills, and behavior challenges in children who demonstrate learning delays (Gothro et al., 2020). In the local community, occupational therapists can provide support to families whose children engage in agricultural work. This support may include safety recommendations and work adaptations for children (National Children's Center for Rural Agricultural Health and Safety & National Farm Medicine Center, 2020).

Adaptation, Coping, and Resilience in Children of Migrant Farmworkers

Health and well-being in children are essential for children's present and future adaptive performance, coping under stress, and building resilience in healthy occupational performance for productive living. Children learn adaptation skills through interacting with the environment in occupations that require change and facilitate personal growth (Grajo, 2019). Children develop coping skills by modifying their cognitive and behavioral responses to challenging tasks or demands (Compas et al., 2001). Children expand their resilience—their adaptive capacity to face adversity such as environmental or interpersonal stress or trauma—through developing intrapersonal capacity with interpersonal supports (Shonkoff, 2019).

Children of migrant farmworkers are likely to face challenges of adaptation, coping, and resilience in everyday life as a result of travel, unstable housing, environmental hazards, inconsistent schooling, and (depending on their age) participating with their

Table 14-1

Occupational Profile: Strengths and Challenges of Migrant Children	
Strengths of Migrant Children	**Challenges Facing Migrant Children**
Adaptable	• Low family income
Hard-working	• Parental long working hours
Education focused	• Multiple annual family moves that interrupt and negatively affect children's educational and social development (Taylor & Ruiz, 2017)
Strong family connections and support	• Inadequate farmworker family housing • Detrimental environmental exposures: lead paint, poor water, sanitation, rodents and insects • Migrant child self-reported loneliness, economic hassles, discrimination (Taylor & Ruiz, 2017) • Teacher-reported child anxiety and depression (Taylor & Ruiz, 2017) • Environmental exposures in and around farmworker fields pose health risks • Occupational exposures and injuries in and around farmworker fields pose health risks • Exposure to violence in migrant farmworker housing poses child physical and psychological risks • Under- and overvaccination due to farmworker family migration for seasonal work • Inconsistent school attendance due to family migration for seasonal work interferes with children's advancement in school • School cultural and language barriers interfere with children's advancement in school

parents in seasonal agricultural work (Figure 14-1). These transitions in activities of everyday living can create challenges to physical, social, and emotional skills (Taylor & Ruiz, 2017) at school, at home, and in the broader community. Occupational challenges of this population can also raise transition change barriers; that is, factors that may impede the adaptation, coping, and resilience necessary for healthy and productive living (Grajo, 2019). Migrant children are at greater risk of facing challenges in adaptation, coping, and resilience than are children who have a stable family and permanent home, school, and community. Migrant children face increased risks of disease, infectious illness, and injuries when housing is unavailable or unsanitary, and are at greater risk for injuries, environmental disease, and infectious illnesses as a result of working on a farm.

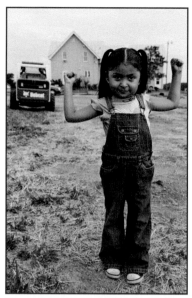

Figure 14-1. Little girl living with farm-worker family. (© www.earldotter.com.)

Migrant children are at risk for not achieving their academic potential because of their frequent school changes as their families move for work, and because some must work to provide family income rather than attend school. Missing school and having to adjust to numerous new schools in a year make learning more difficult and children may fall behind. All these circumstances and factors present significant challenges for the health, education, well-being, and adaptation, coping, and resilience of migrant children, which are not present for children who experience consistent educational opportunities and stable housing that meet their physical and psychological health needs. The following cases illustrate these concerns regarding the adaptation, coping, resilience, and needs of migrant children.

ROLE OF OCCUPATIONAL THERAPY BEST AND EVIDENCE-BASED PRACTICES FOR ASSESSMENT AND INTERVENTION

Occupational therapists aim to aid clients by administering assessment tools and practices specifically selected for each individual. Occupational therapists aid clients with the use of everyday activities for the purpose of enhancing or enabling participation in roles, habits, and routines (AOTA, 2020). It is the goal of the occupational therapist to promote health, well-being, and participation. Occupational therapists provide client-centered care to ensure that personal and meaningful therapy approaches are applied.

Short Case

Hand Injury

Luis is a 9-year-old boy whose family moved to the United States from Mexico. His family now travels between northern California and Florida to take seasonal farm work. Although his family is better off when working the farms, his parents still struggle to put food on the table and access medical care. While harvesting wheat, Luis fell from a wagon and injured his hand, with a break in the metacarpal bone of the index finger of his dominant hand. This injury affects Luis's pincer grasp and limits his abilities to pick in the field. In addition, the break prohibits him from lifting necessary farming equipment and reduces the productivity of the harvest. Luis is also experiencing pain during activities that require movement of the hand, such as showering, brushing his teeth, and getting dressed each day. His lack of productivity on the farm and loss of independence with activities of daily living are causing Luis to feel worthless. He longs to return to helping his family on the farm in order to improve their financial situation. Although Luis is young, he is aware that without the harvest, there will not be enough money for his family to eat or for him to visit the doctor to get his hand fixed.

Migrant children often face unique challenges due to moving from their home country to a new living situation, work conditions, obligations, language barrier, and family responsibilities. These travel experiences can be traumatic and difficult for the entire family, especially the children. Occupational therapists provide therapy for migrant children in schools, in primary and private practices, and in grant-supported community summer programs. Occupational therapists incorporate a trauma-informed care approach (Granado-Villar et al., 2013) with all families they meet in school or community clinical settings for initial family interviews, and in follow-up occupational therapy interventions to address any traumatic episodes that families—and in particular children—have endured during their travels and their migrant work experiences.

Occupational therapists may aid children with the development of adaptive capacity by introducing them to aspects of the new culture in which they may find meaning and, thus, build new health-promoting repertoires of occupational routines and rituals in their new communities. Building an occupational profile for the child and utilizing a client-centered approach allows the occupational therapist to assist children with choosing activities that they will find meaningful. Once engaged in something they find important, children will be able to connect more easily with their surroundings and participate in the new culture. Children are generally resilient, and their minds embrace learning, so occupational therapists can assist children to develop adaptive capacity. Occupational therapists are able to see adaptation, coping, and resilience in a child by their increased participation in new activities. When a child feels disconnected from the environment, they feel like an outlier and often withdraw from activities, such as school, social participation, and play. As a child adapts and copes, they begin to feel more connected and increases participation levels.

Short Case
School

Petra is a bright 7-year-old girl who recently moved to the United States from Mexico (Figure 14-2). At her previous school, she had many friends and flourished in both academics and social interactions. In her previous school, she primarily spoke Spanish but she has some background in the English language from class. She is currently one semester into the second grade at an English-speaking school. Although Petra tries her best to understand the material taught in class, she always feels behind. It takes her a while to process what the teachers are trying to tell her before she can understand the meaning of the new material. Due to poor performance on quizzes and the language barriers, Petra has low self-esteem. This low self-esteem is carrying over into her social interactions. She has trouble connecting with the new students, and her teachers notice that Petra avoids social interactions and is beginning to withdraw into herself in the classroom. After working with an occupational therapist, Petra is better able to adapt to her new culture by finding meaning in the current activities around her. The occupational therapist works with Petra on increasing confidence in the classroom and with peers to help her cope and adapt to her new academic and social life.

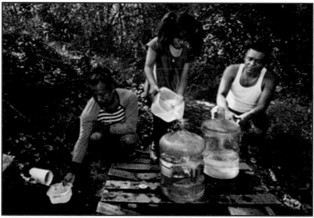

Figure 14-2. Petra collecting water with her family. (© www.earldotter.com.)

Occupational therapists can assist migrant children maintain their cultural identity and help them shape a new identity in the country where their families have moved for work. Nevertheless, these many major life changes can cause stress, confusion, and discomfort for migrant children and their families. Occupational therapists can assess and address adaptation, coping, and resilience to aid this population in finding meaning in their new culture while also maintaining their sense of identity through their cultural heritage (Tables 14-2 and 14-3). For example, if a child was involved with dance in their

Table 14-2

Assessments

Assessments for Building Functional Cognition, Metacognition, and Executive Function

WeeFIM (Granger & McCabe, 1987)	The WeeFIM is a measure used for functional performance with children 6 months to 8 years of age. A 7-point scale is used to assess independence within 18 domains of performance.
PEDI-CAT (Haley et al., 2012)	The PEDI-CAT is a computer-adaptive caregiver report that assesses daily activities, mobility, responsibility, and social and cognitive domains for newborns to 21-year-olds.

Assessments for Building Adaptive Capacity, Coping, Resilience, and Skills for Life

Adaptive Behavior Assessment System, Third Edition (ABAS-3; Harrison & Oakland, 2015)	ABAS-3 is used for classifying various developmental, learning, and behavioral disabilities and disorders in children of any age. This assessment helps to identify a client's strengths and weaknesses; it can also be used to monitor progress in adaptive skills over time.
Hawaii Early Learning Profile (HELP; VORT Corporation, 1995)	The HELP is an ongoing, family-centered assessment for children aged 0 to 3 years. This assessment helps to create goals and developmentally appropriate interventions.
Bayley Scales of Infant and Toddler Development (BSID; Bayley, 1993)	The BSID helps to identify children between the ages of 1 month and 42 months with developmental delay who may require intervention services. This assessment covers cognitive, language, and motor domains.

Assessments for Building Mastery and Competence in Occupational Participation

Canadian Occupational Performance Measure (COPM; Law et al., 2014)	The COPM is a client-centered outcome measure used for children as young as 8 years of age. This assessment focuses on self-perception of performance in everyday living over time.
The Child Occupational Self-Assessment (COSA; Kramer et al., 2014)	The COSA assesses children ranging from 6 to 17 years of age regarding their perceptions of their own sense of occupational competence in everyday activities.
The Participation and Sensory Environment Questionnaire (PSEQ; Piller et al., 2017)	The PSEQ measures the impact of the sensory environment or features of an activity on participation in children ranging from 3 to 10 years of age.

(continued)

Table 14-2 (continued)

Assessments	
Children's Assessment of Participation and Enjoyment (CAPE) and Preferences for Activities of Children (PAC; King et al., 2004)	The CAPE assesses how children participate in everyday activities outside of their mandated school activities. The PAC measures children's preferences for these activities. Both assessments can be completed on children ranging from 6 to 21 years of age.
School Functional Assessment (SFA; Coster et al., 1998)	The SFA measures a student's performance of functional tasks that support participation in academics and social interactions in grades K–6.

Table 14-3

Best Practices List for Assessments and Intervention
Building Functional Cognition, Metacognition, and Executive Function
Educate parents on supporting all aspects of the client's health, including mental and psychosocial.
Assess the client's stress level and sleeping habits and their impact on executive function.
Create supportive readings groups for clients and their parents to promote family learning.
Ensure that assessments are being conducted in appropriate conditions (e.g., make sure that clients have been able to eat before the assessment and have not worked in the past 12 hours in the field before the testing).
Building Adaptive Capacity, Coping, Resilience, and Skills for Life
Work with teachers in the spring to create small groups to support children harvesting in the fields while maintaining educational pursuits.
Work with teachers to make accommodations in the classroom for children with physical injuries and psychosocial issues.
Educate parents on accommodations and adaptive equipment to aid clients working in the field to prevent injury.
Educate clients on creating coping strategies and accommodations for learning challenges.
Provide materials in the appropriate language to increase understanding.
Building Mastery and Competence in Occupational Participation
Inquire about the clients' interests and work toward increasing participation in those areas to increase well-being.
Collaborate with teachers on working toward handwriting and literacy in the new language to build confidence and competence.
Avoid holding expectations about materials and supplies that families have access to.
Plan for continuity of service to ensure that the child does not fall behind and is continuing to build mastery; consider summer programs if schools and families show interest.

previous location, the occupational therapist may encourage them to continue to participate in this type of dance group in the new setting. Latino migrant families continue to honor and continue their family traditions, such as celebrating special holidays, family dinners, and other habits or routines that bring a sense of identity to the members of the family. As the family continues to honor and express aspects of their previous culture, it is possible for them to maintain a sense of identity even as they engage in meaningful activities in their new setting.

This occupational therapy approach will provide support and guidance as children adjust to their new environment. Occupational therapists can help children form a sense of occupational balance by incorporating aspects of both their new and old cultures. Assessments are available to aid occupational therapists in identifying challenges that migrant children may face. Intervention strategies and best practices may be introduced during occupational therapy sessions to enhance functional cognition, metacognition, and executive function, as well as adaptation and coping for life skills. Examples of these include educating the family on the child's mental and psychosocial health, working with teachers to create small groups during the harvest season to support children in the fields while maintaining their educational pursuits, and inquiring about the clients' interests and working toward increasing participation in those areas to increase well-being. It is also important for the occupational therapist to address children's competence in new social and community occupational participation so that they can find support and meaning in their new culture.

COLLABORATIVE APPROACH WITH FAMILIES AND THE SOCIAL ENVIRONMENT

Migrant families often experience new demands and stressors that affect routines and family structure. Occupational therapists play an important role in facilitating a collaborative approach with families, peers, and the social environment to build adaptation, coping, and resilience. By helping families create meaning from challenging family experiences, build personal strength, and work together to increase family strength, occupational therapists can help families adapt, engage, and continue their daily activities with support from one another (Jaffe et al., 2020). For example, a child is stressed about their new learning environment at school and feels that they does not have anything in common with their peers. The occupational therapist can help their child find commonalities and increase the child's sense of belonging. Occupational therapists can utilize a best-practice, trauma-informed care approach by addressing the trauma, identifying current symptoms of the experience, and developing supportive counteracting responses when working with families and children. Taking the family's situation into consideration during the client's treatment will ensure that all aspects of the client's well -being, including physical, behavioral, and mental health, are being addressed. For example, if a family was separated during their travel to their work site and some members of the family remained in another country, children may feel deserted and alone. It is important for the occupational therapist to address these concerns to ensure that the entire person is being treated. Trauma can cause psychological stress that in turn hinders the child's ability to effectively adapt to the new setting.

It is suggested that occupational therapists work with clients at times that fit their needs and their families' needs, to minimize stress as much as possible and encourage participation. This supports families to engage in a balanced life and addresses clients' mental and physical health by taking a client-centered approach. Members of migrant families, including children, are often heavily burdened with stressors of school, work, and adjustment to a new lifestyle, language, and culture. Thus, it may be helpful for occupational therapists to work with family members on transactions with familiar and new environments. For example, occupational therapists can help clients investigate aspects of their new surroundings and find aspects they can connect with and enjoy. Supporting clients' sense of control over their choices and identity, through family routines and rituals such as attending church and family dinners, can facilitate more life satisfaction and meaning in the new aspects of life. This can be done by working with parents to support their children at home and in school by incorporating a variety of ways to adapt and engage in coping activities. Children can identify with their previous culture while also adapting to a new way of life. In addition, opportunities at school and in social situations can increase migrant children's participation and their sense of belonging in the new culture. For example, if some children excel in social situations, they can become peer mentors for other children who are struggling with adapting to their new educational and social environment. This mentoring experience can teach children coping mechanisms and foster resilience.

Occupational therapists can also enhance migrant children's health and well-being by collaborating with other health care providers to facilitate an interprofessional and holistic approach. It is important to consider the social environment in which these children are living when they migrate with their parents. Many migrant children face both social struggles in school and financial challenges at home. Assessing children and their parents for psychosocial issues such as anxiety and depression regarding these challenges can be beneficial for the overall well-being of all family members. Evaluation of children's adaptation, coping, and resilience can yield better understanding and support of the child's performance strengths and areas of concern through more accurate knowledge of how children interact with their surroundings. For example, if it is discovered through assessment that a child has low self-confidence when interacting with peers, occupational therapists can aid the child with coping mechanisms and skill formation to increase self-esteem and participation. Instilling and enhancing a sense of resilience in children within migrant families can increase their confidence and comfort level regarding participation and functioning in their new environment.

BUILDING INTERPROFESSIONAL COLLABORATIONS WITH TEACHERS, HEALTH CARE TEAM, AND COMMUNITY

Occupational therapists can foster a collaborative approach with other disciplinary teams to facilitate adaptation, coping, and resilience in many ways. Occupational therapists can work with teachers to create various school-based programs that support the psychosocial well-being of migrant children. These programs can be formatted in a variety of ways to follow the best client-centered approach. For example, student-focused programs, educational and career support, psychoeducation, peer support, social and emotional instruction, creative expression, and family-focused program activities can aid migrant children with the emotional burdens that often accompany a transition into a new school (Bennouna et al., 2019). These student-focused programs can help therapists and teachers create educational profiles for each child and develop targeted skill sheets for each unique client to direct that client's focus during the school day. According to Bennouna et al. (2019), this type of program allows students to be introduced to the routines and procedures of the school. Occupational therapists and teachers can collaborate to create a mentor program at schools to transition new students into school-day routines and ensure that direct guidance is provided to each migrant child. Promoting peer support allows clients to share their stories with other children and provides opportunities for growth and hope. In addition to peer support, group activities with classmates help build social and language skills. Small-group discussions regarding mental health and psychosocial well-being provide opportunities for students to bond and boost self-esteem. Additionally, occupational therapists can work with teachers to incorporate creative expression into the school day, thereby allowing students to share their personal stories; this practice has been shown to help students who felt that their unique migrant experiences interfered with their friendships, home life, and leisure activities (Bennouna et al., 2019).

Occupational therapists can work with teachers to create a welcoming community where students can share stories and songs from their cultures. This supports understanding from classmates regarding other children's home lives. Bullying can be an issue in the classroom and can drastically affect a child's focus on education, social skills, and mental health (see Chapter 11). Occupational therapists can work with teachers to increase positive psychosocial well-being for migrant children in the classroom by including all students in the process of identifying ways to make new students feel welcomed (Breiseth, 2018). Promoting active participation in the process to include the new students facilitates engagement and investment from the entire class. Similar to how students can build their peers' self-esteem, educators can support migrant students and their families to engage and collaborate with occupational therapists. This interprofessional collaboration can aid students with access to supplies and assistance in navigating the educational process. Teaching children and families how to complete administrative forms and paperwork correctly and how to navigate the school's technology systems can empower parents and facilitate their active involvement in their child's transition to the new school (Free & Križ, 2016). Being cognizant of language barriers, utilizing various communication devices, and providing information sheets in various languages can foster a common understanding among the school administration, staff, and migrant families.

Occupational therapists can also work with health care teams to improve care both within and outside the health care system. Such work often includes expanding migrant families' access within a realm of cultural and linguistic methods of care (Granado-Villar et al., 2013). Occupational therapists can work with health care teams to educate medical personnel on the importance of expanding health literacy programs to increase the migrant family's understanding and feelings of inclusion throughout their medical experiences (National Center for Farmworker Health, 2020). Health programs may include healthy eating, immunization schedules, work safety, and care for common ailments.

Occupational therapists can work collaboratively with the healthcare team to ensure that interprofessional and comprehensive care is provided. Because many migrant children are affected by emotional and health issues, it is crucial for both mind and body to be addressed. Occupational therapists can collaborate with pediatricians on various barriers that migrant children may face, such as family separation, poor living conditions, long work days, repetitive motions required in the field that may cause injury, and difficulty with school work. To ensure that these children are able to participate in meaningful activities such as farming, schooling, and playing with peers, the health care team should use a client-centered approach. It is also necessary for the health care team to conduct screenings regularly and in the child's native language, so as to provide developmental and psychoeducational surveillance and prevent poor health and psychosocial issues. Standard developmental screening tools can be used by occupational therapists. It is important to develop a relationship with pediatricians in order to collaborate with them on inquiring about family beliefs and practices related to health, illness, and disability. Each client has their own health beliefs and values and it is crucial for the health care team to be aware of the migrant's traditional healing practices and medications (Granado-Villar et al., 2013). It is also appropriate for occupational therapists to advocate for culturally relevant programs to address social and economic challenges that affect access to health care. These issues may include food and housing security, language, literacy, and legal services (Granado-Villar et al., 2013). Occupational therapists should also educate the health care team regarding the importance of family social health services. Such services may focus on health literacy, reading skills, and a general understanding of the new language.

When occupational therapists work with the community, overarching care becomes available for migrant children and their families. Community-based health and social centers can provide resources to clients to maintain the migrant family's native language and honor its traditions and individual strengths. Aubé et al. (2019) noted that a community-based health and social center, La Maison Bleue, could be used as a model for providing resources to migrant mothers and children. This center provides support for clients' resilience processes such as building relationships, finding meaning, maintaining identity, problem solving, and gaining independence. Through empowerment and comfort in a safe place, clients build trust and feel supported. Occupational therapists can support community-based health care staff to respect the families' values and culture to help maintain a sense of identity for these clients. In addition, occupational therapists can promote a sense of social community by working with community-based centers to create social groups where child and adult clients can come together and form relationships to foster a sense of belonging in the new community. Holistic care is essential, as both the client's physical and psychosocial needs must be addressed.

Occupational therapists can help advocate for clients' needs and address psychosocial aspects by assisting individuals and families with tasks such as finding housing, completing immigrant paperwork, or looking for employment. It is crucial for clients to be able to interact effectively with their community to form a sustainable life. Facilitating access to coordinated services requires a multidisciplinary approach, requiring occupational therapists to aid with holistic care (Gronski et al., 2013). Occupational therapists can facilitate the connection of clients to community resources such as a group at a local library that connects parents with activities in the community for their children (Aubé et al., 2019). In schools, occupational therapists can assist in identifying and monitoring student needs and connect children to different types of services within the community. School-based occupational therapists can work with children and community members to create an awareness of the challenges of mental health and the services the community has to offer in this area (Bennouna et al., 2019). These programs can also work with clients to identify challenges that migrant children face and address common risk factors that often contribute to an imbalance in psychosocial well-being. Occupational therapists can work directly with the community to help identify these risk factors by offering developmental and mental health screenings at community events such as county fairs or church gatherings. Occupational therapists can provide early-intervention programs, and school occupational therapists can provide summer-kindergarten-readiness programs. It is important for care providers to give emotional support, provide connections with community resources, and assist with activities of daily living as families settle into the new community.

A GLOBAL PERSPECTIVE

Migration for better work opportunities is seen around the globe. In Canada, seasonal farmworkers travel north from Mexico and Central America. Children who travel with these families face challenges similar to those faced by migrants in the United States. Being far from home is difficult for children, and adapting to a new community and school can be a challenge. The French-Canadian language spoken in some provinces can also pose difficulties in acculturation (Aubé et al., (2019). Adjusting to new schools and friends is a process to which some children accommodate quite easily and other children take more time. Each child needs their own personal adjustment support. Occupational therapists can provide support and facilitate teachers' and other school professionals' development of individual child, school, and community plans that help children acclimate to new academic and social routines.

Many migrant workers from the Philippines and Southeast Asia come to Europe to work as child or senior adult caregivers or household workers for families on Europe's western coast in countries such as England, France, Spain, and Portugal (Trovao et al., 2017). In southern Europe, migrant workers come from Africa to work in countries such as Italy or Greece (Trovao et al., 2017). These European workers frequently travel alone to work while their children stay at home with family caregivers. Although these children are cared for by their family members, they are stilled challenged with issues of separation from their parents for long periods of time. This can create problems even when children know that their parents are doing the work away from home to help support the family and allow the children to gain better education opportunities in the future (Lu, 2015). Families cope with separation by communicating by a variety of methods, including writing, phone texts/calls, computer-written emails, and video communication.

Occupational therapists can help migrant children adjust in academic, social, and emotional activities at school. They can help a child whose family is away make a scrapbook of the family; if they have migrated, they might make a scrapbook of the country from which they came and the family and friends they left behind. In each case, the children can, if they wish, share their book with their schoolmates. The occupational therapist can also work to help individual children who are uncomfortable in their new community adjust to the new environment. Occupational therapists can support migrant children's integration by collaborating with health care providers and adult leaders in creating community activities that children can join for health care, sports, arts, and recreational programs.

THE ESSENTIAL CONSIDERATIONS FOR OCCUPATIONAL THERAPISTS

The essential considerations that occupational therapists should take into account when addressing occupational performance concerns in migrant children are broad and comprehensive. Essential considerations should address the child within the family in both the immediate and the long-term timeframe. This is important given the amount of time away from children that many migrant parents experience. A consideration of the child within the community in which the parents work must address housing, health, school, and community activities. Within each of these contact areas, occupational performance and the development of adaptation, coping, and resilience are considered and highlighted. Case Study 14-1 addresses these many issues through the story of one child, Rita, and her family. Table 14-4 provides a list of essential considerations for occupational therapists to build adaptation, coping, and resilience in migrant children. It is hoped that this will help to develop new ideas for occupational therapy programming for this unique and underserved population, not only in the United States but also in countries around the world.

Case Study 14-1

Housing

Rita is a 9-year-old girl whose family has moved to the United States from Panama. Rita's family travels to various states as seasonal farmworkers. Although her family is able to earn income for most of the year in these various locations, their temporary living conditions are far from ideal, with mold and extreme heat in their trailer. Rita began to have breathing problems and a persistent cough. One night, when Rita found it nearly impossible to breathe, her parents decided to take her to the hospital, where she was diagnosed with asthma. Due to a lack of medical insurance and access to affordable care, Rita has not been able to

(continued)

Case Study 14-1 (continued)

keep up with the proper medical attention that she needs. She experiences shortness of breath, a chronic cough, and pressure in her chest. This discomfort is noted especially at night and continues to prohibit Rita from getting an adequate amount of sleep. Because of her symptoms and excessive fatigue, she is unable to keep up with her duties on the farm. The medical condition is leading to a decrease in the harvest output and an increase in stress for both Rita and her parents regarding her well being.

Rita's school nurse identified that Rita would benefit from a visit to a pediatrician and an occupational therapist to address her situation. These professionals' guidance would allow her to control her medical condition and become educated on ways to adapt and cope with asthma in order to fully participate in her desired occupations (e.g., farming). At her first visit, the occupational therapist administered the Canadian Occupational Performance Measure (COPM) to Rita to detect change in her self-perception of occupational performance during farming. With the COPM, the occupational therapist assesses the importance of this activity, Rita's performance of it, and the satisfaction Rita experiences during her time working in the field. The occupational therapist then helps her incorporate adaptations in the field to increase her performance and satisfaction. To address Rita's fatigue, the occupational therapist educates Rita on adaptive equipment that will allow her to work in the field for an extended amount of time, thereby increasing her performance. This adaptive equipment includes a long-handled shovel or picking device to eliminate the need for Rita to continually bend down. By preserving energy and expending it in ways that enhance productivity, Rita is better able to perform and find greater satisfaction in her work. In addition, the occupational therapist addresses Rita's shortness of breath by educating her on breathing techniques to help with her respiratory expenditure. When accessory muscles are used to help raise the chest during breathing, it can be difficult to use those muscles for other activities that require upper extremity movements, such as shoveling, picking crops, and holding farming equipment. Teaching Rita pursed-lip and diaphragmatic breathing techniques helps Rita to steady her breathing and refrain from using accessory muscles of the shoulder girdle to help her breathe. To increase upper extremity function during farming, the occupational therapist also helps Rita use free weights, a TheraBand, and arm ergometers to increase the strength in her shoulder girdle, to improve her ability to breathe, and work on the farm simultaneously. These occupational adaptations allow Rita to engage in her desired farming tasks with a sense of mastery due to adequate environment and person interaction.

Table 14-4

Essential Considerations for Occupational Therapists to Build Adaptation, Coping, and Resilience

Essential Considerations and Reference	Brief Description	Occupational Therapy Essential Considerations	Activity Examples
Physical health considerations (Kroening & Dawson-Hahn, 2019)	Inadequate social determinants often lead to poor health for migrant children. Extreme work conditions and unsanitary housing often cause injuries and illness. Migrant children are at increased risk for physical, developmental, and behavioral health issues. These issues should be considered within an ecological context that includes the family, community, and sociocultural factors.	Occupational therapists should understand the migration history of the child to provide context for infectious disease screening and exposure risk, including trauma. To progress with adaptation and coping, occupational therapists should build rapport and establish trust with parents to work on the child's development within a cultural context.	Activity examples include adapting physical motions utilized in the field when picking crops. For example, bending at the knees rather than at the waist can decrease back pain. Other examples include taking precautions when utilizing farm equipment, managing injuries properly by attending to dressings, and managing edema by elevating the injured limb. These activities will help decrease physical pain and increase productivity on the farm.

(continued)

Table 14-4 (continued)

Essential Considerations for Occupational Therapists to Build Adaptation, Coping, and Resilience

Essential Considerations and Reference	Brief Description	Occupational Therapy Essential Considerations	Activity Examples
Behavioral health considerations (Kupersmidt & Martin, 1997)	Migrant children often experience toxic stress due to drastic life changes and uncertainty. Farmworker children often must engage in work, school, and making friends. It may take children time to adapt to a new lifestyle.	Occupational therapists should consider chronic problems with residential situations, poor school mobility, language barriers in class, work obligations, and peer situations to ensure that a holistic care approach is being used with the child. It is essential for occupational therapists to address the mental and behavioral health of each migrant child to aid the client in finding meaning in new occupations while maintaining their identity and honoring their culture. Given how hard the children work in the field and in school, occupational therapists should stress the importance of play to increase social skill development and facilitate play opportunities with families and schools. Children must be provided time to relax and play to create a balanced lifestyle and serve as a natural coping mechanism. Occupational therapists should communicate with families and teachers about ways to incorporate play into the work day. For example, if a child must go to a water fountain during the workday, the adult may turn it into a skipping game to increase the child's enjoyment. Occupational therapists can benefit children by holding afterschool playgroups to increase playful physical activities and relaxation techniques.	Occupational therapists can administer assessments to inquire about self-confidence and self-esteem. Addressing any reservations children may have about engaging in a new activity can increase their participation.

| Housing and financial considerations (Taylor & Ruiz, 2017) | Large families are often forced to inhabit small living areas that lack necessities such as running water, appropriate temperatures, or electricity for refrigerators and lights. These conditions can lead to a lack of sleep, increase in stress, and mental health issues. In addition, exposure to mold and unhealthy irritants can lead to physical health issues. Taylor and Ruiz (2017) found that economic challenges are linked to teacher reports of children's depressive problems. | Occupational therapists should be aware of each client's economic challenges to ensure that supports can be put in place to benefit the child and lead to a healthier lifestyle. | Activity examples include addressing sleep habits and routines. Sleep has major effects on productivity and mental capacity. Occupational therapists can aid clients in forming good routines before bed. In addition, occupational therapists can aid clients gain occupational balance, ensure that they are still participating in activities they enjoy, and decrease depressive problems. If clients are solely focused on work and financial issues, it can be easy for them to develop great amounts of stress and decrease their overall well-being. |

(continued)

Table 14-4 (continued)

Essential Considerations for Occupational Therapists to Build Adaptation, Coping, and Resilience

Essential Considerations and Reference	Brief Description	Occupational Therapy Essential Considerations	Activity Examples
Social participation and social-skill considerations (James, 1997; Bennouna et al., 2019)	When migrant children move to a new country and leave behind their familiar culture, language, and community, they are at risk for psychosocial issues such as depression, anxiety, drug use, and deviant behavior.	It is essential for occupational therapists to form a trusting relationship with each client and to compile a client-centered profile for each child. Occupational therapists should then inquire about relationships with peers, family, and within the community. Early intervention is a key component for benefiting migrant children at risk for psychosocial issues. Occupational therapists may work with school personnel and health care providers to organize culturally appropriate interventions.	Occupational therapists can administer assessments to children to discover their interests and their sense of belonging with peers. Discovering activities that the child enjoys and ways for them to engage in this activity in the new community will allow the child to meet other children with the same interests. This can increase children's sense of belonging and connection to their new environment.
Language literacy considerations (Farr et al., 2018)	According to Farr et al. (2018), an identity change is noted when clients shift between ethnic identifications with a host and heritage culture to a new language and culture.	It is essential for occupational therapists to consider migrant children's traditions and first language to ensure that they are able to maintain a sense of identity. Families often use their native language within the home, thereby providing a sense of familiar family routines and psychological wellbeing. In addition, it is important for occupational therapists to work with clients and their families to ensure that supports are in place for proper functioning in the new society.	Occupational therapists can advocate for pamphlets in multiple languages to help migrants understand the information being given to them. This is especially essential in health care systems, as many parents struggle to understand medication and admission forms and other paperwork.

| School considerations (Bennouna et al., 2019; Havlik et al. (2018); Merry et al., 2019) | Adjusting to a new schooling system can be a difficult transition for migrant children. They may have a difficult time comprehending the material because they are also trying to understand and learn a new language. In addition, they may feel excluded from peer groups and struggle to fit in. | It is crucial for occupational therapists to assess children's social inclusion and participation in the classroom. These important aspects affect the mental health and psychosocial well-being of all children. Occupational therapists should screen for isolation and depression and encourage inclusive activities. Participating in class and with peers in healthy ways can help create positive behavior support. Occupational therapists should work with students throughout the school day on inclusion of all students, and provide supplemental support to migrant children. | Occupational therapists can aid children in a school setting by helping migrant children understand the material in a new language. Sometimes, it can take children a little bit longer to comprehend the material because it is being delivered to them in a new fashion/language.

Occupational therapists should educate teachers regarding this concept to ensure that they are addressing each child's needs. In addition, occupational therapists can address handwriting with the children. Occupational therapists can also assess for self-esteem in the classroom and work with children to increase their sense of self-worth by working individually with a child to organize their school materials in a manner that allows the most effective learning. For example, matching a different color of notebook to each school subject can help the child stay organized. |

REFERENCES

American Academy of Pediatrics. (2005). Providing care for immigrant, homeless, and migrant children: Policy statement. *Pediatrics, 115*(4, pt. 1), 1095-1100. https://doi.org/10.1542/peds.2005-0052

American Occupational Therapy Association. (2020). Occupational therapy practice framework: Domain and process (4th ed.). *American Journal of Occupational Therapy, 74*(Suppl. 2), 7412410010. https://doi.org/10.5014/ajot.2020.74S2001

Aubé, T., Pisanu, S., & Merry, L. (2019). La Maison Bleue: Strengthening resilience among migrant mothers living in Montreal, Canada. *PLoS One, 14*(7), 1-20. https://doi.org/10.1371/journal.pone.0220107

Bayley. (1993). Bayley scales of infant development (BSID) [measurement Instrument]. http://www.healthofchildren.com/B/Bayley-Scales-of-Infant-Development.html

Bennouna, C., Khauli, N., Basir, M., Allaf, C., Wessells, M., & Stark, L. (2019). School-based programs for supporting the mental health and psychosocial wellbeing of adolescent forced migrants in high-income countries: A scoping review. Social Science & Medicine, 239. https://doi.org/10.1016/j.socscimed.2019.112558

Breiseth, L. (2018). How to provide social-emotional support for immigrant students. https://www.colorincolorado.org/immigration/guide/student

Compas, B. E., Connor-Smith, J. K., Saltzman, H., Thomsen, A. H., & Wadsworth, M. E. (2001). Coping with stress during childhood and adolescence: Problems, progress, and potential in theory and research. *Psychological Bulletin, 127*(1), 87-127. https://doi.org/10.1037//0033-2909.127.1.87

Coster, W., Deeney, T., Haltiwanger, J., & Haley, S. (1998). School function assessment [measurement instrument]. https://www.pearsonassessments.com/store/usassessments/en/Store/Professional-Assessments/Behavior/Adaptive/School-Function-Assessment/p/100000547.

Council on Community Pediatrics. (2013). Providing care for immigrant, migrant, and border children. *Pediatrics, 131*(6), e2028-e2034. https://doi.org/10.1542/peds.2013-1099

Farr, J., Blenkiron, L., Harris, R., & Smith, J. A. (2018). "It's my language, my culture, and it's personal!" Migrant mothers' experience of language use and identity change in their relationship with their children: An interpretative phenomenological analysis. *Journal of Family Issues 39*(11), 3029-3054. https://doi.org/10.1177/0192513X18764542

Free, J. L., & Križ, K. (2016). "They know there is hope": How migrant educators support migrant students and their families in navigating the public school system. *Children and Youth Services Review, 69*, 184-192. https://doi.org/10.1016/j.childyouth.2016.08.003

Gothro, A., Hanno, E. S., & Bradley, M. C. (2020). Challenges and solutions in evaluation technical assistance during design and early implementation. *Evaluation Review.* https://doi.org/10.1177/0193841X20911527

Grajo, L. (2019). Occupational adaptation as a normative and intervention process: Schkade and Schultz's legacy. In L. C. Grajo & A. Boisselle (Eds.), *Adaptation through occupation: Multidimensional perspectives*. SLACK Incorporated.

Granger, C. V., & McCabe, M. A. (1987). WeeFIM® instrument [measurement instrument]. https://eprovide.mapi-trust.org/instruments/weefim-r-instrument

Gronski, M. P., Bogan, K. E., Kloeckner, J., Russell-Thomas, D., Taff, S. D., Walker, K. A., & Berg, C. (2013). Childhood toxic stress: A community role in health promotion for occupational therapists. *The American Journal of Occupational Therapy, 67*(6), e148-e153. https://doi.org/10.5014/ajot.2013.008755

Haley, S. M., Coster, W. J., Dumas, H. M., & Fragala-Pinkham, M. A. (2012). Pediatric Evaluation of Disability Inventory Computer Adaptive Test (PEDI-CAT) [measurement instrument]. https://www.pearsonassessments.com/store/usassessments/en/Store/Professional-Assessments/Behavior/Pediatric-Evaluation-of-Disability-Inventory-Computer-Adaptive-Test/p/100002037.html

Harrison, P. & Oakland, T.. (2015). Adaptive Behaviour Assessment System, Third Edition (ABAS-3) [measurement instrument]. https://paa.com.au/product/abas-3

Havlik, S. A., Rowley, P., Puckett, J., Wilson, G., & Neasen, E. (2018). "Do whatever you can to try to support that kid": School counselors' experiences addressing student homelessness. *Professional School Counseling, 21*(1), 47-59. https://doi.org/10.5330/1096-2409-21.1.47

Jaffe, L., Cosper, S., & Fabrizi, S. (2020). Working with families. In J. C. O'Brien & H. Kuhaneck, *Case-Smith's occupational therapy for children and adolescents* (8th ed., pp. 46-75). Mosby/Elsevier.

James, D. (1997). Coping with a new society: The unique psychosocial problems of immigrant youth. *Journal of School Health, 67*(3), 98-102. https://doi.org/10.1111/j.1746-1561.1997.tb03422.x

Kim, J. (2020). Homelessness as difficult knowledge in early childhood education. *Early Childhood Education Journal, 48*, 815-823. https://doi.org/10.1007/s10643-020-01045-5

King, G., Law, M., King, S., Hurley, P., Rosenbaum, P., Hanna, S., Kertoy, M., & Young, N. (2004). Children's Assessment of Participation and Enjoyment and Preferences for Activities [measurement instrument]. https://www.pearsonassessments.com/store/usassessments/en/Store/Professional-Assessments/Behavior/Adaptive/Children%27s-Assessment-of-Participation-and-Enjoyment-and-Preferences-for-Activities-of-Children/p/100000481.html

Kramer, J., ten Velden, M., Kafkes, A., Basu, S., Federico, J., & Kielhofner, G. (2014). The Child Occupational Self-Assessment [measurement instrument]. https://www.moho.uic.edu/productDetails.aspx?aid=3

Kroening, A. L. H., & Dawson-Hahn, E. (2019). Health considerations for immigrant and refugee children. *Advances in Pediatrics, 66*, 87-110. https://doi.org/10.1016/j.yapd.2019.04.003

Kupersmidt, J. B., & Martin, S. L. (1997). Mental health problems of children of migrant and seasonal farm workers: A pilot study. *Journal of the American Academy of Child and Adolescent Psychiatry, 36*(2), 224-232. https://doi.org/10.1097/00004583-199702000-00013

Law, M., Carswell, A., Baptiste, S., McColl, M. A., Polatajko, H., & Pollock, N. (2014). Canadian Occupational Performance Measure [measurement instrument]. https://eprovide.mapi-trust.org/instruments/canadian-occupational-performance-measure

Lu, Y. (2015). Internal migration, international migration, and physical growth of left-behind children: A study of two settings. *Health and Place, 36*, 118-126. https://doi.org/10.1016/j.healthplace.2015.09.008

Markowitz, D. L., & Cosminsky, S. (2005). Overweight and stunting in migrant Hispanic children in the USA. *Economics and Human Biology, 3*(2), 215-240. https://doi.org/10.1016/j.ehb.2005.05.005

Merry, L., Hanley, J., Ruiz-Casares, M., Archambault, I., & Mogere, D. (2019). Migrant families with children in Montreal, Canada and transnational family support: A protocol for a focused ethnography. *BMJ Open, 9*(9), e029074-e029074. https://doi.org/10.1136/bmjopen-2019-029074

Migrant Clinicians Network (MCN). (2020). https://www.migrantclinician.org

National Center for Farmworker Health. (2020). www.ncfh.org

National Children's Center for Rural Agricultural Health and Safety & National Farm Medicine Center. (2020). www.cultivatesafety.org

Piller, A., Fletcher, T., Pfeiffer, B., Dunlap, K., & Pickens, N. (2017). Reliability of the Participation and Sensory Environment Questionnaire: Teacher version. *Journal of Autism and Developmental Disorders, 47*, 3541-3549. https://link.springer.com/article/10.1007/s10803-017-3273-3

Sandra, L. M., Todd, E. G., & Janis, B. K. (1995). Survey of exposure to violence among the children of migrant and seasonal farm workers. *Public Health Reports (1974-), 110*(3), 268.

Shonkoff, J. P. (2019). Toxic stress: Issue brief on family separation and child detention. https://immigrationinitiative.harvard.edu/toxic-stress-issue-brief-family-separation-and-child-detention

Taylor, Z. E., & Ruiz, Y. (2017). Contextual stressors and the mental health outcomes of Latino children in rural migrant-farmworker families in the Midwest. *Journal of Rural Mental Health, 41*(4), 284-298. https://doi.org/10.1037/rmh0000082

Trovao, S., Ramalho, S., & Ines, D. (2017). Mental health among Asian and African migrant working mothers: New vulnerabilities and old religious coping resources. *Mental Health, Religion and Culture, 20*(2), 162-174. https://doi.org/10.1080/13674676.2017.1329816

VORT Corporation. (1995). The Hawaii Early Learning Profile [measurement instrument]. http://keanyassociates.com/programs/hawaii-early-learning-profile

15

Children and Youth of Color

Douglene Jackson, PhD, OTR/L, LMT, ATP, BCTS

CHAPTER OBJECTIVES By the end of this chapter, the reader will be able to:
- Define adaptation, coping, and resilience as it relates to children and youth of color.
- Identify occupational challenges faced by children and youth of color.
- Illustrate best practices for assessment and interventions to support occupational performance and participation of children and youth of color.

OVERVIEW OF THE POPULATION

The population of the United States is becoming increasingly multicultural, highlighting the importance of occupational therapy practitioners possessing the skills to work with diverse individuals. The most dramatic population shifts are occurring in children. Estimates for 2020 by the United States Census Bureau (2019) projected that children and youth under 18 years of age would comprise 22.3% of the population. For 2020, the racial and ethnicity projected makeup was: Non-Hispanic white, 49.8%; Hispanic, 25.5%; Black/African American, 15.2%; American Indian & Alaska Native, 1.6%; Asian, 5.5%; Native Hawaiian & Other Pacific Islander, 0.3%; and two or more races, 5.8%. Additionally, it was forecasted that the majority of children would identify as a race other than non-Hispanic white by 2020, with this accounting for two out of three children by 2060 (Vespa et al., 2020). These projections indicate that the majority of the pediatric population will be children and youth of color, making it essential to understand different cultures in order for occupational therapy practitioners to provide culturally responsive client-centered care in efforts to improve functional outcomes.

Grajo L. C., & Boisselle, A. K. (Eds.). *Adaptation, Coping, and Resilience in Children and Youth: A Comprehensive Occupational Therapy Approach* (pp. 361-385).
© 2022 Taylor & Francis Group.

Figure 15-1. An adolescent seated on the lawn, meditating.

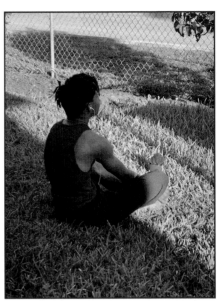

Terminology and Racial Identities

People of color is a socially constructed inclusive term applied to imply a relationship among minority groups, including individuals of African, Latinx/Hispanic, Native American, Asian, or Pacific Island descent (Vidal-Ortiz, 2008; Figure 15-1). Differences in customs and norms vary with each of these populations, also being unique to each family. The term "people of color," when used consciously so as not to collectively lose individual identities, represents racial and ethnic groups who differ from those identifying as white (Jeong, 2019; Vidal-Ortiz, 2008). This identity is assigned to subgroups of people who represent a minority population that might be marginalized or oppressed, with the aim of intentionally affirming such identities through self-determination and acknowledgment of individuality (Alvarez, 2020; Jeong, 2019). It is also important to recognize the differences within each race, as country of origin and place of residence shape culture.

Self-determination and individual identification, rather than having a racial identity assigned, is important, especially in a multicultural society as more people embrace belonging to more than one race (Foner & Fredrickson, 2005; Jeong, 2019). The fastest growing population over the next few decades is expected to be that of people belonging to two or more races, followed by Asians and Hispanics (Vespa et al., 2020). With race being a social construct and the continual change in societal composition, such identities may be in constant flux, especially as a result of immigration and multiracial individuals (Foner & Fredrickson, 2005). As the U.S. population shifts, it is important to understand the terminology used to describe different races and how individuals self-identify. Throughout this chapter, we use the term *children of color* when discussing children and youth who would not identify as non-Hispanic white.

Culture and Occupational Therapy Practice

Client-centered service is foundational to occupational therapy practice, which would not be effective without consideration of culture (American Occupational Therapy Association [AOTA], 2020). The increased diversity projected by population estimates has direct implications for multicultural occupational therapy practice (U.S. Census Bureau, 2019; Vespa et al., 2020). Cultural competence, awareness, humility, and responsiveness are all concepts explored by professionals in efforts to be effective in working with diverse populations (Bernal & Sáez-Santiago, 2006; Substance Abuse and Mental Health Services Administration, 2014). As our clients become more diverse, occupational therapy practitioners need to be knowledgeable about different cultures and exercise cultural humility in the delivery of conscious, culturally-centered practice.

Lack of competence in delivering client-centered services with respect to culture can result in poor outcomes and negatively affect access and use of services (Bartgis & Bigfoot, 2010). In order to provide services to diverse populations, professionals have sought education and training in cultural competency. However, the term *competence* connotes an end goal that is not attainable; professionals are now moving to embrace practices rooted in cultural humility (Agner, 2020). Cultural humility is a lifelong learning process involving active engagement in self-assessment while gaining the skills needed to engage and partner with diverse populations and communities for effective service delivery and advocacy (Tervalon & Murray-Garcia, 1998). This requires that occupational therapy practitioners commit to ongoing self-reflection to understand their personal beliefs and implicit biases, as well as acknowledging systemic policies and practices that negatively affect marginalized populations.

Culture is a reflexive process inherent in occupational therapy practice, as the interplay of context and the individual cultures of the client and practitioner shape the therapeutic relationship. Professional reasoning for occupational therapy is driven by context, in addition to the personal and professional self of the therapist, and personal and client self of the child and the child's family network (Schell & Schell, 2018). Context, including specific personal and environmental factors unique to each individual, influences occupational engagement and participation (AOTA, 2020). This includes multicultural variables such as language, values, spirituality, and other customs. When working with children and youth of color, we seek to understand their context, occupations, client factors, performance skills, and performance patterns (AOTA, 2020). As occupational therapy practitioners engage with clients from diverse backgrounds, they bring aspects of their own personal and professional experiences into the therapy process. This dynamic interplay (Figure 15-2) between the occupational therapy practitioner and the client holds culture at its center. We must consider various multicultural aspects of the therapeutic relationship when working with diverse populations as we strive to deliver conscious, culturally-centered occupational therapy practice.

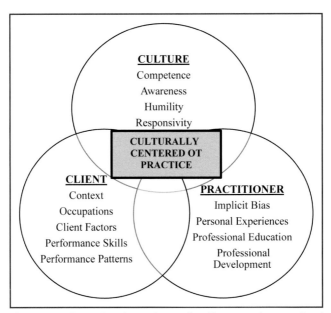

Figure 15-2. Dynamics of conscious, culturally-centered occupational therapy practice.

DEFINING ADAPTATION, COPING, AND RESILIENCE IN CHILDREN AND YOUTH OF COLOR

Adverse childhood experiences (ACEs) have been studied over time and are associated with increased risk for mental health challenges and negative adulthood outcomes (Dunn et al., 2017; Elkins et al., 2019). Experiencing such trauma can result in various internalization, emotional, and behavioral disorders, including post-traumatic stress disorder, oppositional defiant disorder, depression, and anxiety (D'Andrea et al., 2012; White et al., 2015), with resultant occupational engagement challenges. Occupational adaptation in the face of adverse childhood experiences is where occupational therapy practitioners can be instrumental in providing intervention to children and youth of color (Grajo et al., 2018). Through promotion of protective factors and facilitation of coping strategies and resilience, the effects of adverse childhood experiences can be mitigated to improve occupational performance and participation.

Adverse Childhood Experiences

Trauma can occur as the result of abuse, neglect, natural disasters, warfare, and other individual, social, or political factors, with children being more susceptible to experiencing traumatic events related to abuse and violence (International Society for Traumatic Stress Studies, 2015). For a more expansive discussion of ACEs, see Chapter 13. Children and youth of color have been found to have increased exposure to traumatic experiences, which can alter psychological, social, cognitive, and biological development (D'Andrea et al., 2012; Rosenthal et al., 2020). Parent-reported adverse childhood experiences, including divorce, drug abuse, incarceration, violence, and racism, are also positively correlated with poor childhood social-emotional and health outcomes (Health Resources and Services Administration's Maternal and Child Health Bureau, 2020). Considering trauma through a family-unit lens, the impact of childhood experiences becomes apparent in relation to potential detriments to occupational engagement.

Exposure to increased adverse childhood experiences, specifically of persons of Black/African American and Hispanic background, also carries an associated negative stigma and diminished positive outlook for outcomes as these persons transition into adulthood (Elkins, 2019). Health and educational disparities, systemic racism, and other social, cultural, and economic factors present unique challenges for children and youth of color. Racial injustice and systemic inequities further perpetuate childhood trauma, as children and youth of color encounter discrimination and oppression due to their racial identities (Alvarez, 2020; Elkins, 2019; Foner & Frederickson, 2005). There is a continued trend of children and youth of color being over-represented in the juvenile justice systems, as they constitute 62% of incarcerated youth in the United States (Children's Defense Fund, 2020; Robles-Ramamurthy & Watson, 2020; United States Department of Justice, Office of Justice Programs, 2019). Black youth are also more likely to be identified as having an intellectual disability, emotional disorders, or behavior disorders. They have increased rates of school expulsion, and those with disabilities are more likely to drop out of school (Fish, 2019; Office of Special Education Programs, 2020). However, it is also noted that early diagnosis is a challenge, as Black and Hispanic children and youth continue to be diagnosed with autism later than Non-Hispanic white children (Centers for Disease Control and Prevention, 2020). Diagnostic delays in early childhood limit opportunities to receive early intervention, and misdiagnosis leads to inappropriate care. The intersectionality of diagnostic and health disparities, along with adverse childhood experiences, positions children and youth of color at increased risk for resultant occupational engagement challenges.

Adaptation, Coping, and Resilience

Children and youth of color, through transaction with their environment and engagement in various occupations, may experience trauma along with health and educational inequities (Alvarez, 2020; Cahill et al., 2020). Adverse childhood events are known to be detrimental to childhood development and function (National Scientific Council on the Developing Child, 2015). Human development and adaptation arise as a function of occupational engagement and environmental interaction, at the individual, family, and societal levels (Grajo et al., 2018; Masten & Monn, 2015). When faced with adversity, some children are able to overcome these obstacles, whereas others struggle under similar circumstances and present with occupational performance and participation challenges. This variance has been attributed to several factors, including when the trauma occurred, as well as the type, duration, and severity of adversity (Jaffee & Maikovich-Fong, 2011; Racine et al., 2020).

Being adaptive involves navigating the environment, selecting and engaging in meaningful occupations, and being able to respond to adversity with resultant positive outcomes (Grajo et al., 2018). Resilience, often defined as an individual trait, process, or outcome, takes into account a dynamic systems approach, including the family and other societal factors within the context of efforts to overcome adversity (National Scientific Council on the Developing Child, 2015). Protective factors at the individual, family, and community level have been identified as supports to mediate the response to and effects of adversity and trauma (Afifi & MacMillan, 2011). However, prolonged or sustained exposure to adversity and trauma cannot be overcome through protective factors alone; they are detrimental to overall development and functional outcomes (National Scientific Council on the Developing Child, 2015; Racine et al., 2020).

Having endured trauma and a history of adverse events, children and youth of color can benefit from occupational therapy intervention aimed at supporting development of coping strategies and other skills necessary for occupational adaptation. Key protective factors for supporting child development, increasing family strengths, and preventing abuse and neglect have been researched and found to be effective: (1) parental resilience, (2) social connections, (3) knowledge of parenting and child development, (4) concrete social support in times of need, and (5) social and emotional competence in children (Center for the Study of Social Policy, 2017). Access and connection to resources and other supports, in addition to family and social networks, parental knowledge, and personal child factors, help to mitigate factors related to adverse childhood experiences. At the individual level, protective factors include personal traits and characteristics, such as perception of the experience and coping, as well as available resources. Family protective factors include religion, social supports and relationships, and opportunities to access community resources and support beyond the immediate family network (Afifi & MacMillan, 2011). Figure 15-3 lists some common challenges of and supports for children and youth of color.

Occupational therapy practitioners can be instrumental in supporting resilience in the face of adverse childhood experiences. In acknowledging the various races, ethnicities, and cultures within society and the social determinants of health and well-being as a result of such identities, we are uniquely positioned to promote adaptation and foster coping skills to support occupational engagement and positive outcomes. Implementing best and evidence-based practice approaches for screening in early childhood can help to address diagnostic disparities. We can also employ assessment and intervention practices rooted in evidence to guide our professional reasoning, implementing practice-based evidence strategies when evidence is emerging (Chorzempa et al., 2019; Schell & Schell, 2018). Our aim and distinct value when working with children and youth of color is to facilitate occupational adaptation for improved outcomes through conscious, culturally-centered occupational therapy practice. Table 15-1 illustrates an understanding of the occupational profile of a child of color.

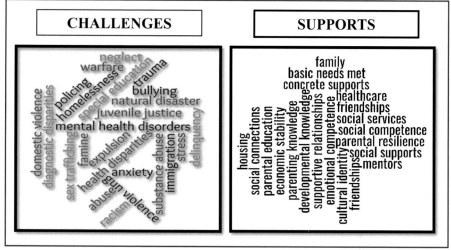

Figure 15-3. Challenges of and supports for children and youth of color.

BEST AND EVIDENCE-BASED PRACTICES FOR ASSESSMENT AND INTERVENTION

Occupational therapy practitioners working with pediatric populations often provide services in homes, schools, clinics, hospitals, and other community-based settings, with assessment and interventions being guided by best and evidence-based practices. As discussed previously, children and youth of color can present with various occupational performance and participation challenges resulting from numerous factors. When working with children and youth of color, we must operationalize our distinct value in helping to improve quality of life and overall health through using culturally appropriate client-centered approaches to achieve positive outcomes (AOTA, 2016).

Best and Evidence-Based Practices for Assessment

With assessment being the gateway to intervention, a strength-based approach is important to identify supports and challenges to occupational adaptation. This begins with an occupational profile, which includes information on developmental and social history, performance patterns, values, interests, and occupational needs (AOTA, 2017; AOTA, 2020). A holistic approach to assessment involves obtaining input from various performance-based and informative self, caregiver, and teacher reports. Synthesis of this information helps guide intervention planning to support occupational performance and participation. With children and youth of color, it is important to approach assessment with consideration of context and the influence of culture so as to ensure conscious, culturally-centered occupational therapy practice. Common assessments used to identify occupational performance and participation challenges related

Table 15-1

Occupational Profile of Jada		
Client Report		
Reason for seeking service and occupational engagement concerns	Jada is a 3-year-old girl with reported hyperactivity, communication delays, and fine motor challenges. She has difficulty communicating with peers and teachers. Jada has difficulty engaging other peers in play and is difficult to understand, as she primarily communicates using short phrases and does not enunciate well. Additionally, Jada holds writing utensils with immature grasp patterns; struggles with pre-writing strokes, and coloring; and is described as a picky eater who dislikes being messy. Jada does not engage well in noisy environments (e.g., church, parties) and demonstrates poor group-play skills.	
Successful occupations	Jada enjoys music, running, and swimming. She can sit to watch preferred television shows and use a tablet to play games. Jada can feed herself using a spoon and drink from an open cup.	
Interests and values	Jada's family values spending time together on weekends, watching television, eating meals together, attending church, and going to activities in the community.	
Occupational history	Jada was adopted from Haiti when she was 6 months old, and achieved gross motor milestones within expected timeframes. There has been a concern with fine motor, communication, and self-regulation skills. Her family speaks both English and Haitian Creole in the home, and expects Jada to be bilingual.	
Performance patterns	Jada does not have any siblings, but does have a 4-year-old cousin who visits often. When on the playground, she runs around the perimeter and prefers to play alone. Her home has a fenced yard and backyard swing-set, and she visits the swimming pool in the neighborhood park on weekends. Jada's mother works full time as a preschool teacher and is Jada's primary caregiver, with the maternal grandparents and an aunt living nearby. Jada attends a full-day preschool program 5 days per week.	
Environment	**Supports**	**Barriers**
Physical	Fenced backyard, outdoor playset, and nearby neighborhood park.	Shares a room with her siblings.
Social	Supportive extended family locally, including aunts and maternal grandparents.	Single mother; limited social engagement with peers.

(continued)

Table 15-1 (continued)

Occupational Profile of Jada		
Context	Supports	Barriers
Cultural, personal, temporal, virtual	Family routines for mealtimes and bedtime; attends church; attends a full-day preschool; multigenerational family, and grandparents who only speak Haitian Creole; enjoys playing on tablet to watch videos.	Mother is a single parent; family recently relocated; recent loss of father; difficulty transitioning from preferred tablet activities; unable to participate in Sunday-school church activities.
Client Goals		
Improve social participation with family and peers; improve fine motor skills; participate in age-appropriate community-based activities; connect to community-based social supports.		
Adapted from American Occupational Therapy Association. (2017). Occupational profile template. https://www.aota.org/profile.		

to adaptive behavior and occupational engagement are listed in Table 15-2 (Kramer et al., 2020; O'Brien & Kuhaneck, 2020; Reed, 2014).

The choice of an appropriate assessment should be informed by best and evidence-based practice approaches. Occupational therapists can make informed decisions to select appropriate assessments by gaining an understanding of the evidence regarding reliability and validity for a particular measure, as well as cultural appropriateness. This information can be found in the respective assessment manual or in research literature pertaining to assessment development, standardization, and pilot data. Additionally, determining cultural appropriateness and standardization processes for inclusivity and representation of the general population is key. The World Health Organization (2018) developed the Adverse Childhood Experiences International Questionnaire (ACE-IQ) for adults to gather global perspectives regarding childhood trauma and its association with health and well-being in later life.

As children and youth of color have been known to go undiagnosed or have delays in diagnosis, it is important to engage in screening practices when possible (Jackson, 2015). For example, proactively administering the Modified Checklist for Autism in Toddlers, Revised with Follow-Up when working with young children of color who have suspected developmental delays and potential risk for autism would be warranted (Robins et al., 2009). Early detection through the use of screenings and ongoing assessment throughout the intervention process are instrumental to informing therapy practices and improving outcomes for children and youth of color.

Table 15-2

Best and Evidence-Based Practices: Assessments	
Tool	Overview
Adaptive Behavior Assessment System-3 Ages: birth to 89 years (various forms) (Harrison & Oakland, 2015)	Rating scale across the lifespan for identification of strengths and weaknesses in adaptive skills for communication, community use, functional academics, health and safety, home or school living, leisure, motor, self-care, self-direction, social, and work.
Behavior Rating Inventory of Executive Function Ages: 2 to 18 years (various forms) (Gioia et al., 2013)	Executive functioning rating scale for inhibition, shift, emotional control, initiation, working memory, planning/organizing, organization of materials, and monitoring.
Child Occupational Self-Assessment Ages: 6 to 17 years (Kramer et al., 2014)	Self-report of personal sense of occupational performance and activity importance.
Children and Adolescent Scale of Participation Ages: Children and youth (Bedell, 2011)	Caregiver report of participation in home, school, community, and home/community living activities.
Children's Assessment of Participation and Enjoyment Ages: 6 to 21 years (King et al., 2004)	Self-report of activity participation outside of school activities with consideration of diversity, intensity, location, and enjoyment.
Developmental Behavioral Checklist-2 Ages: 4 to 18 years; 18 years to adult (Gray et al., 2018)	Rating scale of emotional and behavioral challenges.
Parenting Stress Index Ages: birth to 12 years (short form available) (Abidin, 2012)	Parental report to identify at-risk concerns related to child and parent behaviors.
Pediatric Evaluation of Disability Inventory Computer Adaptive Test Ages: birth to 20 years (Haley et al., 2020)	Caregiver report of performance in daily activities, mobility, social/cognitive, and responsibility in children and youth with behavioral or physical concerns.
Resiliency Scales for Children & Adolescents: A Profile of Personal Strengths Ages: 9 to 18 years (Prince-Embury, 2006)	Rating scale to measure personal attributes for resilience related to sense of mastery, relatedness, and emotional reactivity.

(continued)

Table 15-2 (continued)

Best and Evidence-Based Practices: Assessments	
Tool	Overview
Risk Inventory and Strengths Evaluation Age: 9 to 25 years (Goldstein & Herzberg, 2018)	Rating scale to compare strengths and risk factors at the individual level, as well as family and social supports.
Sensory Processing Measure, Second Edition Ages: 4 months to 87 years (various forms) (Parham et al., 2021)	Rating scale to assess sensory processing difficulties at home, school, and other environments; offers additional intervention strategies (QuickTips).
Sensory Profile-2/Infant-Toddler Sensory Profile-2 Ages: birth to 14 years (Dunn, 2014)	Rating scale to assess sensory processing patterns in home, school, and community-based activities.
Short Child Occupational Profile Ages: birth to 21 years (Bowyer et al., 2008)	Assesses strengths and challenges related to volition, habituation, performance skills, and environmental factors.
Strengths and Difficulties Questionnaire Ages: 2 to 17 years (Goodman, 2002)	Behavior screening questionnaire to assess emotional symptoms, conduct, hyperactivity/inattention, peer relationships, and prosocial behaviors.
Vineland Adaptive Behavior Scales-3 Ages: birth to 90 years (Sparrow et al., 2016)	Rating scale and structured interview to assess adaptive functioning in daily living skills, communication, and socialization.
Note: Editions may vary from those listed here as assessments are updated.	

Best and Evidence-Based Practices for Intervention

Intervention provided to address mental health challenges, in an effort to promote occupational adaptation, can be provided through a three-tiered approach: universal, targeted, and intensive (AOTA, 2016). Information gathered throughout the assessment process is used to guide intervention approaches rooted in best and evidence-based practice. Frames of reference are also foundational to our approach to intervention, serving as theories and used in conjunction with evidence-based practice (Kramer et al., 2020). Examples relevant when working with children and youth of color, especially those who experience adverse childhood events, might include the following:

- Occupational Adaptation (Schkade & Schultz, 1992)
- Behavior (Stein, 1983)
- Developmental (Llorens, 1976)
- Cognitive-Behavior (Kramer et al., 2020)

- Model of Human Occupation (Taylor, 2017)
- Social Participation (Kramer et al., 2020)
- Sensory Integration (Dean et al., 2017).

Using the premises of these frames of reference (in addition to others) to guide intervention, occupational therapy practitioners can develop client-centered interventions that are respectful of culture while addressing the needs identified through the assessment process.

Children and youth of color, as a result of experiencing adverse childhood events, present with various occupational performance and participation challenges. Recommendations are to use a continuum of services aimed at promotion, prevention, and intervention to foster adaption, coping, and resilience (AOTA, 2015; Bazyk & Arbesman, 2013). *Every Moment Counts*, an initiative to help children and youth with mental health challenges succeed across contexts, includes practical resources for occupational therapy practitioners and families for building capacity to promote positive mental health and implement effective strategies (Bazyk, 2014; Bazyk, 2017). Additionally, there are other evidence-based intervention approaches for improving social-emotional learning, promoting positive behavior, and facilitating occupational engagement (AOTA, 2016; Kingsley et al., 2020; Kramer et al., 2020; O'Brien & Kuhaneck, 2020).

Individual and group interventions are primarily aimed at improving social-emotional learning, executive function, and self-regulation. Such interventions combine approaches with a foundation in trauma-informed care, cognitive-behavior therapy, positive behavior intervention strategies, and sensory-based approaches (AOTA, 2016; Kingsley et al., 2020; Kramer et al., 2020; O'Brien & Kuhaneck, 2020). Self-regulation interventions, such as Zones of Regulation and The Alert Program for Self-Regulation of Arousal, and bodywork practices, including yoga, mindfulness, and meditation, are often used to teach individual coping strategies (AOTA, 2015; Bazyk & Arbesman, 2013; Kramer et al., 2020). Peer-mediated approaches, such as the Program for Education and Enrichment of Relational Skills (Laugeson, 2017), are structured curricula effectively implemented in groups to promote social participation in older children and youth (AOTA, 2016; Kramer et al., 2020). Parents are also integral to the intervention process, as practitioners employ coaching practices and help connect families to community resources and social support. Best and evidence-based practices to foster occupational adaption are those that are family-centered, culturally appropriate, and tailored to meet individual needs.

COLLABORATIVE APPROACH WITH FAMILIES AND THE SOCIAL ENVIRONMENT

Children are a part of a unit, with the family being a dynamic system that influences childhood development (Jaffe et al., 2020). Occupational therapists employ a client- and family-centered approach when working with children and families (AOTA, 2020). This requires awareness of individual, familial, and cultural factors to help to guide intervention approaches. Whether providing services in clinical or natural environments,

Case Study 15-1

Marco

Marco (Figure 15-4) was born premature at 30 weeks gestation, with his mother experiencing gestational diabetes during her pregnancy and preeclampsia. He was delayed with walking and was beginning to use words and short two- to three-word phrases with increased consistency in Spanish and English. Marco has a history of feeding difficulties, being averse to various textures, and was fed through a nasogastric (NG) tube for the first 6 months of life. Currently, Marco dislikes various textures of foods and being messy, and recently transitioned from eating only pureed foods. Marco lives with his father and maternal grandparents, as his mother was recently deported. Since his mother has been gone, Marco has regressed in his self-feeding skills and communication skills, has difficulty sleeping through the night, and cries frequently throughout the day. His family is struggling emotionally and financially as they adjust and cope with his mother's recent deportation. Incorporating family customs, including cuisine, and promoting engagement in identified family routines is instrumental for providing client-centered care for Marco.

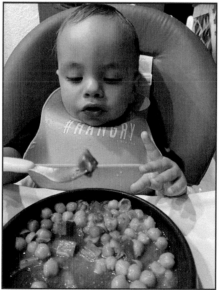

Figure 15-4. Marco eats a traditional dish provided by his family to promote self-feeding skills.

considerations for generalization of skills across contexts are critical to maximize benefit and promote optimal performance. The social environment, cultural practices, and various dynamics of the family network are important considerations to guide occupational therapy practice (Jaffe et al., 2020; Kramer et al., 2020).

Family customs, values, and practices—including those related to adverse childhood experiences—shape a child's development. Family stress can have multi-level and multigenerational effects on childhood experiences; these stressors, including divorce, drug abuse, and domestic violence, can perpetuate cycles of trauma and cause shifts in family dynamics over time (Masten & Monn, 2015). The family dynamic of children and youth of color can vary, ranging from single-parent households, divorced families, and those with extended families directly involved in care (Kramer et al., 2020). When providing intervention, it is important to collaborate with parents and other caregivers involved in the child's life, because building rapport and trust is critical for effective service delivery.

Collaborative approaches for working with families include engagement in training to improve parenting competencies and connecting to community supports; these have strong evidence for effectiveness (Child Welfare Information Gateway, 2015; National Scientific Council on the Developing Child, 2015; Racine et al., 2019). Occupational therapy practitioners, when working with families, can promote protective factors to support adaptation, coping, and resilience through such efforts. Building caregiver knowledge of parenting practices and child development, as well as supporting parents' well-being, have been shown to be beneficial for mitigating adverse childhood experiences (Child Welfare Information Gateway, 2015; Children's Defense Fund, 2020).

BUILDING INTERPROFESSIONAL COLLABORATIONS

Occupational therapy practitioners working with children and youth often engage with other professionals in the context of their service delivery. Whether working in schools, clinics, hospitals, or community-based settings, service provision involves working as part of a network of professionals providing care to children and their families (O'Brien & Kuhaneck, 2020). The makeup of the team of professionals will be contingent on the context where services are provided, such as hospitals, clinics, early intervention, and other community-based settings.

Interprofessional Collaborations

Adverse childhood experiences result in various developmental and behavioral challenges, which require intervention from various professionals (Ryan et al., 2017). Professionals commonly providing services include psychologists, pediatricians, mental health professionals, educators, occupational therapists, and other rehabilitation professionals. When children experience abuse and neglect, law enforcement and child protective service agencies might become involved to help facilitate changes in the child's care.

Case Study 15-2

Shane and Shayna

Shane and Shayna live in an inner-city neighborhood with high gun violence and policing that is undergoing gentrification and recovering from a hurricane that occurred 6 months ago. They recently lost one of their closest childhood friends due to a drive-by shooting and have been struggling to cope.

Shane has a history of attention deficit/hyperactivity disorder (ADHD) and a learning disability; he has received special-education services since he was 8 years old. He is now a sophomore in high school, has established vocational goals to study music production, and was recently suspended due to a fight.

Shayna was recently diagnosed with autism and has difficulty with executive functioning skills, as well as with making friends. She is now being bullied by peers, as she often sits alone and sometimes cries while at school. Shayna enjoys reading, listening to music, and spending time outdoors.

Occupational therapy practitioners can work with children and youth who have experienced trauma, promoting adaptation, coping, and resilience through individual and group intervention approaches, while also providing supports to families (Figure 15-5).

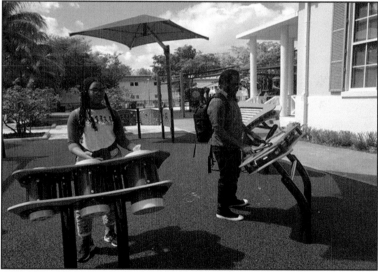

Figure 15-5. Two adolescents engage in playing percussion instruments at a neighborhood park.

As various professionals work to supply and guide interventions, they must work closely together as a team to promote those skills needed for occupational adaptation.

Ryan et al. (2017) described a multidisciplinary team approach to address childhood trauma, involving an occupational therapist, educators, and mental health therapists. They worked collaboratively to guide interventions rooted in play therapy for a 4-year-old boy living with an adoptive family. Access to qualified care, family financial resources, and other barriers might influence the form of professional collaborations afforded to marginalized populations and people of color. What is most important is that evidence-based approaches serve as the foundation of any interventions and that providers work collaboratively with families to best meet their needs.

A GLOBAL PERSPECTIVE

The notion of challenges faced by people of color is not restricted to the United States; it can be considered through various political-cultural perspectives across the globe. Globally, marginalized populations encounter adverse events that are known to pose challenges to developmental and functional outcomes (Bellis et al., 2014; Matheson et al., 2019). Incidents of racism, violence, famine, warfare, natural disasters, and other adverse societal and personal experiences contribute to trauma, and all of these are known to have detrimental effects on the growth and development of children and youth (Bellis et al., 2019; Hughes et al., 2017; Matheson et al., 2019). Adaptation, coping, and resilience in the face of such challenges are the qualities that determine and shape future outcomes, as adverse childhood experiences can negatively affect education and, later, employment (Hughes et al., 2017).

Racism has been at the forefront globally, with the World Federation of Occupational Therapy (WFOT, 2020) publishing a position statement on systemic racism and naming it as a global priority. This has called attention to the social inequities and human right infringements faced by Blacks and other marginalized populations. Discrimination occurs globally and has been associated with traumatic experiences that have negative effects on outcomes (Matheson et al., 2019; WFOT, 2020). With racism being just one factor associated with trauma, multiple adverse childhood experiences further confound occupational performance and lead to externalizing behaviors, such as suicide, risky sexual activity, and drug abuse (Bellis et al., 2019; Hughes et al., 2017). Addressing the maltreatment of children and the global health problems associated with adverse childhood experiences is an initiative to be embraced by occupational therapy practitioners and various international organizations worldwide.

Global Implications for Occupational Therapy

Trauma and adverse childhood experiences occur across the globe, presenting as a costly global public health problem (Bellis et al., 2019). Occupational deprivation can occur as a result of warfare, pandemics, natural disasters, migration, sex trafficking, and other traumatic experiences, all of which disrupt occupational engagement for children and youth. This knowledge presents unique opportunities to engage with children and families in refugee camps, shelters, and other non-traditional settings to help mitigate the effects of childhood trauma and support protective factors (Matheson et al., 2019; Siddiqui et al., 2019). Intervening from a public health perspective, such as by ensuring nurturing and safe childhoods, can provide not only developmental benefits, but also economically beneficial results for systems of care (Bellis et al., 2019).

Occupational therapy practitioners across the globe have an opportunity to make a difference in the lives of children and youth of color and other marginalized populations. Occupational therapy educational programs are subject to minimum standards established by the World Federation of Occupational Therapy (WFOT, 2016). In addition, WFOT publishes statements on inclusion, diversity, and culture to guide practice from an international perspective for service provision with marginalized children and youth (WFOT, 2010). Advocacy efforts and promotion of human rights and occupational justice to address systemic racism and other social determinants of health are encouraged (WFOT, 2020). Through training, resources, and intentional collaborations, the international workforce of occupational therapy practitioners can collectively address issues faced by children and youth of marginalized populations.

ESSENTIAL CONSIDERATIONS FOR OCCUPATIONAL THERAPISTS

Occupational therapy practitioners working with diverse populations need to be well versed in various aspects related to context and culture. The *Occupational Therapy Practice Framework* (AOTA, 2020) equips occupational therapy practitioners with foundational knowledge to identify the strengths and challenges of children and youth of color as we strive to provide client-centered services. The field of occupational therapy has models and frameworks to provide theories and inform intervention developed through our professional reasoning skills (Kramer et al., 2020; O'Brien & Kuhaneck, 2020; Reed, 2014). Our professional training and experiential knowledge together provide us with the skills to deliver effective assessment and intervention when working with children, youth, and their families. It is imperative that we further our training to include those centered on moving beyond cultural competency to embodying cultural humility (Agner, 2020; Tervalon & Murray-Garcia, 1998). See Table 15-3 for considerations regarding culturally-centered practice). Engaging in ongoing self-assessment and intentional self-improvement through professional development and seeking additional resources is essential for best and evidence-based practice with diverse populations (AOTA, 2015; AOTA, 2016; WFOT, 2020).

Table 15-3

Culturally Centered Occupational Therapy Practice Considerations and Resources
Practice Considerations
• Promote self-determination and individual identity, respecting these within the context of service delivery
• Consider the impact of adverse childhood events on development and occupation
• Consider context and the child as a member of their family and community when providing conscious culturally-centered services
• Employ therapeutic use of self, empathy, and collaboration to provide client-centered services
• Use professional reasoning to guide selection of culturally appropriate assessments and interventions
• Engage in ongoing self-reflective practices and seek professional development regarding service to diverse populations
• Promote occupational justice and advocate for educational, health, and social equity
• Refer to resources on diversity, equity, and inclusion available through professional organizations/associations
Resources
• AUCD Diversity & Inclusion Toolkit (Association of University Centers on Disabilities, 2020) http://www.implementdiversity.tools
• Harvard Project Implicit (Harvard University, 2011) https://implicit.harvard.edu/implicit/index.jsp
• Stanford SPARQtools RaceWorks Toolkit (Stanford University, 2020) http://sparqtools.org/raceworks-instructions
• World Federation of Occupational Therapy https://www.wfot.org/resources

Case Study 15-3

Jada

Jada (Figure 15-6) was adopted from Haiti at the age of 6 months following a natural disaster. Her mother, Judith, is a preschool teacher and has relocated to live closer to family, as her husband recently died while serving in a war overseas. Prior to the move, Judith indicated to Jada's previous pediatrician several times that she suspected delays with communication and fine motor skills, with all other developmental milestones being achieved within expected timeframes. However, she was frequently told, "Jada will grow out of it" and "She just needs time to adjust." Judith changed to a new pediatrician when she relocated, who finally referred Jada to have evaluations for occupational and speech therapy to receive the services she needed. Judith has also sought grief support for her family. She continues to advocate for Jada's needs while adjusting to the recent move and loss of her husband.

Diagnostic delays are common with children of color, resulting in missed opportunities for receiving timely early intervention. Empowering families to advocate for their needs is important, as is connecting them to resources and fostering trusting, supportive relationships with community providers.

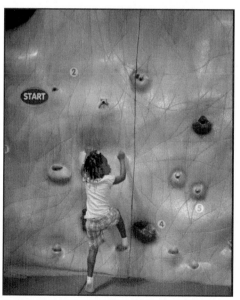

Figure 15-6. Jada attempts climbing a rock wall.

Case Study 15-3 Continuation

Jada

Jada (Figure 15-7) is a 3-year-old who was adopted from Haiti at the age of 6 months following a natural disaster. Her mother, Judith, is a single parent after the recent death of her husband; Judith has just relocated to be closer to her family. Jada was referred for an occupational therapy evaluation and treatment, as delays in development were expressed since she was 2 years old, but were dismissed by her previous pediatrician. To begin the holistic strength-based assessment process, an occupational profile was completed based on an interview with Judith, identifying strengths and challenges for occupational performance and participation. Judith has requested a provider who is Black and preferably fluent in Haitian Creole, due to past dissatisfaction and mistrust of providers not of her family's culture.

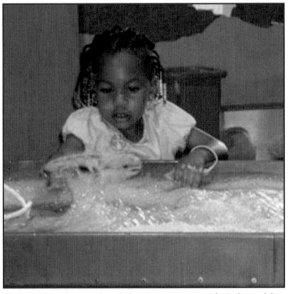

Figure 15-7. Occupational therapy process with Jada and her family.

What would you need to consider to conduct an evaluation that respects Jada and her family's culture and preferences? What personal factors might affect the areas identified as priorities for intervention?

What cultural factors would you need to consider in order to provide appropriate interventions to Jada and her family? How will you address linguistic barriers and learn about the family's culture? What resources would be ap-

(continued)

Case Study 15-3 Continuation (continued)

propriate for this family? Determine any additional training and self-reflection activities that would help you provide culturally-centered occupational therapy services.

Assessment

An occupational profile was completed alongside a structured interview with Jada's mother, Judith (see Table 15-1). Jada was assessed using the following standardized assessments: Sensory Processing Measure-Preschool (Home and Teacher Forms), Peabody Developmental Motor Scales-2, Adaptive Behavior Assessment System-3, and the Short Child Occupational Profile-Parent Report Form. Clinical observations included assessment of neuromuscular skills (gross and fine motor, oculomotor, tone), structured observations of sensory integration, and independent play. Results indicated delays in fine motor, visual motor integration, self-care, social participation, and self-regulation skills, so goals were established to address these concerns. Family intervention priorities included eating family meals, learning to write her name, and participating in church activities.

Intervention

Primary frames of reference used to guide intervention included developmental theory, sensory integration, and ecology of human performance. A client-centered approach was used, including various family members and employing cultural humility throughout. Occupational therapy services were recommended in the natural environment twice per week, for 60-minute sessions, with one provided at Jada's preschool and the other at home. A coaching model was employed in the home setting, with all family members joining sessions, and routine consultation was provided for Jada's teacher. Community resources were discussed with Jada's family, including play, parent, and grief support groups. A referral was also made to seek speech therapy services.

Implementing principles of cultural awareness, humility, and responsivity is critical for effective occupational therapy with children and youth of color. Promoting adaptation, coping, and resilience are essential for improved functional outcomes.

REFERENCES

Abidin, R. R. (2012). *Parenting stress index* (4th ed.). Psychological Assessment Resources.

Afifi, T. O., & MacMillan, H. L. (2011). Resilience following child maltreatment: A review of protective factors. *The Canadian Journal of Psychiatry, 56*(5), 266-272. https://doi.org/10.1177/070674371105600505

Agner, J. (2020). Moving from cultural competence to cultural humility in occupational therapy: A paradigm shift. *American Journal of Occupational Therapy, 74*(4), 7404347010. https://doi.org/10.5014/ajot.2020.038067

Alvarez, A. (2020). Seeing race in the research on youth trauma and education: A critical review. *Review of Educational Research, 90*(5), 583-626. https://doi.org/10.3102/0034654320938131

American Occupational Therapy Association. (2015). *Childhood trauma: Occupational therapy's role in mental health promotion, prevention, and intervention with children & youth.* https://www.aota.org/-/media/Corporate/Files/Practice/Children/Childhood-Trauma-Info-Sheet-2015.pdf

American Occupational Therapy Association. (2016). *Occupational therapy's distinct value: Mental health promotion, prevention, and intervention across the lifespan.* https://www.aota.org/-/media/Corporate/Files/Practice/MentalHealth/Distinct-Value-Mental-Health.pdf

American Occupational Therapy Association. (2017). Occupational profile template. https://www.aota.org/profile

American Occupational Therapy Association. (2020). Occupational therapy practice framework: Domain and process (4th ed.). *American Journal of Occupational Therapy, 74*(Suppl. 2), 7412410010. https://doi.org/10.5014/ajot.2020.74S2001

Association of University Centers on Disabilities. (2020). *AUCD diversity & inclusion toolkit.* http://www.implementdiversity.tools

Bartgis, J., & Bigfoot, D.S. (2010). *The state of best practices in Indian country.* http://www.icctc.org/Bartgis-Bigfoot%20The%20State%20of%20Best%20Practices%20in%20Indian%20Country%20(2).pdf

Bazyk, S. (2014). *Every moment counts: Promoting mental health throughout the day.* http://s3.us-east-2.amazonaws.com/s3.everymomentcounts.com/wp-content/uploads/2020/12/17192809/EMC_Info_Brief_2020.pdf

Bazyk, S. (2017). Occupational therapy: Everyday strategies for promoting positive mental health. https://vota.wildapricot.org/resources/Pictures/Bazyk%20-%20Keynote.pdf

Bazyk, S., & Arbesman, M. (2013). *Occupational therapy practice guidelines for mental health promotion, prevention, and intervention for children and youth.* AOTA Press.

Bedell, G. (2011). The child and adolescent scale of participation. http://sites.tufts.edu/garybedell/measurement-tools

Bellis, M. A., Hughes, K., Ford, K., Rodriguez, G., Sethi, D., & Passmore, J. (2019). Life course health consequences and associated annual costs of adverse childhood experiences across Europe and North America: A systematic review and meta-analysis. *Lancet Public Health 2019, 4*(10), E517-E528. https://doi.org/10.1016/S2468-2667(19)30145-8

Bellis, M. A., Hughes, K., Leckenby, N., Jones, L., Baban, A., Kachaeva, M., Povilaitis, R., Pudule, I., Qirjako, J., Ulokol, B., Raleva, M., & Terzic, N. (2014). Adverse childhood experiences and association with health-harming behaviors in young adults: Surveys in eight eastern European countries. *Bulletin: World Health Organization, 92*, 641-655. http://dx.doi.org/https://doi.org/10.2471/BLT.13.129247

Bernal, G., & Sáez-Santiago, E. (2006). Culturally centered psychosocial interventions. *Journal of Community Psychology, 34*(2), 121-232. https://doi.org/10.1002/jcop.20096

Bowyer, P. L., Kramer, J., Ploszaj, A., Ross, M., Schwartz, O., Kielhofner, G., & Kramer, K. (2008). *Short child occupational profile (version 2.2).* The University of Illinois at Chicago.

Cahill, S. M., Egan, B. E., & Seber, J. (2020). Activity- and occupation-based interventions to support mental health, positive behavior, and social participation for children and youth: A systematic review. *American Journal of Occupational Therapy, 74*(2), 7402180020. https://doi.org/10.5014/ajot.2020.038687

Center for the Study of Social Policy. (2017). *Strengthening families: A protective factor framework.* https://cssp.org/resource/about-strengthening-families-and-the-protective-factors-framework

Centers for Disease Control and Prevention. (2020). *Spotlight on closing the racial and ethnic gaps in the identification of Autism Spectrum Disorder.* https://www.cdc.gov/ncbddd/autism/addm-community-report/spotlight-on-closing-racial-gaps.html

Child Welfare Information Gateway. (2015). Promoting protective factors for in-risk families and youth: A guide for practitioners. https://www.childwelfare.gov/pubPDFs/in_risk.pdf

Children's Defense Fund. (2020). The state of America's children: 2020. https://www.childrensdefense.org/wp-content/uploads/2020/02/The-State-Of-Americas-Children-2020.pdf

Chorzempa, B. F., Smith, M. D., & Sileo, J. M. (2019). Practice-based evidence: A model for helping educators make evidence-based decisions. *Teacher Education and Special Education, 42*(1), 82-92. https://doi.org/10.1177/0888406418767254

D'Andrea, W., Ford, J., Stolbach, B., Spinazzola, J., & van der Kolk, B. (2012). Understanding interpersonal trauma in children: Why we need a developmentally appropriate trauma diagnosis. *American Journal of Orthopsychiatry, 82*(2), 187-200. https://doi.org/10.1111/j.1939-0025.2012.01154.x

Dean, E., Little, L., Tomchek, S., & Dunn, W. (2017). Sensory processing in the general population: Adaptability, resiliency, and challenging behavior. *American Journal of Occupational Therapy, 72*(1), 7201195060. https://doi.org/10.5014/ajot.2018.019919

Dunn, E. C., Nishimi, K., Powers, A., & Bradley, B. (2017). Is developmental timing of trauma exposure associated with depressive and post-traumatic stress disorder symptoms in adulthood? *Journal of Psychiatric Research, 84,* 119-127. https://doi.org/10.1016/j.jpsychires.2016.09.004

Dunn, W. (2014). *Sensory profile-2/Infant-toddler sensory profile 2* (2nd ed.). Pearson.

Elkins, J., Briggs, H. E., Miller, K. M., Kim, I., Orellana, R., & Mowbray, O. (2019). Racial/ethnic differences in the impact of adverse childhood experiences on posttraumatic stress disorder in a nationally representative sample of adolescents. *Child and Adolescent Social Work Journal, 36,* 449-457. https://doi.org/10.1007/s10560-018-0585-x

Fish, R. (2019). Standing out and sorting in: Exploring the role of racial composition in special education. *American Educational Research Journal, 56*(6), 2573-2608. https://doi.org/10.3102/0002831219847966

Foner, N., & Frederickson, G. (2005). Immigration, race, and ethnicity in the United States: Social constructions and social relations in historical and contemporary perspective. In N. Foner & G. Fredrickson (Eds.). *Not just Black and White: Historical and contemporary perspectives on immigration, race, and ethnicity in the United States* (pp. 1-19). Russell Sage Foundation.

Gioia, G. A., Isquith, P. K., Guy, S. C., & Kenworthy, L. (2013). *Behavior rating inventory of executive function* (2nd ed.). Psychological Assessment Resources.

Goldstein, S., & Herzberg, D. (2018). *Risk inventory and strengths evaluation.* Western Psychological Services.

Goodman, R. (2002). *Strengths and difficulties questionnaire.* https://www.sdqinfo.org

Grajo, L., Boisselle, A., & DaLomba, E. (2018). Occupational adaptation as a construct: A scoping review of literature. *The Open Journal of Occupational Therapy, 6*(1). https://doi.org/10.15453/2168-6408.1400

Gray, K., Tonge, B., Einfeld, S., Gruber, C., & Klein, A. (2018). *Developmental behavioral checklist* (2nd ed.). Western Psychological Services.

Haley, S. M., Coster, W. J., Dumas, H. M., Fragala-Pinkham, M. A., & Moed, R. (2020). *Pediatric evaluation of disability inventory computer adaptive test.* Pearson.

Harrison, P., & Oakland, T. (2015). *Adaptive behavior assessment system* (3rd ed.). Western Psychological Services.

Harvard University. (2011). *Project implicit.* https://implicit.harvard.edu/implicit

Health Resources and Services Administration's Maternal and Child Health Bureau. (2020). *Adverse childhood experiences: National Survey of Children's Health data brief.* https://mchb.hrsa.gov/sites/default/files/mchb/Data/NSCH/nsch-ace-databrief.pdf

Hughes, K., Bellis, M. A., Hardcastle, K. A., Sethi, D., Butchart, A., Mikton, P., Jones, L., & Dunne, M. P. (2017). The effect of multiple adverse childhood experiences on health: A systematic review and meta-analysis. *Lancet Public Health, 2*(8), E356-E366. https://doi.org/10.1016/S2468-2667(17)30118-4

International Society for Traumatic Stress Studies. (2015). *A public health approach to trauma: Implications for science, practice, policy, and the role of ISTSS.* https://istss.org/getattachment/Education-Research/White-Papers/A-Public-Health-Approach-to-Trauma/Trauma-and-PH-Task-Force-Report.pdf.aspx

Jackson, D. (2015). *A mixed methods study of diagnostic and adaptive functioning challenges in African American preschool-aged children with Autism Spectrum Disorder* (Publication No. 1851) [Doctoral dissertation, Walden University]. Walden Dissertations and Doctoral Studies.

Jaffe, L., Cosper, S., & Fabrizi, S. (2020). Working with families. In J. O'Brien & H. Kuhaneck (Eds.), *Case-Smith's occupational therapy for children and adolescents* (pp. 46-75). Elsevier.

Jaffee, S. R., & Maikovich-Fong, A. K. (2011). Effects of chronic maltreatment and maltreatment timing on children's behavior and cognitive abilities. *Journal of Child Psychology and Psychiatry, 52*(2), 184-194. https://doi.org/10.1111/j.1469-7610.2010.02304.x

Jeong, B. (2019). A people yet to come: "People of color" reconsidered. In E. S. Lee (Ed.), *Race as phenomena: Between phenomenology and philosophy of race* (pp. 1-14). Rowman & Littlefield.

King, G., Law, M., King, S., Hurley, P., Rosenbaum, P., Hanna, S., Kertoy, M., & Young, N. (2004). *Children's assessment of participation and enjoyment*. Pearson.

Kingsley, K., Sagester, G., & Weaver, L. (2020). Interventions supporting mental health and positive behavior in children ages birth-5 yr: A systematic review. https://doi.org/10.5014/ajot.2020.039768

Kramer, J., Kafkes, A., Basu, S., Federic, J., & Kielhofner, G. (2014). *Child occupational self-assessment (version 2.2)*. The University of Illinois at Chicago.

Kramer, P., Hinojosa, J., & Howe, T. (2020). *Frames of reference for pediatric occupational therapy*. Wolters Kluwer.

Laugeson, E. (2017). *PEERS® for young adults: Social skills training for adults with autism spectrum disorder and other social challenges*. Routledge. https://doi.org/10.4324/9781315297057

Llorens, L. A. (1976). *Application of a developmental theory for health and rehabilitation*. American Occupational Therapy Association.

Masten, A., & Monn, A. (2015). Child and family resilience: A call for integrated science, practice, and professional training. *Family Relations, 64*(1), 5-21. https://doi.org/10.1111/fare.12103

Matheson, K., Foster, M. D., Bombay, A., McQuaid, R. J., & Anisman, H. (2019). Traumatic experiences, perceived discrimination, and psychological distress among members of various socially marginalized groups. *Frontiers in Psychology, 10*. https://doi.org/10.3389/fpsyg.2019.00416

National Scientific Council on the Developing Child. (2015). *Supportive relationships and active skill-building strengthen the foundations of resilience: Working paper 13*. http://www.developingchild.harvard.edu

O'Brien, J., & Kuhaneck, H. (2020). *Case-Smith's occupational therapy for children and adolescents*. Elsevier.

Office of Special Education Programs. (2020). *OSEP fast facts: Black or African American children with disabilities*. https://sites.ed.gov/idea/osep-fast-facts-black-or-african-american-children-with-disabilities-20

Parham, L. D., Ecker, C., Kuhaneck, H. M., Henry, D. A., & Glennon, T. J. (2007). *Sensory processing measure/sensory processing measure-preschool*. Western Psychological Services.

Prince-Embury, S. (2006). *Resiliency scales for children & adolescents: A profile of personal strengths*. Pearson.

Racine, N., Eirich, R., Dimitropoulos, G., Hartwick, C., & Madigan, S. (2020). Development of trauma symptoms following adversity in childhood: The moderating role of protective factors. *Child Abuse & Neglect, 101*, 104375. https://doi.org/10.1016/j.chiabu.2020.104375

Reed, K. (2014). *Quick reference to occupational therapy*. Pro-Ed.

Robins, D., Fein, D., & Barton, M. (2009). *The modified checklist for autism in toddlers, revised with follow-up (M-CHAT-R/F)*. https://mchatscreen.com/wp-content/uploads/2015/09/M-CHAT-R_F_Rev_Aug2018.pdf

Robles-Ramamurthy, B., & Watson, C. (2020). Examining racial disparities in juvenile justice. *Journal of the American Academy of Psychiatry and the Law Online, 48*(3). http://jaapl.org/content/early/2019/02/13/JAAPL.003828-19.abstract

Rosenthal, A., Meyer, M., Mayo, D., Tully, L., Patel, P., Ashby, S., Titone, M., Carter, C., & Niendam, T. (2020). Contributions of childhood trauma and atypical development to increased clinical symptoms and poor functioning in recent onset psychosis. *Early Intervention in Psychiatry, 14*(6), 755-761. https://doi.org/10.1111/eip.12931

Ryan, K., Lane, S. J., & Powers, D. (2017). A multidisciplinary model for treating complex trauma in early childhood. *International Journal of Play Therapy, 26*(2), 111-123. https://doi.org/10.1037/pla0000044

Schell, B., & Schell, J. (2018). *Clinical and professional reasoning in occupational therapy*. Lippincott Williams & Wilkins.

Schkade, J. K., & Schultz, S. (1992). Occupational adaptation: Toward a holistic approach for contemporary practice, part 1. *American Journal of Occupational Therapy, 46*(9), 829-837. https://doi.org/10.5014/ajot.46.9.829

Siddiqui, S., Said, E., Hanna, B., Patel, Natasha, N. H., Gonzalez, E., Garrett, S. L., Hilton, C. L., & Aranha, K. (2019). Addressing occupational deprivation in refugees: A scoping review. *Journal of Refugee & Global Health, 2*(1), art. 3. https://doi.org/10.18297/rgh/vol2/iss1/3

Sparrow, S., Cicchetti, D. V., & Saulnier, C. A. (2016). *Vineland adaptive behavior scales* (3rd ed.). Pearson.

Stanford University. (2020). Stanford SPARQtools RaceWorks toolkit. http://sparqtools.org/raceworks-instructions

Stein, F. (1983). A current review of the behavioral frame of reference and its application to occupational therapy. *Occupational Therapy in Mental Health, 2*(4), 35-62. https://doi.org/10.1300/J004v02n04_03

Substance Abuse and Mental Health Services Administration. (2014). A treatment improvement protocol: Improving cultural competence. https://store.samhsa.gov/sites/default/files/d7/priv/sma14-4849.pdf

Taylor, R. (2017). *Kielhofner's model of human occupation: Theory and application* (5th ed.). Wolters Kluwer.

Tervalon, M., & Murray-Garcia, J. (1998). Cultural humility versus cultural competence: A critical distinction in defining physician training outcomes in multicultural education. *Journal of Health Care for the Poor and Underserved, 9*(2), 117-125. https://doi.org/10.1353/hpu.2010.0233

United States Census Bureau. (2019). *Quick facts: United States.* https://www.census.gov/quickfacts/fact/table/US#

United States Department of Justice, Office of Justice Programs. (2019). *OJJDP statistical briefing book.* https://www.ojjdp.gov/ojstatbb/crime/qa05104.asp?qaDate=2017

Vespa, J., Armstrong, D. M., & Medina, L. (2020). Demographic turning points for the United States: Population projections for 2020 to 2060. *Current Population Reports* 25-1144. https://www.census.gov/content/dam/Census/library/publications/2020/demo/p25-1144.pdf

Vidal-Ortiz, S. (2008). People of color. In R. Schaefer (Ed.), *Encyclopedia of race, ethnicity, and society* (pp. 1037-1039). Sage Publications.

White, J., Pearce, J., Morrison, S., Dunstan, F., Bisson, J., & Fone, D. (2015). Risk of post-traumatic stress disorder following traumatic events in a community sample. *Epidemiological and Psychiatric Sciences, 24*(3), 249-257. https://doi.org/10.1017/S2045796014000110

World Federation of Occupational Therapy. (2010). *Position statement: Diversity and culture.* https://www.wfot.org/resources/diversity-and-culture

World Federation of Occupational Therapy. (2016). Minimum standards for the education of occupational therapists. https://www.wfot.org/assets/resources/COPYRIGHTED-World-Federation-of-Occupational-Therapists-Minimum-Standards-for-the-Education-of-Occupational-Therapists-2016a.pdf

World Federation of Occupational Therapy. (2020). *Resources.* https://www.wfot.org/resources

World Health Organization. (2018). Adverse childhood experiences international questionnaire (ACE-IQ). https://www.who.int/violence_injury_prevention/violence/activities/adverse_childhood_experiences/en

16

The Lived Experience of Adaptation, Coping, and Resilience by Children and Youth and Their Families

Angela K. Boisselle, PhD, OTR and
Lenin C. Grajo, PhD, EdM, OTR/L

> **CHAPTER OBJECTIVES** By the end of this chapter, the reader will be able to:
> - Describe the lived experienced of adaptation, coping, and resilience from the perspective of pediatric clients and their caregivers.
> - Examine common factors, such as sense of self, contexts, and social connections, that may positively or negatively influence client and caregiver perspective of adaptation, coping, and resilience.
> - Develop a self-awareness of personal adaptation, coping, and resilience, and be reflective about the delivery of pediatric occupational therapy services through practice, education, and research.

In this chapter, we conclude our journey of deep understanding of adaptation, coping, and resilience through the lens of occupational therapy scholars and clinicians on many pediatric considerations and factors. We now provide a voice for those who lived and continue to live with adversity and their perspectives on how to respond to and overcome challenges. We developed a series of guiding questions involving the themes of adaptation, coping, and resilience and chose three youth and their families to respond. The respondents were given the opportunity to answer the questions of their

Grajo L. C., & Boisselle, A. K. (Eds.). *Adaptation, Coping, and Resilience in Children and Youth: A Comprehensive Occupational Therapy Approach* (pp. 387-399).
© 2022 Taylor & Francis Group.

choosing. The following presents reflections of the three families: Daniel and his mother, Elizabeth, and MJ's aunt and brother. We edited their responses for brevity but allowed each respondent to have their own tone and unique voice in the narratives. The reader may notice this contrast in the style of responses. We wanted to portray the authenticity of responses based on the age, role, and viewpoint of the respondents; therefore, only minor edits were made to establish themes, clarity, and grammatical flow within the chapter. Edits and final responses were sent back for review and were approved by the three families. In this chapter, we also reflect on and support the primary themes from this book on how to understand adaptation, coping, and resilience: a shift to a strength-based approach, a highlight on strong social supports, and a focus on mastery and competence in participating in meaningful daily occupations. The perspectives from the three youth and families in this chapter further strengthen and also give heart to many of the dense discussions that have been presented in the various chapters in this text.

DANIEL AND HIS MOTHER: RESILIENCE THROUGH CO-OCCUPATION

Daniel is 13 years old and has been diagnosed with spastic quadriplegia and dystonia. He lives with his parents and brother. His story, as told by Daniel and his mother, demonstrates how Daniel and his family learned to cope with challenges and develop adaptive capacities to remain positive that ultimately allowed him to develop into a resilient adolescent (Figure 16-1). Daniel's own words are presented in interview format, as written by him on his augmentative communication device. His mother's responses follows as a narrative.

Figure 16-1. Daniel enjoying a swim in the pool.

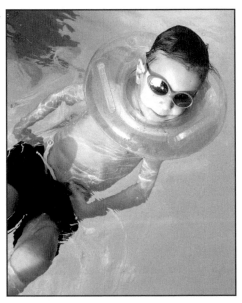

Daniel's Perspective

In what ways do you do your daily activities differently than your peers?
A para. Device talk. Wheelchair drive around.

Why do you think you do these activities differently?
Brain hurt born. Cerebral palsy.

What activities do you find most challenging to do every day?
Power chair.

When you try to do these activities, what do you do when you reach a point that it becomes overwhelming or challenging for you to do?
Ask mom drive.

What are activities you have never tried before but always wanted to?
Football.

Explain an activity or task that needed to be changed or adjusted for you to be able to do them.
Swimming use float ring.

Tell us about the strong emotions you may have experienced because of the challenges you experience as a result of this condition.
Feel different. Sad. Power chair drive happy drive.

Relative to hospitalizations, what things have medical professionals done to make your experience easier and/or more difficult? What did you find was helpful for you? What did you find was not helpful for you?
DBS [Deep brain stimulation] help body. Botox shots hurt help body.

Have you experienced bullying?
No.

What is something that gives you purpose or gets you excited about life?
People, TV, Go Target, look dvds.

What is one characteristic or personality trait of yours that you have that you think made you become a tough person and overcome daily life challenges?
Nice, happy.

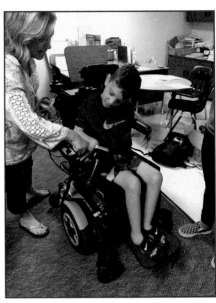

Figure 16-2. Daniel learning to use his power wheelchair.

A Mother's Perspective

As a result of a traumatic birth, Daniel experienced hypoxic ischemic encephalopathy (HIE). Due to the lack of oxygen, he has brain damage, which led to a diagnosis of cerebral palsy. Daniel requires assistance for all his self-care needs, as well as help to access his environment. At school, he has a paraprofessional to help him access the classroom and school materials, as well as to help him with anything else he needs. Daniel is nonverbal, but he does use an augmentative communication device via eye gaze to communicate, as well as a lot of head gestures and facial expressions. He also uses a power wheelchair that he can control with a head array (Figure 16-2).

Coping

It takes a lot of physical and mental energy for Daniel to do everyday tasks. It takes a lot of processing time for his brain to tell his body how to move. He uses his head and his eyes to control so many things in his environment. Because of this, he becomes fatigued easily. He is in his wheelchair using his communication device from the time he gets up until the time he goes to bed. Not only does he access his device to talk, but he also uses the eye gaze for schoolwork, to access the internet, to watch videos, and to operate the television. That takes a lot of energy. He also gets a lot of headaches, which I'm assuming is from eye fatigue. Driving his power chair with his head array just adds an extra layer of energy output. When we are in public and he becomes too tired to drive the chair, he will ask me to drive it with the attendant mode. This frees up some of his energy so that he can continue using his communication device.

Context and Connection

Since Daniel needs help to access his environment, there is usually an adult around. I think this has played a role in how Daniel is treated by peers. Daniel has also been included in the general education classroom since he was in pre-K. Inclusion plays such a significant role in the socialization. The kids Daniel is in school with have known him for many years. They see him in their classrooms, the hallways, the lunchroom, and in the community. They understand he has a disability, but they don't shy away from that. He is well known in school and people are always speaking to him. Unfortunately, this doesn't equate to true friendships, but it does support an environment of acceptance. I think that being included and taking part in activities with kids who both do and don't have disabilities have played a role in Daniel not being made fun of or bullied.

Daniel has a device called Deep Brain Stimulation (DBS), which are wires that are implanted in his brain and connected to a battery in his chest. The wires are programmed to activate different parts of his brain that, in turn, affect his body movements. Because of the DBS, Daniel has much better trunk control and his arm movements are more fluid. It also decreases his salivation and helps with swallowing. We both notice a significant difference in how his body works when the battery dies. Daniel doesn't like to charge the battery, which is implanted—he says it hurts—but he knows that it helps his body work better. The same goes for the Botox shots. They hurt in the moment, but the relief he gets in his muscles is beneficial, so he continues to get them on a regular basis. All of his doctors and nurses in the hospital and in the clinic work very well with him. They always ask him for his thoughts directly instead of talking through me. I believe Daniel appreciates this. He has his own thoughts and opinions about what is happening to him.

Adaptation Through Occupation and Resilience

Daniel didn't answer directly how he feels about changing activities. I asked him if he likes using the float ring to swim and he said, "Yes." I asked him if it bothers him that he has to use a float to swim by himself, and he said, "Yes." I asked him if he wished he could swim by himself and he said, "Yes." Unless Daniel is being held, he is not able to be in the pool on his own. We have a float that can go around his neck that keeps him upright in the pool. With this ring around his neck, he can float independently. Because of his cerebral palsy, he still can't freely move his arms and legs to swim, but the neck ring does give him a little independence in the pool and do something that is meaningful to him—something he likes to do.

By nature, Daniel is a very happy and joyful kid. He rarely expresses sadness, so it was surprising for me to hear that his challenges make him sad. Although I was surprised, this is a feeling I would expect. We try as much as possible to adapt experiences to make sure Daniel can be included. We go on vacations, to theme parks, water parks, swimming, hiking, etc. But as he is getting older (age 13 now) these outings get more difficult. I explored a little about why he says his power chair makes him happy. He said that he likes it because he can go places on his own and he doesn't need help.

Daniel has a pretty simple life, but he seems to enjoy it a lot. Because he has limited mobility and functional use of his arms and hands, it's always been very difficult finding activities that he likes and can engage in independently. I think that's one reason he enjoys TV so much. He can search and find things that interest him. A few years ago, he somehow discovered gymnastics. He finds old gymnastics videos on YouTube, and they can entertain him for hours. He gets physically excited when he watches gymnastics. He even extends his body as if he's attempting to do the routines. He's also found a few YouTubers who go to Target and other stores to shop and review DVDs. Some other YouTubers do movie reviews. This is his outlet and hobby, so to speak. He also enjoys going to Target and looking at all the different DVDs on his own. He's able to take off through the store on his own using his power chair, and he directs me to the DVD section, and we spend time looking at all the different DVDs. It's one of his favorite things to do. It seems a little unusual to me, but I'm thrilled that he has something that he enjoys so much, and it truly brings him happiness. I hear so much laughter coming from his room when he's watching these channels. I'm also glad that this is something he can do with such independence. I'm hopeful that as he matures, so will his interests, and he'll find ways to explore these interests with independence.

Daniel also loves people! Even if he can't always participate in all the physical activities, just being in the presence of people makes him happy. He enjoys listening to everyone talk and laugh. And he absolutely loves getting attention. We have a big extended family in Virginia and going to Virginia for vacation is something he looks forward to twice a year.

When I asked Daniel what was the best part of his personality, he told me that he is nice and that he is happy. This is so true. Daniel is such an easygoing kid and he truly exudes joy and happiness. I am told all the time by people, especially teachers, that they look forward to seeing Daniels's smile every day. It's truly infectious, and it can light up a room. I think his happiness and laughter put people at ease when they meet him. Instead of focusing on the disability, he makes it so easy for them to focus on the smile and laughter. Having such an easygoing personality makes life challenges and obstacles a lot easier to deal with. Daniel is also very resilient and determined. Since he was little, he has always found ways to make things work for him. He tries and tries without giving up. For instance, when the iPad first came out, he couldn't activate it with his hands. He somehow realized that he could make it work with his forehead! Before he was able to use a communication device, he found very effective ways to communicate with his eyes and small head gestures. As he grows older and moves toward adulthood, I hope this determination carries over to a meaningful job and meaningful relationships, and of course, a more independent life.

ELIZABETH: IN HER OWN VOICE

Elizabeth is 16 years old and diagnosed with spastic diplegia. She lives in a blended family with her mother, brother, stepfather, and two stepsisters. Her perspective is presented as her own narrative.

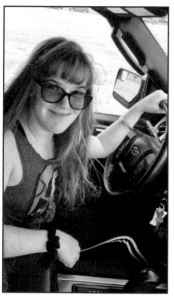

Figure 16-3. Elizabeth practices driving.

Adaptation Through Occupation

I get dressed differently; I usually have to sit down to put my pants on. When I shower, I use a seat. I think I do these things differently because as I grew up, I had to adapt to do things differently, and as I grew up, I had to adjust. Sometimes when I can't put food in the trash, I have to have my mom help me.

I want to be able to play in a soccer game because it seems like it would be fun to kick a ball around. They would add an adaptation, like make wheelchair soccer a more common sport. It looks like fun because I see my sister doing it all the time. I feel strongly about it because it's one of my favorite sports to watch and it's not very well adapted for people like me.

To do activities, I just usually advocate. I wish they had more things that could adapt better to what people's needs are. I would like to play soccer and eventually drive (Figure 16-3). Not many other people have helped me adapt activities besides my parents. Well, my best friend helps me get materials for class when I'm going to be late. I vocally express and tell multiple people about my needs prior to going. Like school, for instance; I let people know about my needs, but if I need things fixed, I will advocate for myself.

Coping

When I was younger it angered me a lot because I would see kids do certain things that I couldn't do. I definitely felt anger, feeling left out and helpless, and also dumb. I've realized that I think people are constantly staring at me even if they aren't really, and I've tried to ignore it. One time, a kid took away my walker because I told him I can walk, which is true, but he forced me to walk unassisted and I had to go to the ER [emergency room] because he made me walk down a ramp chasing my walker and I tripped on a crack in the sidewalk and busted my eyebrow open. Another time in eighth grade, I was walking to go to another class at school and this kid specifically waited until I got one of my back wheels of my walker right next to his foot and he stuck his foot out and I tripped and dropped all of my stuff. And then there was a wasp incident that everyone made fun of me for. In the eighth grade, I saw a wasp in a light fixture cover and seeing it made me feel like I was having an anxiety attack. They all made fun of me because of that. Someone even drew a picture of me and put it on my walker. I sought out administration and I told my friends so they could be a witness to it if needed.

Now, I've learned to accept my differences and embrace it and I just try to fit in to the best of my ability. I've overcome not feeling smart by realizing other people feel the same way as I do. I've overcome feeling helpless by realizing that sometimes I need help even when I don't want help. I do feel a pressure to fit in, and I can't really cope with it because it happens so often. But one thing I try is to stop thinking about not fitting in and instead, I look ahead to the future. When people stare at me, I just say "hi" and stuff, or when I was younger and little kids would stare at me I would just explain to them what I had. Other times, I just ignore it. I just learned recently from a good guy friend of mine that people's opinions don't matter and if they can't see past my disability, then they have a disability called Ignorance.

Sense of Self and Connection

Some things that help me cope are just vegging out and watching YouTube or Netflix or eating and also, accomplishing things that people wouldn't expect me to accomplish. Like every day, I wake up and try to say, "I'm going to bring my grades up." School, in general, gives me purpose because it gives me a way to show people that I can work just as hard and accomplish just as much as they do. I do wish that medical professionals and teachers, in general, talked about us in a way that made us seem as normal as possible and not seem so different. Like, talk about us in a way that didn't make us seem so alienated.

When I get stressed, I try to think about other things that don't get me as worked up. My ability to have a positive outlook on life has made me stronger. One thing I can tell other kids is that if someone asks about their disability, just explain it to them. I also found out that you may think you're alone in this world, but you're really not, and in the future, you won't feel as excluded as you once felt. My best friend helps because we both have a disability and it made me realize that I'm not as alone as I once thought I was. And since she understands what it's like to have a disability, she helps me a lot. I definitely say that it has made me have a more positive outlook on life because it makes me see that people have it rough just like I do, but everyday there are new things to overcome. Being tough doesn't necessarily mean you're strong, it means you are able to overcome the hardest things in your everyday life and still being able to wake up in the morning and still have a positive outlook on life.

MJ: CAREGIVER PERSPECTIVES

This response is a combination of reflections and insights from MJ's aunt and brother. She is now 22 years old but was diagnosed with attention deficit hyperactivity disorder (ADHD) and learning disability (LD) at around age 5. MJ's aunt is a retired professional who took the primary responsibility of taking care of MJ, along with her brother who is an occupational therapist. MJ and her aunt live in the Philippines.

Adaptation

When MJ was in her early elementary years, her difficulties were not as challenging as when she was in high school. We have always found her attention span to be limited, [she] had challenges with math and reading comprehension activities, and had difficulty following the rules. As early as kindergarten, we would get reports from teachers about misbehaviors. The reports started "mild," then increasingly became worrisome. Initially, we would get a remark from a teacher that she couldn't stay still, always chatting with classmates, needed more help following multistep instructions. Then, there came the reports about grabbing school materials from other kids, which later became reports of fighting back when taunted or teased by peers.

MJ's first formal preschool was a Catholic private school where her brother also went from elementary to high school. That was an eye-opening experience for us. We knew the principals and many of the teachers and head teachers, as some of them of them were the same teachers when her brother went to that school. We were essentially told MJ wouldn't be successful there, with a big class size, one teacher, and a traditional, discipline-strict, Catholic-school style of teaching. It was heartbreaking. That's when we decided to have her assessed by a developmental pediatrician who gave the ADHD diagnosis. We moved MJ to a very small, Montessori-style program with a small, pod-style learning environment with several teachers and teacher aides for preschool, then to a private school with smaller class sizes and more flexible teaching styles. MJ enjoyed that style of school, and she has always enjoyed and looked forward to going to school.

Performing self-care is always a challenge, and we have always needed to help her out with constant reminders, assistance and cues throughout, even to this day as an adult. School homework is a completely different process. While MJ enjoyed going to school, she always disliked doing homework. I [MJ's aunt] have a different style of working with MJ than her OT brother. Her brother always worked on ways and strategies to make her understand and complete her homework as independently as possible (Figure 16-4). This can take much time and frustrates MJ frequently. My approach was to do as much prep work for her as possible, doing the research, answering the math problems, so most of what MJ needs to do is to copy them or put them all together. These different styles were both helpful but also sometimes challenging. Her brother's method really helped her understand the homework, but caused her a lot of frustration, avoidance, and frequent disappointments. My approach got the job done, but sometimes I worry that I am spoon-feeding her too much. This is something her brother and I always have to discuss.

Figure 16-4. Young MJ and her brother.

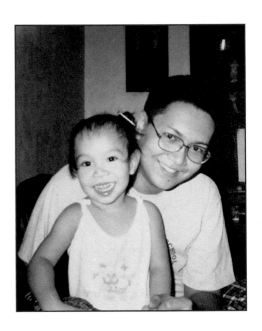

From my perspective [aunt], this caregiving process was a completely different experience. It was very challenging and caused a lot of heartaches. I raised and was primary caregiver for MJ's brother, as well. He has always been so independent, consistently top of the class, and never had behavioral or academic issues. I never had any experience taking care of a child that has very different parenting needs. It was helpful that her brother is a pediatric occupational therapist, but sometimes, when he gets home having worked all day, he is also tired of having to deal with the issues MJ is experiencing. We had to figure out ways on how to constantly get her to complete schoolwork, and not avoid doing long assignments. Preparing for written exams are most challenging. MJ's brother and I would both be frustrated when we ourselves don't know how to best explain and simplify complex math concepts and reading comprehension questions to prepare her for exams. She has always received some form of accommodation and support from teachers. One adaptive strategy we have learned is to be upfront to her teachers every school year, talk to them about her special learning needs, and always be in constant communication with them. This can be hit or miss. There are grade levels where she would have a more flexible, responsive teacher who will be willing to work with her one-on-one, and some that are more traditional in approach and can be very strict with classroom discipline. Every school year is just another surprise; and we would celebrate each March when school ends in the Philippines for barely making it through every year.

Coping

I would say that we both coped with the diagnosis pretty well, but this was new to our family. No one has ever had such challenges, although we know there was a strong family history of developmental and learning disability from MJ's mother's side of the family. The day-to-day coping with the teacher reports of misbehaviors, struggling with schoolwork, teachers not being as accommodating, and avoidance with structured tasks can be challenging and overwhelming at times.

What we were not really prepared for was when MJ reached adolescence and started high school. That's when the bullying started. Male classmates just started ganging up on her. As MJ's female classmates became more refined and finessed as teenage girls, MJ kept her "rough on the edges" personality. She had one friend, a student with an unspecified developmental disability that became her close friend. But other than this friend, MJ frequently hung out with the boys, many of whom ended up being bullies. We really didn't know the scope of the bullying until MJ started acting out. She became more aggressive, at one point hitting a classmate and making verbal remarks that warranted a suspension for a few days and a strongly worded letter from the principal. She was almost expelled from the school, and there was even an accusation made that she was being abused at home. This was particularly heartbreaking and overwhelming. MJ was never the communicative and expressive type. So, we would never really know the scope of how much the bullying hurt her emotionally, how she was bullied, who were her aggressors, and what really happened that caused her to snap and fight back. This became a bigger issue later on, when the high school principal put all of the blame of the situation on MJ and accused her as the primary aggressor and troublemaker in class. At that time, MJ's brother had immigrated to the U.S. and most of our communication was via Skype. We saw a drastic change in MJ. Despite her challenges, she was always excited to go to school and would never want to miss school even if she was sick or when school was cancelled due to bad weather. She always had a cheerful and positive disposition, always helpful to her teachers. But during the bullying days and after her suspension, she started not wanting to go to school. It was very heartbreaking for me, as I felt helpless and didn't know how to address this. I didn't know how to talk to the principal and what to say so that they wouldn't expel her. If she gets expelled from this school, we wouldn't know where else to send her to. Not having her brother here to navigate all this for us on a day-to-day basis was another contributing factor to the stress and difficulty. Worse, the accusation that MJ was being abused at home made it much more painful. We give so much of our love, energy, and attention to singularly address all her needs, only to be accused of such!

We needed to learn how to self-advocate. MJ's brother fought back and crafted a very strongly worded letter to the principal, how they have been unhelpful, accusatory, and almost discriminating of her special learning needs. It caused tension; I was worried that such a strong letter might just cause the school to fight back even harder and I would have to worry about all the repercussions later on. However, this strategy helped us well. Learning to self-advocate and assert MJ's needs rather than looking at ourselves as victims of the situation helped MJ and us make it through. The entire case was brought up to the board of directors and trustees of the school, who eventually rescinded the suspension and created an educational plan for her. That's when the dynamics at school shifted, and we felt some level of protection and better support for MJ. We made it through, and MJ graduated from high school.

MJ still has difficulties understanding her strengths and challenges. When everyone else from her high school started going to college, she was worried why she couldn't go. We couldn't find an area or field she was particularly interested in, and we decided college is not really something she will be successful at. We've had plenty of arguments about this. She thought that college is something she had to do because all her peers are doing it, and had difficulty identifying where she could go, what she could study, and what she could do.

Resilience

Since MJ graduated from high school, she has mostly been at home exploring options for what comes next. Her interests are very limited and her attention span on doing anything is very limited. She has been doing some e-commerce, selling food items in our neighborhood, that earns her a little money. Her interest in that also ebbs and flows. One thing that has allowed her to flourish is her interest in music and singing, and we have allowed her to explore that. She did a few guitar lessons and joined the community church as a member of the choir. Since then, she has found a sense of community and purpose, and something to look forward to every week. The COVID-19 pandemic took that away, and she has been insisting on going back to church, but it's just too risky right now, and that frustrates her. She has also flourished and is feeling more connected on social media where she would post videos of her singing and love all the reactions from family and high school friends.

Resilience for us is that day-to-day facing up to the challenge. We know that life will not be easy for her, and as I am growing older and less able to have the stamina to always support her and assist her, she will need to learn to be more self-reliant and independent. But we know that with the support of our extensive family and her strong faith, that we will rally through.

One thing we have learned from this journey is the power of self-advocacy. Working with MJ's therapists through the years, and especially with her teachers, we needed to be upfront about her challenges, communicate about strategies that work for her, and how best to explore her interests. We hope that service providers (therapists, teachers, school administrators) are more open to conversation and problem solving, rather than merely imposing strategies that they think will work, or what they think best needs to be done. Every child is unique and has very different contexts and circumstances, and a cookie-cutter approach won't work. We were fortunate that MJ's brother is an OT who specialized in child development. If not, we don't think we would have known how to handle all this. I wish there were more programs for parents on how to cope and support children with special learning needs. We hope there were more resources on how we can be more resilient and face these daily life challenges.

CONCLUDING THOUGHTS FROM AN OCCUPATIONAL THERAPIST

To be very candid, throughout the beginning of my career [Angela, first author], I designed treatment plans *for* my patients, not *with* my patients. It was not until I began to *listen* and *observe* that I began to transform my practice. I often say that the children, youth, and caregivers whom I encountered throughout my career taught me far more than I have taught them. They taught me to adapt my thinking, overcome challenges, and develop an art for solving everyday problems in order to facilitate a transactive process of adaptation through occupation. They taught me that every child has a voice, regardless of age, background, or level of disability. They taught me that failure and frustration are part of the process—but more importantly, so are determination and resilience.

I am sure most therapists may share similar personal accounts toward their own development of coping skills and resilience. As occupational therapists, along with our clients and their caregivers, we may take steps forward and backward; we grieve losses, and celebrate the small everyday successes that make the lives of our clients better. What we hope that you take away from this book is a new understanding of how each of us (clients, caregivers, and health care providers alike) are influenced by each other, our contexts, and our own ability to cope, adaptively overcome obstacles, and promote positive factors related to long-term resilience.

FINANCIAL DISCLOSURES

Dr. Susan L. Bazyk has no financial or proprietary interest in the materials presented herein.

Dr. Angela K. Boisselle has no financial or proprietary interest in the materials presented herein.

Dr. Tammy Bruegger has no financial or proprietary interest in the materials presented herein.

Dr. Susan M. Cahill has no financial or proprietary interest in the materials presented herein.

Dr. Catherine Candler has no financial or proprietary interest in the materials presented herein.

Dr. Anne Cronin has no financial or proprietary interest in the materials presented herein.

Rebecca Crossland has no financial or proprietary interest in the materials presented herein.

Dr. Elaina DaLomba has no financial or proprietary interest in the materials presented herein.

Dr. Lenin C. Grajo has no financial or proprietary interest in the materials presented herein.

Dr. Lisa Griggs-Stapleton has no financial or proprietary interest in the materials presented herein.

Dr. Julia M. Guzmán has no financial or proprietary interest in the materials presented herein.

Dr. Douglene Jackson has no financial or proprietary interest in the materials presented herein.

Kathleen Kauper has no financial or proprietary interest in the materials presented herein.

Dr. Karrie L. Kingsley has no financial or proprietary interest in the materials presented herein.

Dr. Lauren E. Milton has no financial or proprietary interest in the materials presented herein.

Dr. Kristie K. Patten has no financial or proprietary interest in the materials presented herein.

Dr. Jennifer S. Pitonyak has no financial or proprietary interest in the materials presented herein.

Dr. Debra Rybski has no financial or proprietary interest in the materials presented herein.

Dr. Jessica Sparrow has no financial or proprietary interest in the materials presented herein.

Dr. Laura Stimler has no financial or proprietary interest in the materials presented herein.

Dr. Christine Urish has no financial or proprietary interest in the materials presented herein.

Index

Printed in the United States
by Baker & Taylor Publisher Services